The SEXUAL HERBAL

Prescriptions for Enhancing Love and Passion

BRIGITTE MARS, A.H.G.

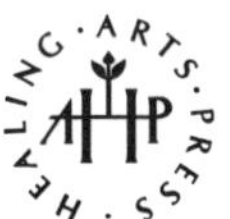

Healing Arts Press
Rochester, Vermont • Toronto, Canada

Healing Arts Press
One Park Street
Rochester, Vermont 05767
www.HealingArtsPress.com

Healing Arts Press is a division of Inner Traditions International

Originally published as *Sex, Love, and Health: A Self-Help Guide to Love and Sex* by Basic Health Publications

Note to the reader: *This book is intended as an informational guide. The remedies, approaches, and techniques described herein are meant to supplement, and not to be a substitute for, professional medical care or treatment. They should not be used to treat a serious ailment without prior consultation with a qualified health care professional.*

Library of Congress Cataloging-in-Publication Data
Mars, Brigitte.
The sexual herbal : prescriptions for enhancing love and passion / Brigitte Mars.
p. cm.
Rev. ed. of: Sex, love & health. c2002.
Includes bibliographical references and index.
ISBN 978-1-59477-286-3 (pbk.)
1. Hygiene, Sexual. 2. Sex instruction. 3. Sexual disorders—Alternative treatment. I. Mars, Brigitte. Sex, love & health. II. Title.
RA788.M336 2010
613.9'5—dc22

2009035776

Printed and bound in the United States by Lake Book Manufacturing

10 9 8 7 6 5 4 3 2 1

Cobra photograph, Bow photograph, and Fish photograph on page 124, and Yab Yum photograph on page 194 by David Paul
Lotus photograph on page 124 by adidas
Tree pose photograph on page 124 by Howard Wise
The model for all yoga photographs on page 124 is Rainbeau Mars; the models for the Yab Yum photograph on page 194 are Rainbeau Mars and Carlo Marzano
Clothing in all yoga photographs on page 124 from Rainbeau Mars Signature Line by adidas
Foot reflexology illustrations on pages 162 and 185 by Sierra Swan Palermo, Gretchen Grace, and Trish Cooke

Text design by Virginia Scott Bowman Text layout by Virginia Scott Bowman and Peri Swan
This book was typeset in Garamond Premier Pro with Bauer Text Initials and Gil Sans as display typefaces

Contents

Acknowledgments ix

Introduction: The Healing Power of Sex and Love 1

PART ONE
Love Therapies

1 Diet: Setting the Table for Passion 11

2 Herbs: Supporting Natural Sexual Vitality 49

3 Nutritional Supplements: Balancing and Rebuilding Sexual Health 106

4 Sexercises: Strengthening the Love Muscles 117

5 Aromatherapy: Essential Oils for Love 126

6 Homeopathy: A Dose for What Ails You 140

7 Flower Essences: The Blossoming of Sexual Harmony 146

8 Feng Shui: Creating a Pleasure Palace 150

9 Massage and Acupressure: An Energetic Connection 158

10 Hydrotherapy: Waters of Love 166

PART TWO

HOW TO BE A FANTASTIC LOVER

11 Improving Your Techniques 173

12 Controlling and Intensifying Orgasms 205

13 Adapting to Special Circumstances 217

14 Practicing Safe Sex 224

PART THREE

ACHIEVING AND MAINTAINING SEXUAL HEALTH

15 Women's Health 245

16 Men's Health 312

17 Menstruation and Menopause 335

18 Fertility and Infertility 378

19 Sexually Transmitted Diseases 394

PART FOUR

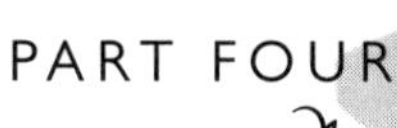

LOVE AND RELATIONSHIPS

20 The Fine Art of Flirting and Attracting a Mate 421

21 Keep Your Love Alive: The Twenty-five Principles of a Strong Relationship 432

22 Healing from Trauma 443

23 Healing the Spirit from a Broken Heart 450

24 Is It Love or Addiction? 456

APPENDIX 1 The Chemistry of Love 460

APPENDIX 2 Anatomical Terms 469

APPENDIX 3 Herbal Vocabulary 474

Resources 477

Bibliography 482

About the Author 487

Index 489

To Tom Pfeiffer,
Eternal beloved.
You are forever my hero!

I met you one cold January night.
You gave me a ride home.
You had a mandala on your Jeep.
I took it as a sign
You were meant to keep.
And keep you did
And keep you well
It's been heaven.
It's been a bit of hell.
We've endured
We've delight
Weave our love
We walk in light.
Thank you for saving me
Believing in me
Asking me
your bride to be.
Thank you Tom
Om
Home
Shalom
We go on!
DNA strands
Sharing a destiny.
Why even our angels are friends!
Through universe journey
what the future may bring
This has been more than a fling
Thank you for
your
Kiss of bliss.
Namaste.

THE HEART CHAKRA: COMPASSION

Scarlet

Can you float through the universe of your body . . .
And not lose your way?
Flow with fire-blood through each tissued corridor?
Can you let your heart pump you down long red tunnels?
Stream into cell chambers?
Love with your heart?
Let your heart become central pump-house
For all human feeling . . . pulse for all love . . .
Beat for all sorrow . . . throb for all pain . . .
Thud for all joy . . . beat for all humankind . . .
Burst . . . bleed . . . into warm compassion
Flowing . . . flowing . . . pulsing . . . out . . . out

Life
Scarlet
Drum

—Dr. Timothy Leary,
The Psychedelic Prayers

THE SEX CHAKRA: FUSION

Rainbow

Can you float through the universe of your body
and not lose your way?
Lie quietly engulfed in the slippery union of male and female?
Warm wet dance of generation?
Endless ecstasies of couples?
Offer your stamen trembling in the meadow
for the electric penetration of pollen While birds sing?
Writhe together on the river bank While birds sing?
Can you coil serpentine While birds sing?
Become two cells merging?
Slide together in molecule embrace?
Can you . . . lose . . . all fusing
Rainbow

—Dr. Timothy Leary,
The Psychedelic Prayers

ACKNOWLEDGMENTS

A heartfelt thank-you to Inner Traditions, especially to Jon Graham for his belief in this project and to Laura Schlivek, Gail Rex, and Nancy Ringer, editors extraordinaire.

Tom Pfeiffer, beloved husband of more than thirty years, none of this would be possible without you. You were so brave to take on a young single mother and love her children as your own. I love you forever and find you beautiful and wise.

My daughters—Sunflower Sparkle Mars, firstborn, always bright, child delight, and awakener of my heart, and Rainbeau Harmony Mars, child of fortune and constant source of inspiration—how I love you both!

To the midwives and herbalists of days of futures past. Thank you for helping to preserve the time-tested techniques of healing with nature's allies.

Thanks to my teachers on the path of healing sexuality: Light and Bryan Miller, Charles and Caroline Muir, and Margo Anand and Annie Sprinkle.

I am so grateful for my raw inspirations: Juliano, Tonya Zavasta, the Boutenkos, Happy Oasis, and David Wolfe.

Many thanks to the Garlic Queens: Rosemary Gladstar, Mindy Green, Diana De Luca, Kathi Keville, Beth Baugh, Sara Katz, Cascade Anderson Geller, Pam Montgomery, Jane Bothwell, Linda LeMole, Rosita Arvigo, Margie Flint, Chanchal Cabrerra, and Rebecca Luna. Herb sisters in my life, you are beloved! Susun Weed, Amanda McQuade Crawford, Debra St. Claire, Feather, Farida, Lilja Oddsdottir, and Gitte Lassen, you inspire!

Marjy Berkman and Briggs Wallis, your spirit of adventure is refreshing.

To Laura Lamun for joy, laughter, and song. To friends and celestial artisans Bob Venosa and Martina Hoffmann. To Steve McIntosh and Tehya Jai, always on the path of truth, beauty, and goodness. Rebecca and Robbie Gordon—such amazing friends you are. Elysabeth Williamson and Kate Bullings you have great healing gifts. To Mo and Jennifer Siegel and Chris Halverson for *Urantia* study groups. Thank you my beloved friends at Pharmaca, Kimba Arem, Jirka Rysavy, Alana, Richard Rose, Donna Eagle, Alex and Allyson Grey, Alicia Bay Laurel, Jeane Marie Swalm, Deb and Eddie Shapiro, you all bring wonderful contributions to the planet.

Matthew Becker, herbalist extraordinaire, you always comfort and heal with your kindness and wisdom. Thanks to herbalists Michael and Lesley Tierra, Christopher Hobbs, Roy Upton, "Herbal Ed" Smith, David Winston, David Hoffmann, Ed Bauman, Mark Blumenthal, Stephen Buhner, James Green, Paul Bergner, Rick Scalzo, Ryan Drum, and the late and great ones: Rosemary Woodruff (and the good doctor) Leary, Jeannine Parvati Baker, William LeSassier, and Terence McKenna. Thanks also to Miss Hall's School for young ladies.

Bob Ramey, you are extraordinary, as is your ability to heal on so many levels! Norm Allard—you'll go down in history! Much gratitude to Dr. Jia Gottlieb for his knowledge of medicine, and great thanks to Dr. Ann Mattson for her ob/gynecological and holistic medicine wisdom. *Merci mes amis.* Thank you Adam and Eve for coming to this isolated planet about 38,000 years ago from the star system Edentia, and doing your best.

Mom and Dad, I am so grateful for all the wonderful blessings you created in my life. Dominique Roberts and Rachel Tufunga, so glad to have you as my sisters.

I am grateful for *The Urantia Book,* which has answered so many of my questions about life on Earth and beyond. Thank you, Universal Father and Mother Spirit. Thank you for this beautiful planet, for the gift of love that heals, and for the passion that makes life worthwhile. Blessed be!

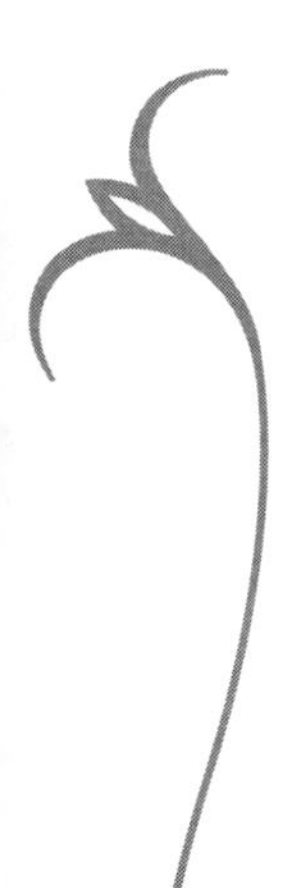

INTRODUCTION
The Healing Power of Sex and Love

WARM GREETINGS! Sex is an extraordinary form of communication (usually) between two people. When sex is joyous, body, mind, and spirit bond together as one. In its highest form, sex leads to a transcendent, mystical experience and simple, total bliss. How do you bring that kind of joy to sex? Tend your relationship as if it were a garden. Treat your body as a temple. And practice making love as if it were a sacred adventure.

A natural, healthy lifestyle is one of the fundamental ways of honoring the sacred temple of our bodies; it brings us greater health and a vastly deeper awareness of our connection to all beings. As we become more in tune with the world that grows outside our doorsteps, we begin to recognize that plants have even more to offer us than basic sustenance. In fact, "green medicine" is one of the ways the plant world shares with us its vibrant, fertile good health.

This book is intended to embrace the vitality of plant medicine as it relates specifically to sexuality; it is an herbal compendium of botanical blessings that have long served humanity. It is also a modern guide to dietary supplements, exercises, and practices for supporting your sexual health and vitality through the many stages of your life. It includes much information that I want to share with my brothers and sisters, providing many ways of tending to your body and your relationship so that you can continue to discover new paths of sacred sexual adventure.

THE BODY: HOLY TEMPLE OF CONSCIOUSNESS

Our incredible biological complexity is a sacred miracle; evidence, perhaps, of that Greater Mystery that people of different faiths (but similar beliefs) have loved, traded, argued about, and fought over for centuries. Yet awareness of and appreciation for the physiological beauty of the human body seems to have been lost from modern culture. We are affected by waves of technological ingenuity. It is interesting that there are sixty-four hexagrams of the I Ching, the ancient Chinese book of fortunes, and sixty-four codons of the DNA code. We now have the ability to take ancient information and combine it with modern research. We come to realize that nature has long held wisdom.

We can reclaim our bodies as sacred vessels and renew our commitment to experiencing their delights in a conscious, heartfelt way. One of the first things we can do is reinvent linking sex and swearing vocabulary. Think of all the sexual words that are also used for cussing (*fuck, cunt, mother fucker—you get the picture*). These are not words of love, but what is said when *fucking pissed off!* Let go of anger and embrance the highest vibrations of voice.

To heal sexual vocabulary, you and your lover might make a list of all the possible terms for sexual acts and anatomy and see what seems the most friendly and romantic to you. Throughout this book I use the terms *yoni* and *lingam* to describe the vagina and penis. *Yoni* is a term for the vagina that comes from Sanskrit; its meaning translates as "origin" or "source." *Lingam* is another Sanskrit term that is used to describe the penis; its literal meaning is a "mark" or a "sign." Choosing a name of honor blesses these tools of creativity.

The bone at the base of the spine is called the sacrum. Its name has its roots in the Latin *sacer,* meaning "sacred." The term reflects the high honor that sexual union can have. Let us restore that sense of sacredness in sexuality. Let us investigate, test, research, and learn all we can about human anatomy and physiology, but let us not forget to honor the sheer marvel of it all. Let us love each other with a sense of gratefulness for being here, on this planet, in this body, capable of love, sex, soulful union, and shimmering pleasure.

The grand design of the human body is a truly wondrous mandala filled with patterns of multiplicity. Men and women mirror and complement each other, their bodies reflecting the dance of creation. We find that even in our reproductive systems, where the differences between male and female are truly manifest, we are patterned from the same mold. In scientific terms, male and female bodies are filled with homologues—structures or tissues of common origin. The penis develops from the same tissue that produces the clitoris. Testicles and ovaries are homologues, as are the labia majora and the scrotum. Cowper's glands are the male equivalent of the female Bartholin's glands. The prostate gland and uterus both develop from the same embryonic cells. When we make love, we are much more alike than we realize!

SEXUAL ENERGY

Sex lifts the spirits, stimulates the immune system, boosts circulation, lowers cholesterol, gets creative juices flowing, and much, much more. It is also aerobic exercise, and much more fun than riding a stationary bike. It can even be yogic. When you are making love, your heart rate increases, your muscles get a workout, your cardiovascular system gets pumping, and *chi* (life force) moves through your vital organs.

Sex can help to clear a man's backed-up prostate gland and regulate a woman's menstrual cycles, even improving many of the symptoms associated with premenstrual syndrome. By increasing estrogen levels, sex can also help protect menopausal women from heart disease and bone loss and keep vaginal tissues moist and healthy. For both genders, sex can help relieve pain by stimulating the release of cortisone and endorphins. Regular monogamous sex has even been proved to extend our life spans. What a lovely gift to enjoy!

In the Hindu tradition, sex is said to stimulate *kundalini,* the dormant energy or life force that lies coiled at the base of the spine. When awakened, kundalini floods up the spinal column to the brain, where it can stimulate a higher state of consciousness and bring enlightenment. When combined with the joys of true love, we can have a partner on the path to creating a beautiful life on our planet, also known as Urantia.

Of course, not all sex can be described as a journey toward enlightenment. But you must admit that sometimes, every once in a while, just maybe, you find that spark of magic. That sense of losing yourself and finding yourself all at once. The feeling of having touched Spirit. That sense of "wow." At one-ment. No wonder we sometimes say "Oh God!" (*"What's the hardest thing about being an atheist? There's no one to talk with when you are having an orgasm!"*)

Sex and love stimulate the brain to release all sorts of chemicals, ranging from feel-good endorphins to libido-boosting DHEA. The brain—controller of hormones, neurotransmitters, and other physiological compounds—is the ultimate sexual organ: things that improve brain function generally improve sex, too, and vice versa. Brain function and sexual activity are natural cohorts; after all, the most basic human drive is to procreate—whether you want to or not!

During orgasm there is an intense discharge of electrical energy in the limbic cortex or "hind brain." The limbic system helps to arouse emotions and relay nerve messages, relieving tension and promoting psychological well-being. Orgasm relaxes the muscles and leads brain waves into an alpha state that encourages dreaming and creativity, or sometimes a theta state of deep sleep that leaves you feeling powerfully energized when you awaken.

Levels of hormones, neurotransmitters, and other physiological chemicals rise and fall in the body like tides in the ocean and the motions of the Moon. The sexual impulse and reproductive ability are dependent on body chemistry, as are most physiological processes. Researchers are still in the early stages of learning about these compounds and their effects upon the body and the psyche. For an overview of the chemicals of love, see appendix 1.

SEXUAL ENERGY: AN EASTERN VIEW

Oriental medicine has its own way of describing sexual chemistry and energies, relating our activities to those in the natural world.

The Five Elements

In the Eastern worldview, human beings are microcosms of the universe, dwelling within the macrocosm. Just as nature is ordered by five primordial powers—Wood, Fire, Earth, Metal, and Water—so, too, is the human body infused with these five elements. Each element corresponds to a particular organ or bodily system. Note that when an organ system is referenced in the context of Oriental medicine, its initial letter is often capitalized. This helps differentiate, for example, the Western understanding of the liver (the singular organ) from the Oriental understanding of the Liver (the organ, the system it is associated with, and its energy).

- Wood—Liver and Gall Bladder
- Fire—Heart and Small Intestine
- Earth—Stomach and Spleen
- Metal—Lungs and Large Intestine
- Water—Kidneys and Bladder

These elements are the foundation of physiological harmony. An imbalance in one element can cause imbalance in others.

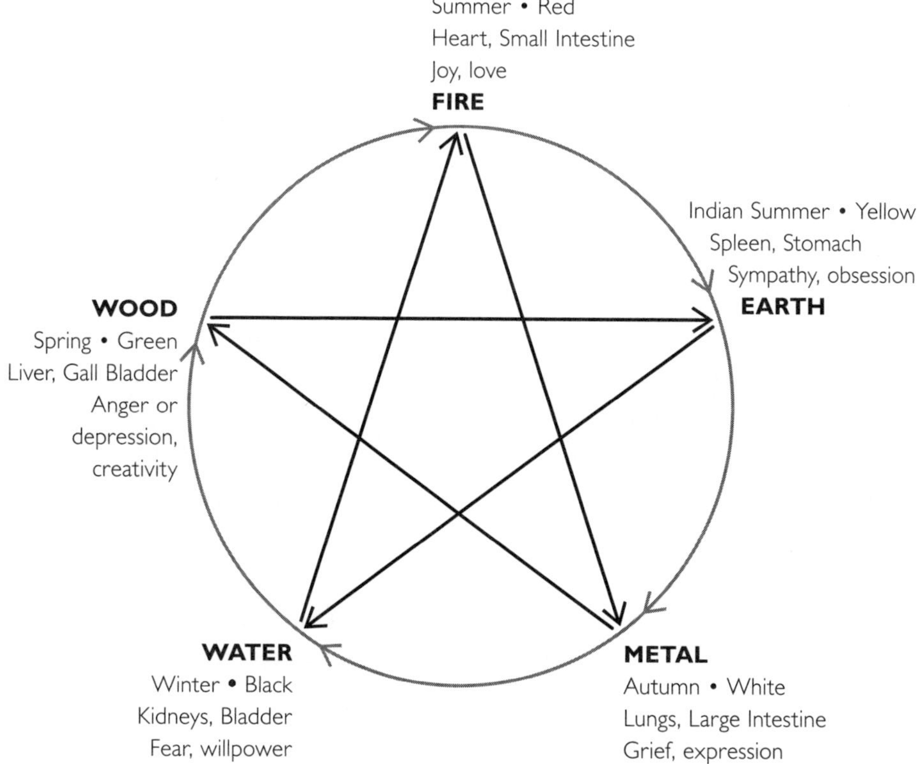

The five elements

The Flow of Energy

The human body is infused with *chi,* which translates as "breath" and means "life force" or "vital energy." Chi flows throughout the body in meridians, or energy pathways, bringing life force to each of the organs and bodily systems that contribute to health. When chi is excessive, deficient, or blocked (stagnant), health is negatively impacted.

Certain points along the body's meridians may be stimulated to affect the flow of chi. Acupuncture, acupressure, and massage make use of these vital points to keep chi flowing freely.

Yin and Yang

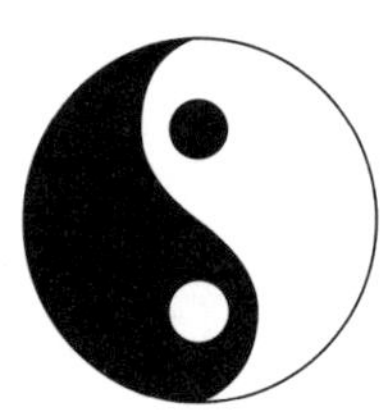

The yin-yang symbol

Yin and yang are the vital polarities that permeate the universe, from the tiniest to grandest dimensions. They are not opposites but different aspects of a continuum, merging into one another. They are yin and yang only in relation to each other; one does not exist without the other. Each contains elements of the other. The black-and-white yin-yang symbol shows a spot of white in the black, and a spot of black in the white. While yin is traditionally associated with feminine attributes and yang with masculine ones, these spots demonstrate that a healthy polarity contains a bit of its opposite. In the same manner, women (yin) have "male" hormones in their bodies, and men (yang) have "female" hormones in their bodies. In some relationships, the male may take on the more yin role, and the female the yang role. Yin and yang are not descriptions of gender; they are patterns of the manifestation of energy.

In traditional Oriental medicine, ailments are often described in terms of a yin-yang imbalance. A yang deficiency, for example, could result in a wet, cold condition, such as lower back pain, lethargy, edema, and a feeling of always being cold. A yin deficiency, on the other hand, could result in a dry, warm condition, such as night sweats, insomnia, nervous exhaustion, and dizziness. Treatment is focused on restoring balance to the affected system or organ.

Nurturing the Kidneys

The Kidneys, representative of the Water element, govern sexual vitality and mental energy. Maintaining yin-yang balance and preventing chi blockage in the Kidneys is imperative to sexual health and libido.

To support Kidney vitality and thereby sexual vitality, avoid stress, overwork, and loud noises. Do not allow your lower back to become chilled, minimize your intake of icy foods and beverages, and get adequate sleep every night. If the Kidney system is depleted, take a nap between 3 and 7 p.m. Even if the nap lasts only a few minutes, it will be a potent restorative. Eat super tonic foods!

KIDNEY YIN

Kidney yin is the aspect of Kidney energy that nourishes, moistens, and restores other tissues and organs in the body. Kidney yin deficiency may manifest as low libido, dry skin (including vaginal dryness), erectile dysfunction, low sperm count, premature ejaculation, seminal emissions (wet dreams), night sweats, constipation, hair loss, constant hunger, aggressive tendencies, loud behavior, insomnia, an aversion to heat, a desire for quick sex with minimal foreplay.

To cultivate Kidney yin, incorporate into your diet sea vegetables, roots, green leafy vegetables, olive oil, and small amounts of raw honey. Yin can also be built by eating fish, swimming, taking baths, listening to the sound of water (fountains, waterfalls, or streams), gardening, being in nature, resting, and absorbing moonlight.

KIDNEY YANG

Kidney yang is the aspect of Kidney energy that warms, enlivens, and activates other tissues and organs in the body. Kidney yang deficiency may manifest as erectile dysfunction, low libido, inability to orgasm, paleness, low energy, poor appetite, timid voice, fluid retention, lack of ambition, aversion to cold, and poor listening skills.

To cultivate Kidney yang, increase the amount of time you spend outdoors in the sun, take saunas, and stay warm—most beneficially from fire, such as a campfire, fireplace, or woodstove. (I have lately been enjoying the infrared heat of my BioMat. It's a good source of heat if you don't have access to fire.) Also eat mineral-rich black foods such as black sesame seeds, sea weeds, wild rice, and sun-cured olives.

SEX, LOVE, AND HEALTH

Sex, love, and health—it's what most of us spend our lives searching for, although not necessarily in that order. My friends, the search may continue, but it is my hope that this book will help you collect wildflowers of wisdom upon your way and brighten your journey.

Of course, there is no single approach to sex, love, and health that will work for everyone. In this book, you'll find a broad range of ideas, drawn from many different cultures, theories, and schools of healing. You will have the opportunity to increase your knowledge about herbal medicine, food, yoga, massage, homeopathy, flower essences, colors, and magic, and you will learn some of the wisdom of the grandmothers and grandfathers, midwives, herbalists, Hildegard, and Hippocrates. Take some of their leads and follow paths to see what works for you, and walk your way better bestowed. If you are in a same-sex relationship, you will find that many concepts in this book will work for you sometimes with a bit of imagination. Blessed be!

Feel free to read this book with a highlighter to cast light upon ideas that suit you and your loved ones. Part 3 of this book, "Achieving and Maintaining Sexual Health," might be something you read as needed, if menopause or prostate health, for example, become issues of importance to you. However you choose to use this collection of lore and lessons, there are many surprises within its pages. My intention is to stimulate new thinking on ways of making love and life more beautiful, sex more pleasurable, health more vibrant, and relationships more connected. Even if you skip over the chapters on sexual health concerns for now, please read ahead to part 4 for ideas on the fine art of flirting, keeping your love alive, healing a broken heart, and much more!

Having a lover—a partner on the path—is truly one of life's great blessings. Cherish this gift. Heal and be healed by each other. Let go of patterns that no longer serve. Honor the aspects of god and goddess that dwell in each of us. Celebrate love, and celebrate life!

May you radiate love to all corners of the universe. Many blessings!

PART ONE

Love Therapies

GOOD SEX both requires and builds good health. You may be fortunate in feeling that you have plenty of both in your life, or you may feel you could use a little boost. In either case, there are many ways to to expand love, sensual awareness, excitement, satisfaction, and health benefits!

Whether you're considering a sexy, healthy dinner, looking for just the right herbs or flower essences to balance a few physical symptoms, or embarking on a new exercise program, a little bit of advance planning goes a long way toward creating desire. A couple can take the path toward good health together, weaving good life practices, a healthy diet, and healthy attitudes toward sex into their lives.

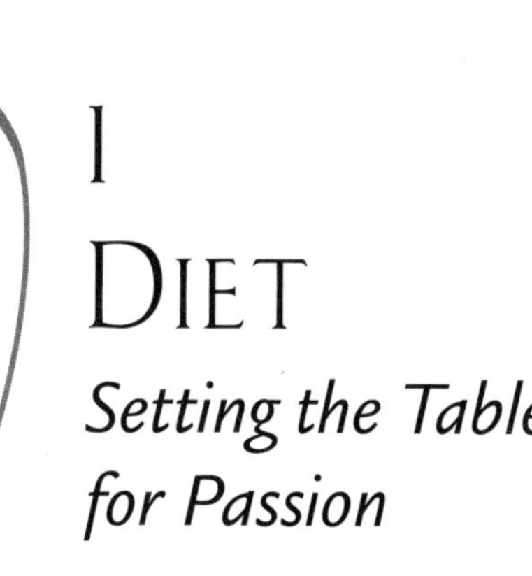

I

DIET

Setting the Table for Passion

> *Fruits are the children of trees.*
>
> JEREMY SAFRON

> *In the plant world, sex provides us with fragrance, flowers, fruits, and seeds. It fills the countryside with varied hues and elixirs. In the animal world, sex provides antlers and plumage, birdsong, and the call of insects.* —*B.M.*

FOOD, MORE THAN a mere filling for the belly, can also pleasure the soul, fuel the body, and promote good health. The ideal food for inciting passion is light, moist, sweet, easily digested, and enzymatically active. Moist foods lend their yin to sexual fluids. Yang comes from their enzymes—the spark of life—and from their seed-reproducing capabilities. Naturally sweet foods, such as fruits and vegetables, provide energy and stamina.

The presentation of food is an opportunity for loving expressions of creativity. Make your food a mandala of love, celebrating the fantastic forms and colors of nature! Serve entrées on a bed of colorful greens, grated carrots, or cabbage. Decorate with colorful garnishes: try cucumber slices, radish roses, cherry tomatoes, cauliflower buds, carrot curls, sprouts, avocados scooped out with a melon baller, buckwheat lettuce, sunflower greens, lemon slices, watercress, almonds, chopped nuts, olives, chopped red pepper, coconut, stuffed celery, berries, slices of citrus, pomegranate seeds, or star fruit slices. Stick a small bundle of green beans or asparagus spears in the round of a red pepper.

Sprinkle food with paprika or cinnamon. You can create beautiful designs by placing a lace paper doily or large maple leaf on top of a dish, then sprinkling your colorful powdered seasoning all around it. When you carefully remove the doily or leaf, you'll have a stunning ornament! Use fresh herbs from your garden (basil, chives, cilantro, dill, fennel, oregano, mint, parsley, or rosemary). Add crunch and color with sesame, sunflower, chia, or poppy seeds. Use nuts, dried fruit, or edible flowers to make designs. Use pretty molds shaped like hearts or butterflies for cakes and pâtés. Set the table with beautiful serving ware. Decorate with edible flowers to cause your chakras to vibrate!

Prepare food with loving intention. Play beautiful music or positive self-help tapes while doing food prep. Remember food magic: When preparing food for you and your beloved, take turns putting a slice or spoonful into each person's bowl. Energetically, you will be sharing of the same fruit.

Burn a red candle (hemp, beeswax, or soy candles are safer than paraffin) in the kitchen while preparing food for sexual vitality. Green can be used to call in love or health. Bless your food and give thanks.

Buying a product at the natural food store doesn't necessarily make it healthy. Organic whole-wheat macaroni and cheese in a box is still a processed food. The best foods are unrefined ones that provide a wide range of colors and satisfy the senses. Make snacks an opportunity for health by letting nuts, seeds, yogurt, fruit, and vegetables replace candy and ice cream. If you allow the media to guide your food choices, the next step will be to ask *your* doctor is if *this drug* is right for you!

Vibrant food helps you feel great and look good in your body. The organic, free range, fair trade, vegetarian, vegan, organic, local, slow food, and raw food movements are all efforts toward improving the way we eat. A healthy diet is better for us and our planet. Now *that* is sexy.

Sexual energy is extra energy. If you are exhausted or ill from trying to digest poor-quality foods, your libido will be one of the first things to diminish so that your body can focus its energy on healing rather than on sexual activity. Enjoy nourishing yourself and your loved ones well to promote sexual excitement.

Exchanging processed foods filled with preservatives for organic foods that are as close as possible to their natural state can effect incredible improvements in your energy levels, emotional stability, mental acuity, and sexual vitality.

Food allergies and sensitivities are also a big problem in our culture. I have seen many people feel amazingly better and discover more energy by going off all gluten products (especially wheat, rye, barley), or all dairy and/or soy products. Yet many people sabotage their health—and therefore their energy and libido—by persisting in eating the very foods they are allergic to.

We often crave the most compromising foods because when we consume ingredients we're allergic to, the body temporarily produces more white blood cells to neutralize the allergen. We feel comforted by the revving up of our immune system. However, if a body is constantly dealing with digestive distress, pain, constipation, and other all-too-common maladies, it will dampen your sex life. Consider keeping a food journal for a few weeks. Record what you eat and how you feel. What can you do better?

Demonstrating the ability to feed one another, whether it is preparing a homemade meal, creating a spontaneous picnic, or dining in nice restaurants, really is a way of showing your love. When a partner or potential partner shows that he or she is capable of feeding and nurturing us, it triggers ancient subconscious programming—a sense of trust that at least some of our primal needs will be met. Many couples connect deeply over food and eating, so why not make the most of the opportunity!

Eat colorful vibrant fresh foods and feel your body come alive!

SEXUAL SUPERFOODS

The term *aphrodisiac* derives from the name Aphrodite, the Greek goddess of love, fruitfulness, and beauty. An aphrodisiac is a substance that puts you in the mood for love, whether it be food, herbs, good conversation, moonlight on the beach, or even lingerie.

Some aphrodisiacs have a direct stimulating effect on the erogenous zones. Some affect the mind, causing relaxation, releasing inhibitions, or inspiring passion. Others endow the user with stamina, allowing longer lovemaking sessions. Still others are simply reminiscent of sex in their shape, texture, or smell. Consider the phallic nature of a banana or the sweet succulence of a ripe persimmon.

Taken as a tonic, aphrodisiacs can be enjoyed thirty to sixty minutes before a lovemaking session. However, they are best put to use as an integral element of daily life, inspiring health, passion, and sensuality throughout the day and offering the utmost of their tonifying properties.

Superfoods are unprocessed foods that pack a wide range of nutrients into a delicious healthful package. They provide powerful healing benefits to the human body. A superfood can be considered an aphrodisiac tonic if it satisfies one or more of the following requirements.

1. It is highly nutritious and makes a significant contribution to overall health, thereby improving libido.
2. It nourishes the liver system, which breaks down toxins and excess hormones in the body, helping maintain the immune system and hormonal balance.
3. It nourishes the kidney system, which governs sexual vitality and libido, and contributes to the ability to bring forth new life should that be on the agenda.
4. It stimulates circulation, which moves blockages from, boosts sensitivity in, and improves the function of the sexual organs. Improved circulation also creates more warmth in the body, fueling the fires of passion.

The foods that follow satisfy one or more of these requirements. To reach and maintain peak sexual vigor, make them a regular part of your diet!*

Apples *(Malus* spp.*)*

Apples, forbidden food of Eve and Snow White, belong to the Rose (Rosaceae) family. Consumed since ancient times, they were considered a gift of perpetual youth to gods and goddesses. Apples symbolize love, peace,

*Since March of 2000, I have adopted a mostly raw food vegan diet, and I've found that a raw food diet has blessed me with incredible energy and happiness, not to mention helping me feel good in my body. I know that raw foods have had a life-changing effect. Raw foods have an incredible potential for supporting health and energy, and of course, sex. I now encourage clients to go raw—and you might want to try it, too. For more information on following a raw food diet, see my book *Rawsome! Maximizing Health, Energy, and Culinary Delight with the Raw Foods Diet* (Laguna Beach, Calif.: Basic Health Publications, 2004).

and health. As part of Yuletide rituals, apples were hung from Yule trees to symbolize the continuing fertility of the earth.

Apples are alkaline, and high in fiber, beta-carotene, vitamin B complex, vitamin C, iron, phosphorus, potassium, silica, and iron. Eating apples stimulates the flow of saliva and cleans the teeth and gums, making your kisses sweet and delectable. Share an apple with your beloved!

Other members of the Rose family known for their sweetness, succulence, and aphrodisiac properties include apricots, cherries, peaches, pears, plums, raspberries, and strawberries. Many of their flowers contain a five-pointed star.

Artichoke *(Cynara scolymus)*

The artichoke, also known as Globe Artichoke, is a member of the Asteraceae (Daisy) family, making it a relative of dandelion, thistle, and sunflower, all plants of the sun. The genus name *Cynara* is from Latin *canina,* meaning "canine"; it refers to the similarity of the leaves to a dog's sharp teeth. The English name artichoke is derived from the Arabic word *khurshuf,* which means "thistle." In Elizabethan England, doctors prescribed artichokes as an aphrodisiac; eighteenth-century French peddlars would cry out, "Artichokes! Artichokes! Heats the body and the spirit. Heats the genitals!" After all, you are consuming an unopened flower ripe with potential.

Artichokes are considered cool, moist, and nourishing to the yin (fluids) of the body and the blood. Considered a choleretic, artichoke promotes bile flow and breaks up fat, thus easing digestion and protecting the body from arteriosclerosis. Artichokes contain beta-carotene, calcium, and potassium. Eat from the same artichoke in sensuous delight.

Asparagus *(Asparagus officinalis)*

This member of the Liliaceae (Lily) family is a relative of garlic, onions, and scallions. Asparagus can grow up to ten inches in a day! Talk about a phallic food!

Cultivated by the ancient Arabs and Greeks as an aphrodisiac, asparagus not only has a suggestive shape but also is a genitourinary stimulant. (It's an effective diuretic due to the presence of the alkaloid asparagine.) The seventeenth-century English herbalist Nicholas Culpepper said that asparagus "stirreth up bodily lust in man and woman." So if you're wondering what to serve that special someone . . .

The fresh young shoots are delicious and rich in beta-carotene, vitamins B, C, and E, iodine, potassium, and zinc. Asparagus is best in the springtime and is delightful eaten in salads, cooked into soups, or as an addition to vegetable dishes. Stalk the wild asparagus.

Avocado *(Persea americana, P. gratissima)*

Avocados are members of the Lauraceae (Laurel) family. The word *avocado* is an Anglicized version of *ahuacacuahatl,* an Aztec word meaning "testicle tree." Holy guacamole!

Avocado is a traditional remedy for erectile dysfunction; it also helps beautify the skin and hair. This is a green ray fruit governed by the planet Venus, the Mother Goddess (also known as Aphrodite and Eve)—symbol of love, beauty, fertility, and healing.

A single avocado has up to 300 calories, in part because it is composed of 20 to 60 percent monounsaturated fat (the varying percentages depend on the variety of avocado chosen). This type of fat helps maintain levels of good cholesterol (HDL, or high-density lipoprotein) in the body. Avocado is cooling and especially beneficial for dry skin and hair. It nourishes the blood, and in cases of cystitis soothes the bladder. It is a traditional remedy for erectile dysfunction, nervousness, and insomnia. It is also recommended for convalescence.

Avocados are rich in protein, beta-carotene, vitamin B complex, vitamin E, lecithin, fluorine, and copper. An avocado has two to three times the amount of potassium found in a banana. Don't worry about the calories in an avocado. This food also contains lipase, an enzyme to help the body digest fats.

An ancient tradition is to hold an avocado in your hand and visualize as strongly as you can your desired appearance. Maintain this as you peel and enjoy the avocado.

Banana *(Musa acuminata, M. sapientum)*

These members of the Musaceae (Banana) family simply make one think of smiles, and penises! Not necessarily in that order. Bananas, a yellow-rayed fruit, are governed by Mars and the Moon. In ancient India bananas were considered a sacred food offered at altars and in marriages; they symbolized love, money, and spirituality.

Rich in carbohydrates, folic acid, B_6, and vitamin C, bananas provide long-term energy and stamina. They moisten the yin fluids of the body and have been used to treat alcoholism, arteriosclerosis, depression, exhaustion, hemorrhoids, and weak muscles.

Bananas stimulate the production of serotonin, a compound that can improve sleep and elevate mood. They are high in calories but low in fat; they are an excellent food for pregnant mothers.

Use bananas as a snack or in puddings, pies, fruit salads, and smoothies. Bananas blended with water make nourishing banana milk. Try a sandwich of banana and almond butter. Freeze peeled bananas and run them through a juicer to make dairy-free "ice cream." Dried banana chips make a tasty sweet snack.

Beets *(Beta vulgaris)*

Beets, of the Chenopodiace (Goosefoot) family, are governed by Saturn and Mars. Corresponding to the energies of Earth, love, and beauty, beets have long been considered a food of beauty and energy. Aphrodite herself is said to have eaten beets to maintain her charms. Folk tradition says that two people who eat from the same beet are likely to fall in love. If only it were so simple!

Beta is from the Celtic, meaning "red." The French term for beets is *betterave,* which is also slang for "penis" or "man root."

Beets, being roots, are said to have a downward energy, affecting the lower organs and the genitals. Beets are blood cleansing and blood building. They increase the production of red corpuscles and have therefore long been used therapeutically to improve anemia. Betaine, the red pigment that gives beets their color, helps increase oxygen intake in the body. Beets are also used to treat irregular menses, acne, and lumbago.

Beets abound with beta-carotene, vitamin B complex, vitamin C, calcium, iron, phosphorus, sodium, and manganese.

Try beets grated raw into a salad, or cook them with a little lemon juice. Visualize beauty while eating beets. Be aware that eating lots of beets may give a red color to your urine or stools. This is normal and not a cause for worry. No need to go to the emergency room!

Berries

The sour flavor of berries is an indicator of their liver-activating potential. Remember that the liver is the organ that breaks down hormones no longer needed by the body. Berries encourage the metabolism of fats and thus improve circulation. They also increase circulation to the brain and extremities. Berries are an excellent source of colorful antioxidants and flavonoids. Red berries like raspberry build the blood and increase passion—but might also increase fertility! Blackberries and blueberries nourish the kidneys and adrenals. Spend an afternoon with your beloved going berry picking: enjoy some straight from the branch and save some for a love snack later. Wild berries. Forest fairies. Careful not to stain the sheets!

Blue-Green Algae *(Aphanizomenon flos-aquae)*

There are several species of edible blue-green algae found in freshwater lakes, though the Upper Klamath Lake in southern Oregon is the only place in the world where large quantities are available in the wild. This plant reproduces at a very fast rate, almost daily in the summer. It is said to contain 65 percent protein, easily digestible because of the algae's soft cell wall. It is also rich in neuropeptides, making it an aid to the brain's neurotransmitters. People enjoy this food in either powder or tablet form for its energizing properties.

Cabbage *(Brassica oleracea)*

Cabbage, a member of the Brassicaceae (Mustard) family is a warming nutritive sexual tonic and a potent alkalizer. It is a circulatory stimulant, a diuretic, and a muscle builder. Cabbage strengthens the eyes, gums, teeth, bones, hair, and nails and has been used to treat depression, fibrocystic breast disease, hearing loss, irritability, kidney and bladder disorders, lumbago, and yeast infections.

Cabbage is a good source of fiber, protein, histamine, beta-carotene, folic acid, vitamins B_1, B_6, C, K, U, bioflavonoids, calcium, fluorine, iodine, iron, potassium, and sulfur. It contains indoles, which may help prevent breast cancer by inhibiting estrogens from stimulating tumor growth, monoterpenes, and antioxidants that give protection against heart disease and cancer.

We use raw cabbage leaves to make taco shells! Cabbage can be juiced or stuffed, diced into cole slaws, or shredded into salads and soups. Fermenting cabbage with the addition of salt makes sauerkraut, which—when unpasteurized—contains microorganisms that promote healthy intestinal flora. In folklore, cabbage is governed by the Moon and corresponds to water, money, and protection.

Cacao, a.k.a. Chocolate *(Theobroma cacao)*

Cacao is a Steruliaceae (Cacao) family member. The genus name *Theobroma* derives from the Greek *theos,* meaning "god," and *broma,* meaning "food," thus "food of the gods." The common name *chocolate* derives from an Aztec name for this plant, *chócolatl.* Cocoa was the "love tonic" of Montezuma II, who is reputed to have drunk some fifty cups daily before visiting his harem of six hundred women. In 1502 the returning crew of Columbus brought cacao beans back to Europe, and in 1550 nuns came up with the idea of adding sugar and vanilla, leading to what we now regard as chocolate. During the 1800s, physicians recommended chocolate to boost libido, and to this day it is well known for its ability to inspire passion.

Cacao is considered aphrodisiac, antioxidant, cardiotonic, diuretic, emollient, laxative, nutritive, and a nervous system stimulant. Its many constituents include B complex and E vitamins, chromium, copper, iron, magnesium, phosphorous, potassium, amino acids (arginine, phenylalanine, tryptophan, tyramine, tyrosine), phenylethylamine, anandamide, dopamine, serotonin, xanthines (caffeine, theobromine, trigonelline), flavonoids (epicatechin, catechin, procyanidins), essential oil, sucrose, glucose, mucilage, oleopalmitostearin, tannins, and natural sugars.

Cacao increases the levels of serotonin and endorphins in your body. It gives a short-term boost to energy and, when consumed in its whole, raw form, is even beneficial for the teeth as the tannins it contains inhibit dental decay. The phenylethylamine in cacao is a compound that also occurs in trace amounts in the brain; it is released naturally when we are in love, especially during orgasm. Cacao's theobromine dilates the coronary artery and increases blood flow to the heart. Cacao is bitter, warm, dry, and yang. It is governed by Mars and Uranus and corresponds to the element of Fire.

Raw cacao is one of my muses and how I get so many books written. Most commercial chocolates today, however, have a low cacao content and contain an abundance of sugar and hydrogenated oil instead. Try to seek out chocolates that have a high cacao content and little added sugar, flavors, or oils. Be sensible and don't overdo it. Chocolate is a strong stimulant for some people.

Carrot *(Daucus carota sativa)*

Carrots are orange-rayed members of the Apiaceae (Parsley) family; they were highly regarded as an aphrodisiac by the ancient Greeks. Carrots are sweet, warm, and alkaline. They are governed by Mars and correspond to the element of Fire.

Carrots contain beta-carotene, vitamin B_6, vitamin C, calcium, phosphorus, potassium, pectin, and fiber. They are an antioxidant, diuretic, galactagogue, and have urinary antiseptic properties. They have been used to treat acne, cystitis, dry skin, eczema, and night blindness.

Carrots are a popular vegetable in salad, soups, cakes, and vegetable medleys. Carrot juice is an excellent remedy to cleanse the liver but should be diluted first with water, as it is very sweet. Organic carrots can be eaten with the peel, which is beneficial for our skin. Choose whole, unwilted, colorful carrots. An old folk saying reports that "a man who likes carrots likes women."

Celery *(Apium graveolens)*

Celery is another member of the Apiaceae (Parsley) family governed by Mercury, the element of Fire, and the energies of sex, psychic protection, peace, and weight loss.

Celery has a long history of use in aphrodisiac recipes. It contains androsterone precursors, a hormone that is released from the human body in sweat and urine. It is rich in beta-carotene, folic acid, vitamin C, calcium, magnesium, potassium, silica, sodium, chlorophyll, and fiber. Celery helps dry damp conditions in the body like yeast overgrowth. It is a traditional remedy for acne, cystitis, and obesity. After exercise drinking celery juice helps replace lost electrolytes.

Celery can be enjoyed in salads and soups and with dips as an alternative to chips. Spread almond butter on celery stalks for an afternoon treat. Celery makes an excellent vegetable juice, especially combined with carrot and apple, but should be used only in moderation during pregnancy as it can promote menses.

Cherry *(Prunus avium, P. cerasus)*

The cherry is a member of the beautiful Rosaceae (Rose) family. Cherries are considered alkaline, warm, and sweet. They make an excellent detoxifying food, helping to eliminate uric acid, cleanse the kidneys, and clear blood stagnation. Cherries are a circulatory stimulant that impart a rosy glow to the complexion; in the Orient, they are known as the "fruit of fire." Cherries are a traditional remedy for anemia, fatigue, obesity, and frequent urination.

Cherries are rich in beta-carotene, vitamin B_1, vitamin C, calcium, copper, iron, manganese, phosphorus, potassium, silicon, flavonoids, and pectin.

Cherries can be enjoyed plain or in fruit salads, pies, jams, puddings, smoothies, and juices. They can be dried for year-round consumption. They are governed by Venus and correspond to the element of Water and the energy of love.

Make a cherry pie while visualizing love. Lightly trace a heart in the bottom of the crust before adding the cherries. Then eat one piece of pie every day while continuing to visualize love. If you have already found the one you love, you can strengthen that love by sharing a piece of pie every day.

Durian *(Durio zibethinus)*

The durian is a member of the Bombaceae (Durian) family. It is the large fruit of one of the world's largest fruit trees, which grows throughout Southeast Asia. The genus name is from the Malaysian *duri,* meaning "spike," in reference to the fruit's sharp spines. The fruit is a preferred food for wild elephants, orangutans, and tigers, while the flowers are a favorite of fruit bats. In Malaysia they say that "when the durians fall, the sarongs rise."

Durian fruit has a strong sulfurous smell, and its species name—*zibethinus*—means "smelling like a civet cat" (an animal with powerful scent glands).

Though the aroma is indeed peculiar, a durian fruit can make very arousing Love Tonic smoothies. Under the dominion of Jupiter, the element of Fire, and having an energy of strength, durians are considered an aphrodisiac and longevity tonic. They are high in oleic fats, vitamin E, and sulfur, and contain more protein than any other fruit.

Figs *(Ficus carica)*

Figs, of the Moraceae (Mulberry) family, are good restoratives; they improve energy levels in those who feel fatigued, boosting fertility and libido. They are rich in vitamin B_6, folic acid, calcium, copper, iron, magnesium, manganese, phosphorus, and potassium.

Figs are warming, sweet, and alkaline in nature. They are governed by Jupiter, correspond to the element of Fire, and are associated with the energies of sexuality and strength.

Enjoy figs as a snack or for dessert. Try them stuffed with almond butter.

Of all the dried fruits, dried figs are considered the healthiest, though you should brush your teeth after eating them as they are also among the stickiest. Soak dried figs overnight in water and blend them for a breakfast compote. Use them as a natural sweetener, like dates, for cookies, pies, and puddings.

Figs are an excellent food for body builders and those wanting to gain weight. They are also used to deter cravings for sugar, alcohol, and drugs.

Fish: Aphrodisiacs of the Sea

Even though I am mostly vegan, I do honor that fish from the sea can be a potent medicinal food and tonic. Where available in healthy abundance, fish are high in minerals, phosphorus, calcium, and iodine. Fish are said to correspond to Neptune, Venus, and the Moon, and to the energies of water, psychic awareness, dreams, and sexuality.

Phosphorus is known to improve sex drive and responsiveness. Calcium is vital for skeletal health, calms the emotions, and promotes restful sleep. Iodine is found in high concentrations in the thyroid gland, which is important in regulating metabolism. A person with an iodine deficiency might feel listless and sluggish and have a diminished libido.

Unfortunately, many fish are factory raised nowadays, consuming processed pellets (including beef by-products) rather than real food, being dosed by antibiotics, and living in crowded cement troughs that erode their fins and scales. Wild-caught fish are generally healthier than farm-raised fish, though they can also be contaminated with heavy metals such as mercury and industrial pollutants. If eating fish is not your thing, you can also reap great benefits from supergreen foods like spirulina and blue-green algae.

ANCHOVIES, SALMON, TUNA

Oily fish like herring, mackerel, sardines, and those listed above are rich in essential fatty acids, which build the body's lubrication systems and promote the production of various hormones. Oily fish support the health of the kidneys, which govern sexuality.

CAVIAR

Caviar—the salted, processed roe of large fish—is a highly valued Russian remedy for restoring potency. Unprocessed fish roe was also considered a potent food by many native communities around the world, including the Inuit of the far north, and native peoples of the Andes. They considered fish roe to be a staple for producing strong healthy babies. Fish eggs contain vitamins A and D, iodine, and essential fatty acids.

EEL

In traditional Japanese culture, eel is considered a supreme sexual tonic, in part because of the long, phallic shape of the fish. Eel also contain essential fatty acids.

NUOC-MAN

Nuoc-man is a spicy fish-based sauce served with dishes from a wide range of Asian cultures. It is rich in essential fatty acids and phosphorus. You can find it in most grocery stores.

OYSTERS

Oysters, which resemble the female genitalia, are rich in zinc, protein, phosphorus, and selenium; they also contain high levels of mucopolysaccharides, which improve the elasticity of tissues and boost output of seminal fluids. Oysters were prized by Casanova (and even those in religious orders) for their seductive effect.

Goji berries *(Lycium barbarum, L. chinense)*

Goji is a member of the Solanaceae (Nightshade) family. The berries are antioxidant, aphrodisiac, hypotensive, nutritive, rejuvenative, and restorative. They are an immune system stimulant and a vasodilator, and in Oriental medicine are considered tonic to the Kidneys, Liver, blood, and yin. Goji stimulates hormones, enzymes, and blood production. It increases levels of the antioxidant superoxide dismutase, nourishes bone marrow, and removes toxins from the blood by strengthening the kidneys and liver.

Goji berries are used to treat anemia, erectile dysfunction, exhaustion, all visual problems, fatigue, hair loss, leukorrhea, low libido, low testosterone levels, lumbago, menopause, night sweats, premature aging, prematurely gray hair, as well as seminal and nocturnal emissions. In Asia the goji berry is traditionally used as a longevity tonic that nourishes the Kidneys and Liver; it is also said to enhance beauty and cheerfulness when taken for long periods.

Goji berries are rich in carotenoids (physalin, zeaxanthin, beta-carotene), vitamin C, vitamins B_1 and B_2, niacin, iron, selenium, zinc, linoleic acid, amino acids (tryptophan, arginine, leucine, isoleucine—they are high in protein!), polysaccharides, phenols, betaine, and beta-sitosterol.

These powerful little fruits correspond to Mars and Venus and to the element of Water and are associated with sexuality and energy. Enjoy them as a tonic food. They can be used like raisins as a garnish, in fruit salads, or soaked then blended into smoothies.

Grains

Whole grains contain both male and female energies and are universal symbols of fertility and abundance. When you plant a whole grain, it sprouts and grows into a grass plant. When you eat a whole grain, you take in that tremendous energy.

Whole grains help keep blood sugar levels stable, which, in turn, keeps us calm. Grains that are especially beneficial for libido include barley, corn, millet, oats, rice (no wonder it's thrown at weddings), and wild rice. However, many people overeat grains, even eating refined and rancid ones that put great stress on the digestive and immune systems.

For many Americans, wheat and wheat-based products make up between one-third and two-thirds of the diet. Yet there is a large population of people with an undiagnosed wheat allergy and/or gluten intolerance; eating wheat causes them to feel fatigued and congested. Wheat, found in bread, muffins, pizza, wraps, cookies, pancakes, waffles, cereals, and many other foods, is one of the most common allergens. Gluten is also found in rye, barley, spelt, and kamut. Interesting that gluten is like the word *glue*. Imagine what it does to your insides. And what is created with glutinous substances? Pastas and pastries sound a lot like *paste*. Pass on them. Expand your horizons, there are other grains out there. Oats as a food do actually encourage people to "sow their wild oats"; they're also a rich restorative food for those who feel depleted. They can even be sprouted if you find some that have never been heated. Be aware that some may be contaminated with gluten.

Because they are not from the Poaceae (Grass) family, quinoa, amaranth, and buckwheat are technically seeds, not grains, and are therefore less likely to be allergenic or inflammatory.

Most people are familiar with grains as cooked food, but many can also be eaten as sprouts, used in cereals, or dehydrated into sprouted breads. Grains that are sprouted are easier to digest. In addition, sprouting increases a grain's enzymatic activity and increases its vitamin C and vitamin E content. My favorite grains and grainlike seeds are millet (alkalizing), wild rice (Kidney yang tonic), quinoa, and buckwheat. All are good sources of protein.

NOT HEALTHY = NOT SEXY

Sugar and wheat are stressors for the liver. In excessive amounts, sugar impairs estrogen metabolism in the liver, promotes yeast overgrowth, weakens the immune system, and aggravates endometriosis. (Sugar = a legal drug for kids.) Wheat is a common allergen and, in excessive amounts, irritates the liver and causes fluid retention. If you are working to improve the health of your liver, limit your intake of or avoid foods that contain sugar and wheat. Just say no.

Grapes *(Vitis vinifera)*

Grapes are members of the Vitaceae (Grape) family and are sweet, sour, neutral, and cooling. They contain beta-carotene, vitamin B complex, vitamin C, boron, calcium, magnesium, potassium, and pectin, as well as malic, citric, and oxalic acids. Grapes stimulate the endothelial cells (those that line the blood vessels) to release nitric acid. They also contain ellagic acid, a compound that scavenges carcinogenic factors and moves them out of the body. Grape skins contain resveratrol, which prevents blood platelet aggregation and elevates levels of HDL (high-density lipoprotein) in the body, which helps protect the arteries and encourages good circulation. Grapes contain the antioxidant quercetin, which is helpful in reducing the symptoms of allergies. They also help improve mental focus. Grape seeds are potent antioxidants. Why should we have to buy them for twenty dollars in a bottle at the health food store? Support heirloom gardening.

The darker varieties (red and purple) are more strengthening, more blood building, and richer in iron than the white or green varieties. Ruled by the Moon, grapes correspond to the element of Water and to the energies of fertility and prosperity.

Grapes are excellent by themselves or in fruit salad, jelly, or juice. Raisins, of course, are made from dried grapes and have many of the same properties. A bowl of washed organic grapes by the bed can be lovely to share with your beloved.

Greens

Green foods are packed with nutrients and are powerfully energizing, detoxifying, and strengthening to the immune system. As green foods grow, they provide oxygen for people and the planet. This oxygenating ability is due to the presence in green foods of chlorophyll, a potent collector of the Sun's energy. Chlorophyll is the green pigment required for photosynthesis. The word is derived from the Greek *chloros,* meaning "greenish yellow," and *phyllon,* meaning "leaf."

Sometimes referred to as "plant blood," chlorophyll is similar to the hemoglobin in our red blood cells, though rather than containing iron at the cell center, as blood does, chlorophyll cells hold magnesium. Found in all green foods, chlorophyll can improve moods and make skin look more beautiful. Greens help relieve pain, decrease stress, and make muscles and joints more flexible. Greens calm the mind and clean the digestive tract. There is no tolerance level that builds up with repeated use of green foods, unlike many drugs that work initially and then require larger amounts.

Greens help build blood, alkalinize the body, and improve energy and mood. The green ray nourishes the heart chakra and strengthens immunity. It is the color of love, healing, and nature. Greens such as collards, kale, spinach, lettuce, arugula, and watercress—and their wild counterparts lamb's-quarters, malva, and dandelion—provide a wide range of minerals. For optimal health, make at least one meal a day a celebration of dark leafy greens. Go green!

Mango (Mangifera indica)

The mango is a member of the Anacardiaceae (Cashew) family. Mangoes are considered by many to be one of the planet's most delicious and fragrant fruits. They have been used to treat anemia, calm the emotions, benefit the brain, strengthen the heart, and provide energy. They are also consumed to promote sexual excitement. Mangoes are governed by Mars and correspond to the Fire element, as well as to energies of love, sex, and protection. They have long been used in Vedic magic.

As a yin tonic, mango provides moistening fluids for the body and quenches thirst. It is cooling, alterative, and diuretic. Some people are allergic to mangoes, especially the juice under the peel. Mangoes are in the same family as poison ivy! Avoid getting mangoes on your skin, where they can cause irritation. Mangoes are rich in beta-carotene, niacin, vitamin C, flavonoids, vitamin E, iron, and potassium.

You can enjoy a mango by itself or add it to fruit salads. Use in pies, ice creams, smoothies, juice, and salsa. Enjoy a mango in the bathtub with your beloved! *Where the woman go, the mango.*

Nuts and Seeds

The word *nut* comes from the Latin *nux,* meaning "to nourish." Technically, all nuts are seeds. Both nuts and seeds contain the spark of life—the design and pattern for new growth. They are infinitely more nutritive raw than roasted. If you plant a raw sunflower seed it has the life potential to grow into an eight-foot-tall flowering fragrant plant. Should that seed be roasted and salted . . . would it grow and bear a yellow flower? What if we prayed over it? Chanted? Played ragas and placed pyramids around it? *Nada*. Go for the life energy!

When we eat nuts and seeds, we ingest all the nourishment and energy that is needed to sustain the new plant, including phytosterols—the plant hormones that have a structure similar to human hormones. Nuts increase sexual desire and fertility in both sexes and are excellent for bodybuilders and others who work their muscles.

Nuts and seeds provide beneficial fats, vitamins, and carbohydrates. Nuts have a higher fat content than seeds, while seeds tend to have more iron. Both contain beta-carotene, B complex, vitamins D and E, and calcium. They are high in trace minerals and help regulate blood sugar. Both contain excellent vegetarian protein per volume—more protein than meat or milk. They are cholesterol free, and eating three ounces of almonds, for example, along with a low-fat diet, can actually help lower LDL (low-density lipoprotein—the undesirable type of cholesterol) within three weeks. Raw nuts contain lipase, an enzyme that actually helps digest fats.

Almonds, hazelnuts, hempseeds, pine nuts, pistachios, poppy seeds, walnuts, pumpkin seeds, sesame seeds, and sunflower seeds are particularly rich in zinc, which helps protect the prostate gland and is a component in vaginal and seminal fluids.

Soak nuts and seeds to remove enzyme inhibitors and bring them into life-force activation. Soaking activates protease, which neutralizes enzyme inhibitors that prevent grains, seeds, nuts, or legumes from germinating at the wrong time (such as in the bulk bins at the store, or in the fall just before the snows come).

Seeds can be soaked in or out of the refrigerator, but in hot climates it is a good idea to refrigerate those that require long soaking times. Use twice as much water as seed, and soak for eight to twelve hours. If you are in a hurry, even twenty minutes of soaking can improve digestibility. If you soak seeds for longer than twelve hours, rinse them and add fresh water every twelve hours. After soaking, rinse, drain, and use in a recipe or store in the refrigerator. You can give the rinse-water to your plants, but don't drink it. Soaked nuts have a creamier texture when blended than unsoaked ones, which tend to be oily and grainy.

Nuts are acid forming, with the exception of almonds. They're also a very concentrated food and should be eaten in small amounts, preferably with alkalizing green leafy vegetables. Digesting nuts into amino acids, fatty acids, and glucose takes several hours. Use nuts for decorating. Enjoy them as a snack, in trail mix, and as an extra crunch added to cookies. One nut can be substituted for another in most recipes. The phrase "gone nuttin'" has long referred to wild and wanton behavior by young people who would go out into the woods to collect nuts.

ALMONDS (*Prunus amygdalus, P. dulcis*)

Almonds, one of the oldest cultivated nuts, are members of the Rosaceae (Rose) family and a relative of peaches and apples. Almonds are anti-inflammatory, antispasmodic, demulcent, emollient, and tonic. They help alkalize the blood and move Liver chi stagnation. Almonds improve energy, strengthen the nervous system, and increase strength and sexual vitality. They are known as brain and bone food. Almonds contain about 18 percent protein, vitamin E, and are a good source of calcium, iron, magnesium, potassium, and zinc.

In Ayurvedic medicine, almond is used to strengthen the *ojas,* the essence that exemplifies intellect and spiritual receptivity. Yogananda said almonds foster "self-control and calmness of the mind and nerves." In folklore, almonds are governed by Mercury, correspond to the element of Air, and are associated with healing and money. Look for almonds that have not been pasteurized as even most almonds labeled "raw" have been heated to high temperatures. Spanish almonds are generally unheated as are nuts that are still in the shell. So consider shelling nuts yourself. Try it as a couple in front of a great movie.

BRAZIL NUTS (*Bertholletia excelia*)

Brazil nuts are native to South America and are members of the Lecythidaceae (Brazil Nut) family. They are a good source of the amino acids cysteine and methionine, making them beneficial in a vegetarian diet. Brazil nuts are also a rich source of selenium. Considered an excellent food for those who work with their muscles or want to increase sexual libido, Brazil nuts are said to be governed by Venus. They correspond to the element of Earth and to the energies of love and money.

CHIA SEED (*Salvia columbariae, S. hispanica*)

The chia seed is a member of the Lamiaceae (Mint) family. *Salvia,* the genus name, is from the Latin *salvere,* meaning "to save." Our word *chia* is from the Mayan *chiabaan,* which means "strengthening." Native communities of the American Southwest have long used chia for endurance. Chia is rich in omega-3 fatty acids and is considered an energy tonic that moistens the yin.

COCONUT (*Cocus nucifera*)

Coconut, from the Palmaceae (Palm) family, is the largest known seed. In Sanskrit, the word for the coconut palm is *kalpa vriksha:* "the tree that supplies all that is needed to live." Coconut is considered an energy tonic, warming with a sweet flavor. It is excellent fare for vegetarians. Coconuts are high in iodine and are a good source of protein, beta-carotene, B complex, and minerals.

Coconuts under six months old have a gelatinous meat that is soft enough to eat with a spoon and is considered a delicacy. It is used to feed babies (often the first food of island children) and to nourish the sick. "Spoon coconut" restores damaged bodily tissues and boosts male and female sexual fluids.

Young green coconuts can contain up to a pint of rejuvenating coconut water. Coconut water takes nine months to develop, traveling through the coconut's fibers, which filter and purify it. Coconut water is a good source of electrolytes, very similar to human blood plasma, for which it has been used as a replacement, especially in Asia. Coconut water is considered a supreme sexual tonic food. Cut one open and offer it to your lover. Drink one to share the love.

Coconut oil can be considered a medicine in its own right. It contains short- and medium-chain fatty acids including the anti-yeast compounds caprylic acid, lauric acid, and myristic acid. It is antibacterial and antifungal and can be eaten to stimulate thyroid function, normalize blood sugar levels, decrease seizures, and improve chronic fatigue. Coconut oil appears in many Asian dishes, as well as in cakes, candies, and salad dressings. Coconut is under the dominion of the Moon. It corresponds to the element of Water and to the energies of purification, love, spirituality, and intuition.

FLAX (*Linum lewisii, L. perenne, L. usitatissimum*)

Flax, of the Linaceae (Flax) family, has been cultivated as a food source for more than seven thousand years. In the eighth century Charlemagne passed a law requiring French citizens to consume flaxseed so they would be healthy subjects. Mahatma Ghandi said that when flaxseed became a regular food, all people would have better health.

Flaxseed has a high mucilage content that nourishes the body's sexual fluids. When consumed with plenty of water, flaxseed is also an excellent laxative. Three tablespoons of freshly ground flaxseed eaten every day will support liver function, improve the metabolism of fats, and reduce inflammation.

Flaxseed moistens and soothes irritated and inflamed conditions due to its demulcent and oily qualities. It is used in the treatment of breast cysts, eczema, and hemorrhoids. In magical traditions, flaxseed is used to attract prosperity.

Flaxseed is sweet, warm, and moist. It is rich in omega-3 and omega-6 fatty acids as well as protein and vitamins A and B. It also has the most vitamin E of any known seed.

Flaxseed oil turns rancid rapidly, faster than other vegetable oils, especially when exposed to light, heat, or oxygen. For this reason, it is wise to store your flaxseed whole in the refrigerator, grinding it only when you are ready to use it. Try making it into flax crackers.

HAZELNUT (FILBERT) (*Corylus avellana, C. maxima*)

Hazelnuts are members of the Corylaceae (Hazel) family. The genus name, *Corylus,* is from the Greek *korys,* meaning "helmet," in reference to the helmet-shaped husk that encloses the nut. Under the dominion of the Sun, the hazelnut corresponds to the element of Air and to the energies of fertility, consciousness, and wisdom.

For the Celts, hazel was regarded as "The Tree of Knowledge." In France and Germany, young women danced under the hazel tree to attract suitors. This event, also known as "nut crack night," helped the young women determine their suitors' desire: if the nuts cracked and flew apart, love might be fleeting. A prolific show of hazel catkins was said to signify fertility, thus the saying "Plenty of catkins, plenty of prams" was taken quite seriously.

HEMP SEED (*Cannabis sativa*)

A member of the Cannabaceae (Hemp) family, hemp seed is one of the best sources of vegetable protein. It is easier to digest than soy and is unlikely to cause allergic reactions. Like flaxseed, hemp contains omega-3 fatty acids, but it has longer shelf stability. By now, most people are aware of the multiple uses of hemp, including as fiber, fuel, and paper. It also can be grown easily without chemicals and helps reclaim marginal soil. Hemp seeds have a sweet and mild flavor, somewhere between a sunflower seed and a pine nut. Unlike many seeds, hemp is free of trypsin inhibitors and does not need to be soaked before use. For more information on delicious hemp fare, see my book called *The HempNut Health and Cookbook,* written with Richard Rose and Christina Pirello (Santa Rosa, Calif.: HempNut, Inc., 2000).

MACADAMIA (*Macadamia tertrphylla, M. integrifolia*)

Macadamia, also known as Queensland Nut, is a member of the Proteaceae (Protea) family and is native to Australia. Macadamias are high in fat (70 percent) and low in protein (8 percent) but also contain carbohydrates, calcium, iron, phosphorus, selenium, and zinc. They are considered rejuvenating to the liver, and have been used to discourage alcohol cravings, improve anemia, and aid convalescence. Under the dominion of Jupiter, Macadamia nuts correspond to Earth and are associated with prosperity.

PECAN (*Carya illinoensis*)

Pecans, from the Juglandaceae (Walnut) family, are about 71 percent fat and a rich source of protein, minerals, and B vitamins—especially B_6 (pyridoxine). They are considered especially nourishing for the nervous system and helpful in repairing damaged cells in cases of heart disease. Governed by Mercury, pecans correspond to the element of Air and to the energies of prosperity; they are said to be beneficial to eat when seeking employment. Pecans are generally steamed to remove them from their shells, so shell them yourself if you want them truly raw.

PINE NUTS *(Pinus species)*

Pine nuts come from trees of the Pinaceae (Pine) family that have seeds large enough to be edible. They are also known as *piñon* or *pignoli*. Pine nuts contain precursors to the human hormones estrone and estradiol, are 14 percent protein, and are most well known for the distinctive flavor they bring to pesto sauce. Under the dominion of Mars, pine nuts correspond to the element of Air and to the energies of love, physical strength, and prosperity. In China they symbolize friendship and loyalty.

PISTACHIO *(Pistacia vera)*

Pistachios are members of the Anacardiaceae (Cashew) family. They are 55 percent fat and 20 percent protein; the green color of the nut is from chlorophyll. Pistachios are neutral, sweet, bitter, and slightly sour. They are similar in nutritional value to almonds but higher in iron and vitamin B_1. In Oriental medicine pistachios are considered lubricating to the Intestines and tonifying for the Kidneys and Liver. Under the dominion of Mercury, pistachio corresponds to the element of Air and to the energy of love.

POPPY SEED *(Papaver rhoeas)*

Poppy seeds are members of the Papaveraceae (Poppy) family. It takes more than ten million tiny poppy seeds to make one pound. In general, black-colored foods indicate a high presence of minerals that strengthen the Kidneys. Poppy seeds have also been used as a mild narcotic and sedative and to reduce anxiety.

Poppy seeds are good to sprinkle on vegetable dishes. They are governed by the Moon and correspond to the energies of Water, love, and fertility. Use in moderation.

PUMPKIN SEEDS *(Curcurbita maxima, C. pepo)*

Pumpkin seeds, also known as *pepitas,* are members of the Curcurbitaceae (Gourd) family. They are warming, rich in omega-3 fatty acids, and contain 29 percent protein, along with vitamin B complex and calcium. Therapeutically, pumpkin seeds help relieve erectile dysfunction. Their high zinc content and anti-inflammatory properties help protect the male prostate gland from enlargement and can also help reduce the formation of calcium oxalate crystals, which can contribute to bladder and kidney stones. I do believe I have seen pumpkin seeds increase growth and sexual maturation in young people who were slow to bloom. Pumpkins correspond to the Moon, the Earth element, and the energy of nurturing.

SESAME SEEDS (*Sesamum indicum*)

Sesame seeds are members of the Pedaliaceae (Sesame) family. They tonify the yin and strengthen the Kidneys, Liver, bones, hair, nails, and teeth. They are considered demulcent, emollient, laxative, and a general tonic. They also stimulate libido in women and men.

Sesame seeds are about 50 percent oil and 25 to 35 percent protein. They also contain vitamin E, calcium, and iron. Black sesames are especially good Kidney tonics and are considered strengthening to the reproductive system. They are used in Oriental medicine to prevent hair from graying and to improve libido. Sesame corresponds to the Sun, to the element of Fire, and to energies of sex, fertility, protection, and prosperity. Alexander the Great is said to have fed his soldiers sesame seeds to increase their willpower, courage, and endurance.

Hulled sesame seeds are used to make tahini and unhulled seeds make sesame butter. Hulled seeds lose much of their fiber, calcium, potassium, B_1, and iron. Grinding the seeds right before use makes them more digestible.

SUNFLOWER SEEDS (*Helianthus annuus*)

Sunflowers are members of the Asteraceae (Daisy) family. The Latin name is derived from the Greek word *helios* for "sun" and *anthos,* meaning "flower." The species name is from the Latin word for annual. Flower heads in some varieties are heliotropic, meaning they follow the sun as it crosses the sky. The Incas considered the sunflower a representative of the sun god, Atahualpa. They carved sunflower images into gold, and solar priestesses wore sunflower crowns. At one time Russian soldiers were given rations of two pounds of sunflower seeds daily, which at times was their only nourishment.

As a medicinal food, sunflower seeds are antioxidant, diuretic, expectorant, and nutritive. Sunflower seeds are considered a tonic for the eyes, decreasing light sensitivity and preventing eye degeneration. They strengthen the fingernails due to their high nutrient content. Sunflower seeds build energy; they are warming and increase sexual vigor in both sexes. Their high B vitamin content makes them excellent for strengthening a debilitated nervous system and for building Kidney strength. Buy sunflower seeds in the shell to quit smoking as they require satisfying oral-manual work to crack open the shell and peel it off before you can enjoy the tender seed. Sunflowers correspond to the Sun and to the element of Fire and are associated with energies of success, protection, fertility, and eternal life.

WALNUT (*Juglans nigra:* Black Walnut, *J. regia:* English Walnut)

Walnuts are members of the Juglandaceae (Walnut) family. The genus name, *Juglans,* is contracted from the Latin *Jovis glans,* or "nut of Jupiter," in the belief that gods and goddesses dined on walnuts. They correspond to the Sun and Jupiter, to the element of Fire, and to energies of consciousness and protection.

The Chinese refer to walnuts as "longevity fruit" because a walnut tree lives for several hundred years. In Oriental medicine walnuts are considered warming, strengthening for the Lungs and Kidneys, and lubricating to the Large Intestine.

Walnuts are about 60 percent fat and 20 percent protein and include vitamin E, calcium, potassium, and zinc. Because of their resemblance to the brain, many cultures consider walnuts a good brain tonic and use them to treat head injuries.

Okra (Hibiscus esculentus)

Okra is a member of the Malvaceae (Malva) family. The stiff vegetable exudes a slimy liquid not unlike sexual fluids. Okra is a powerfully nutritive vegetable for those who feel weak, exhausted, or depressed. It is rich in beta-carotene, vitamin B complex, vitamin C, calcium, iron, phosphorus, potassium, and sodium. It is also an excellent source of electrolytes, which help balance the body's fluids and are necessary for nerve impulse transmission.

Commonly used in Creole cooking, okra can be sliced into wheel-like shapes and added to salads or used in soups as a thickener. It combines well with tomatoes, which minimize its gelatinous consistency. Try okra sliced in salads, used for dips, or added to vegetable soups and juices. Okra is governed by Venus and the Moon. It is associated with the element of Water and with energies of soothing, protection, and comfort.

***Olive** (Oleum europea, O. olviva)*

Olive is a member of the Oleaceae (Olive) family. The olive tree has been a symbol of peace since the days of Noah and is still used this way today at the United Nations. Greek mythology describes the olive tree as a gift from the goddess Athena, who endowed the tree with the ability to nourish and heal. Its leaves were used to crown Olympic champions. Olive is governed by the Sun, is a symbol of the Air element, and associated with the energies of sex, peace, health, and spirituality.

The fruit of the olive tree is sweet, pungent, hot, and moist. Olives contain linoleic acid, linolenic acid, oleic acid, and lecithin. They are an excellent vegan source of protein. Olive fruits are antioxidant, demulcent, emollient, nutritive, and tonic.

Olives are used in salads, pizzas, Mediterranean cuisine, dips, breads, and hors d'oeuvres. Look for sun-cured olives that are not pasteurized, canned, or heated. The black ray nourishes the Kidneys, which govern sexuality in Oriental medicine.

***Peaches** (Prunus persica, P. vulgaris)*

Peaches are members of the Rosaceae (Rose) family. In the Taoist tradition, peaches are considered a fruit of immortality and to this day are a most sacred plant, often served at birthdays. The flowers are a symbol of love, springtime, virginity, fertility, and wishes, and are often worn by brides. Peaches correspond to the element of Water, the planet Venus, and the Sun. The fruit has traditionally been consumed to enhance wisdom.

There is a legend that tells of the peach tree of the gods, which belonged to the Royal Mother in China and which bloomed only once every three thousand years. Touching its sap made the body luminous and granted health, happiness, virility, wisdom, and immortality to those who ate of it. Ho Hsien-Ku, a famous Chinese heroine, was said to have been transformed into a fairy after eating a celestial peach. Thereafter she lived on moonbeams and mother-of-pearl.

Peaches are rich in beta-carotene as well as lycopene and lutein, flavonoids including quercetin, vitamin C, niacin, calcium, boron, magnesium, phosphorus, potassium, and zinc. Peaches are warm, alkalizing, antioxidant, aromatic, digestive, diuretic, and emollient. Being of the orange ray, which combines the red ray of passion with the yellow ray of wisdom, they bestow warming and strengthening properties to the Kidneys and Lungs.

Enjoy peaches alone or in fruit salads, cold soups, salsas, ice creams, and pies. You can also find them dried or preserved in jams, syrups, and liqueurs. Many dried peaches are treated with sulfur dioxide, however, so buy organic. Lovers might enjoy eating sliced peaches off each other!

Persimmons *(Diospyros virginiana, D. kaki)*

Persimmons are of the Ebenaceae (Ebony) family. The genus name, *Diospyros,* is from the Greek and means "born of Zeus."

Persimmons are sweet and cooling and help tonify the yin (moistening fluids) of the body. Corresponding to the Sun, the element of Water, and the energy of happiness, persimmons are a good source of beta-carotene, vitamin C, calcium, magnesium, phosphorus, and potassium. Enjoy persimmons by themselves, peeled and added to salads, or used in jams, chutneys, puddings, and pies. Suck the sweet orange flesh out of a perfectly ripe persimmon for a totally sensuous experience.

Plums *(Prunus domestica)*

Plums, of the Rosaceae (Rose) family, provide energy and are considered a tonic food for the brain, nerves, and blood. Plums are rich in vitamins C, B_1, calcium, iron, phosphorus, and potassium.

When dried, of course, they are called prunes. Add plums or soaked prunes to fruit salad, puddings, pies, jams, and sauces or eat them by themselves as a tangy snack.

In Chinese mythology, plums symbolize wisdom, longevity, and resurrection. In traditional Oriental medicine, plums are thought to help people open up emotionally. They correspond to the planet Venus, the element of Water, and to energies of sexuality and protection. Prunes were served to customers in Elizabethan brothels for free to stimulate libido. Imagine that!

Pomegranate *(Punica granatum)*

Pomegranate is a member of the Lythraceae (Henna) family. The word *pomegranate* comes from the Latin term for "apple of many seeds." The pomegranate was the food of Persephone during her journey into the Underworld. With its blood-red color, the pomegranate has long been a symbol of fertility, birth, and sexuality. In Oriental medicine pomegranate is considered a yin tonic that builds the Kidneys, Liver, Urinary Bladder, and the blood. Pomegranate exhibits anti-aging properties and helps encourage creativity. It is a rich source of vitamin C and potassium. The seeds contain phytoestrogenic compounds; eating half a pomegranate daily is said to improve fertility. Pomegranates also contain pelleterine, an alkaloid that is similar to the hallucinogen mescaline and is associated with spiritual states of consciousness. Under the dominion of Mercury, pomegranate corresponds to the element of Fire and to the energies of creativity, fertility, and prosperity.

To eat a pomegranate, try rolling the fruit on a hard surface; then make a hole in one end and suck out the juice. You can also slice open the fruit and scoop out the seeds; they're great in fruit salad. Or try pomegranate sorbet. Best of all is to eat one with your lover. On Halloween or Samhain, an ancient tradition is to share a pomegranate in silence with your beloved, then make love.

Sea Vegetables

Sea vegetables, also known as seaweeds, grow in the rich brine of the ocean and transform its fifty-six known minerals into nutrients that we can assimilate, including calcium, iodine, iron, potassium, and magnesium. In fact, sea vegetables contain ten to twenty times more minerals than land-grown plants. Their abundant mineral content makes seaweeds an important element in any diet. They nourish the thyroid gland and the entire endocrine system, thereby supporting libido and improving metabolism. They also strengthen the Kidneys and beautify the skin and hair.

Energetically, seaweeds are cool and wet. They correspond to the Moon, the element of Water, and the energies of release (such as letting go of weight and old emotions). They can help old programming to resurface, allowing negative memories to come to light and have the opportunity to be resolved.

Seaweeds such as arame, dulse, hiziki, kelp, kombu, nori, sea palm, and wakame are usually available in dried form at natural food stores. Crush and sprinkle them over salads, eat them plain as snacks, add them to soups as flavorings, or use them as wrappers to hold other delights. If you need to soften dried seaweed, soak it for twenty minutes in room-temperature water, then rinse and drain. Use a bit of oil in preparing seaweeds to enhance the absorption of minerals and vitamins A and D. Different types of edible seaweeds are described below.

BROWN ALGAES

Arame (*Eisenia bicyclis*) supports the Spleen, Stomach, and Pancreas. Arame is rich in beta-carotene and potassium.

Hiziki (*Hizikia fusiforme*) strengthens the Intestines and enhances the assimilation of nutrients. It is rich in calcium, iron, and vitamins B_1, B_2, and C.

Kombu (*Laminaria* species) is especially strengthening to the Kidneys and reproductive system. It is high in calcium, iron, potassium, and sodium.

Sea palm (*Postelsia palmaeformis*) resembles a palm tree, grows on rocky shores, and is almost constantly pounded by the surf, enduring more hardship than most plants. It contributes greatly to stamina and supports glandular function.

Wakame (*Undaria pinnatifida*) helps support the Liver and nervous system as well as mental flexibility. It is rich in protein, trace minerals, beta-carotene, and vitamin B complex.

RED SEAWEEDS

Dulse (*Rhodymenia palmetta*) is soft, flat, and delicate, resembling gloves or mittens. It is rich in iron, beta-carotene, and vitamin E, and it benefits the Heart and Spleen.

Nori (*Porphyra tenera*) stimulates circulation and gives short bursts of energy, relieving fatigue and loneliness. It is high in protein, beta-carotene, and minerals. Black nori sheets are raw, and the green ones have been roasted.

Shiitake (*Lentinus edodes*) (syn. *Lentinula edodes*)

Shiitake mushrooms belong to the Polyporaceae (Polypor) family. Shiitake is considered an aphrodisiac, chi tonic, and rejuvenative. For thousands of years shiitake mushroom, known as "the mushroom of immortality," has been used to prevent premature aging. Amino acids (lysine, arginine), polysaccharides (lentinan), eritadenine, vitamin C, vitamin D, vitamin B_2, vitamin B_{12}, calcium, potassium, and purines can all be found in this super immune tonic.

According to traditional Oriental medicine, shiitake mushrooms can make women more open to love. Mushrooms are governed by the Moon, and correspond to the element of Earth and to energies of immune health and psychic awareness.

Spirulina (Spirulina platensis)

Spirulina is a spiral, multicelled blue-green algae. It is rich in protein and was considered a "sacred power plant" by the Aztecs and Mayans. Spirulina grows in warm alkaline or salty water. One acre of spirulina yields twenty times more protein than an acre of soybeans. It is 65 percent protein and also contains GLA (gamma linoleic acid) and vitamin B_{12}. It is easy to digest due to its soft-wall cell structure. Popular with dieters, this superfood is packed with nutrients, including the amino acids phenylalanine and tyrosine, which suppress appetite and help you feel satisfied. Governed by Venus and the Moon, spirulina corresponds to the element of Water and is associated with love and healing. Try sprinkling the powder into salads, dressings, smoothies, soup, or guacamole.

Truffles (Tuber melanosperm, T. magnatum)

Truffles are members of the Polyporaceae (Polypor) family. The underground fruiting body of particular forest fungi, the truffle is a rare delicacy. Truffles also have a long history of use as an aphrodisiac. Interestingly, they have been found to contain a particular phytosterol, or plant hormone, that is similar to a hormone found in boars' testicles and secreted in female wild boars' saliva when they are in heat. Truffles are also rich in minerals, especially iron. Unfortunately, they are becoming rare in the wild due to climate changes.

Watermelon (Citrullus lannatus, C. vulgaris)

Watermelon is a member of the Curcurbitaceae (Gourd) family. It is cold, sweet, and alkalizing. Watermelon is a rejuvenating blood tonic and has antibacterial, antioxidant, diuretic, and laxative properties. It has an affinity for the Bladder, Kidneys, and Heart and can help lift the spirits from depression. Watermelon has been used in treatments for halitosis, hangover, mouth sores, and urethral pain and also makes an ideal food during a cleanse.

Watermelon is a good source of beta-carotene, vitamin C, potassium, and silicon. Watermelon is best enjoyed on its own, but you can also try it with other melons in a fruit salad, juice it, or freeze the puree for a cool watermelon sorbet. The inner rind of watermelon contains chlorophyll and can be eaten with the pink flesh or run through a juicer; it will help build blood and strengthen the glands. The red ray of watermelon denotes passion and energy. Watermelon is governed by the Moon and corresponds to the energies of Water, healing, energy, and sexuality.

Black watermelon seeds are a traditional remedy for strengthening the Kidneys and for use as a sex tonic. For a truly invigorating watermelon tonic, try juicing the seeds, juice, and pink flesh all together. Finding watermelons with seeds can be difficult in these days of hybridization and genetic modifications, but it's worth it. I promise your libido will grow, but a watermelon will not grow in your stomach.

Today, most fruits and vegetables are grown with the assistance of pesticides and herbicides, and livestock are injected with a wide range of hormones to force them to grow quickly, to achieve a larger size, and to increase their resistance to disease. Trace amounts of those pesticides, herbicides, and hormones make their way into the food on our tables, and they can cause the liver extreme stress as it works to remove these toxins from the body.

Therefore, choose organic produce whenever it's available, and make sure that any meat, dairy products, and eggs you purchase derive from animals that were raised on organic feed and without the "assistance" of hormone treatments. Should you choose to eat animal foods, some of the better alternatives are goat's milk cheese and yogurt, wild-caught fish from deep clean waters, and wild game (though chronic wasting disease is a growing problem that has arisen because wild animals have gained access to commercial cattle feed that has been contaminated with infected animal by-products).

In the past, many native cultures awarded a hunter the honor of eating the still-beating heart of the elk or deer he had killed so that he could absorb its courage and strength. What might be the effects today of eating the factory-farmed animals that live in such a hellish existence? Could that not be a factor in the depression and anxiety so many people experience today?

If you eat healthy organic foods, you can feel good about taking them into your body, and the pure energies they contribute to your well-being will keep you feeling wonderful!

CULINARY HERBS

Most classic culinary herbs are considered aphrodisiacs, after all, they stir the senses. The herbs in the following list have a warming, stimulating effect on the body and help improve circulation. Use lavish amounts of them in your cuisine. Spicing up your love life never tasted so good!

Anise seed (*Pimpinella anisum*) is a member of the Apiaceae (Parsley) family that has long been considered an aphrodisiac as well as a breath freshener. In Oriental tradition, anise warms the Kidneys. Historically, the seed was added to wedding cakes to stimulate "wedding night vigor."

Anise seeds are used to relieve menstrual cramps. Stuffed in a sachet and taken to bed, they are said to prevent nightmares. Some believe that hanging a sprig of anise on one's bedpost promotes youthfulness.

Cardamom seed (*Elettaria cardamomum*) is a member of the Zingiberaceae (Ginger) family. It has been used in Asian countries as an ingredient in love potions and in Arabic cultures as a sign of hospitality. The seed is sometimes added to smoking blends and, like anise, is used as a breath freshener; people chew it after drinking alcohol or eating garlic to conceal their indulgence.

Cayenne pepper (*Capsicum frutescens*) is a member of the Solanaceae (Nightshade) family. It improves circulation, producing a feeling of warmth throughout the body, and also stimulates the production of endorphins. Paprika, a milder version of this red-hot plant, adds colorful flavonoids when sprinkled on prepared dishes.

Cinnamon bark (*Cinnamomum species*), a golden-rayed member of the Lauraceae (Laurel) family, has been used as a warming spicy aphrodisiac since ancient times. A vasodilator and a yang tonic, cinnamon's prolonged use is known to beautify the skin and promote a rosy complexion. It is especially helpful for people who are always cold and have poor circulation. It is used in the treatment of dysmenorrhea, erectile dysfunction, fatigue, flatulence, halitosis, irregular menses, lumbago, poor circulation, and vision problems.

Cinnamon is often included in massage oils for its warming and sexually arousing properties and in toothpastes for its ability to freshen breath. The aromatic scent of cinnamon stimulates the senses yet calms the nerves. In love magic, cinnamon encourages love, success, and prosperity.

Clove bud (*Syzygium aromaticum*), in the Myrtaceae (Eucalyptus) family, has long been considered an aphrodisiac and is a common remedy for premature ejaculation, especially when included in topical lotions. Clove stimulates circulation and digestion, warms the body, and is used to treat candida, depression, erectile dysfunction, flatulence, halitosis, and poor circulation. Folklore says that sucking on two whole cloves without chewing or swallowing them helps curb the desire for alcohol.

Coriander seed (*Coriandrum sativum*), a member of the Apiaceae (Parsley) family, is mentioned as an aphrodisiac in *The Arabian Nights*. It was an important ingredient in love potions of the Middle Ages. Coriander seed tea is used to treat amenorrhea, anxiety, cramps, cystitis, flatulence, and halitosis.

Coriander seeds are a common spice used in preparing dishes from a wide range of cuisines, including Latin American, Indian, Ethiopian, Arabic, and Thai and other Asian cuisines. The leaves of the plant, known as cilantro, are also a popular flavoring used in Asian, North African, and Mexican cooking. The root is also edible and may be prepared as a vegetable.

Cumin seed (*Cuminum cyminum*), another member of the Apiaceae (Parsley) family, improves peripheral circulation to the body's extremities—including the genitals—and has long been used in love potions.

Curry. The various blends of herbs known as curries are warming and beneficial to the circulatory system, providing another possibility for spicing up your love life.

Fennel seed (*Foeniculum officinale*), yet another member of the Apiaceae (Parsley) family, improves energy, freshens the breath, and increases libido. Being antifungal, galactagogic, and phytoestrogenic, fennel is also used in the treatment of various ailments, including amenorrhea, endometriosis, fatigue, fever, menstrual cramps, and premenstrual syndrome.

Garlic (*Allium sativum*) is part of the Lilliaceae (Lily) family and is one of the most studied herbal medicines on the planet. It is only medicinal when raw, and in this state it increases testosterone levels, increases sperm production, and elevates libido. It also improves circulation and warms the body. In ancient Rome, garlic was a favorite herb of Ceres, the goddess of fertility. Excess amounts of garlic can be irritating to the stomach and kidneys; some people find that even small amounts of raw garlic can cause heartburn. Avoid large doses during pregnancy and while nursing, as it may cause digestive distress in the mother and baby. Excessive use can provoke anger and emotional irritability.

SWEETENING GARLIC BREATH

Garlic breath—a result of garlic consumption—can last for as long as ten hours. Some simple remedies for it include chewing anise, caraway, cumin, or fennel seeds; chewing pieces of cinnamon or sprigs of parsley; or taking one drop of pure peppermint oil in a cup of water. Enjoy garlic with your beloved when you can be in for a few hours; if you eat it together, neither will smell it on the other's breath.

Gingerroot (*Zingiber officinale*) is a member of the Zingiberaceae (Ginger) family. The genus name, Zingiber, and common name, ginger, derive from the ancient Greek word for the plant, *zingiberi,* which is itself thought to be from the Indo-Aryan and possibly to mean "shaped like a horn." Ginger warms the body and has been used for centuries to treat amenorrhea, delayed menses, low libido, and low sperm motility. Ginger is an antifungal, antioxidant, circulatory stimulant, diaphoretic, and emmenagogue. In magic practices, ginger attracts love, prosperity, and success.

Mustard seed (various species). Various seeds in the Brassicaceae (Cruciferous) family are all warming to the body, improving circulation and enhancing libido.

Nutmeg (*Myristica fragrans*), part of the Myristaceae (Nutmeg) family, contains an essential oil called myristicin, which is chemically similar to MDMA, also known as the "love drug" Ecstasy. Nutmeg is best when grated fresh onto food. It is known to make alcoholic beverages even more intoxicating. Nutmeg has long been used in magical traditions to attract love and prosperity. It can be burned as incense, and the essential oil is often an ingredient in perfumes, soaps, toothpastes, and massage oils. Nutmeg is also sometimes added to smoking mixtures and snuff.

Parsley (*Petroselinum crispim*), of the rich, green ray, is related to anise, coriander, cumin, and fennel. It is an antioxidant, aphrodisiac, blood builder, emmenagogue, and galactagogue. Eating fresh parsley is an ancient remedy to strengthen the vision, regulate delayed menses, improve fertility, and freshen the breath. Use its fresh curly greenness to garnish your food.

Rosemary *(Rosmarinus officinalis)* is a member of the Lamiaceae (Mint) family. It has long been considered a symbol of friendship, loyalty, and remembrance. In some traditions brides wear a wreath of rosemary and carry it in their bridal bouquet as a symbol of their remembrance of their families and their marriage vows. The leaves are valued as antidepressant, antifungal, anti-inflammatory, antioxidant, antiseptic, antispasmodic, aromatic, astringent, diuretic, emmenagogic, rejuvenative, rubefacient, stimulant, and tonic to the yang energies of the body.

Rosemary tonifies the nervous system, improves peripheral circulation, promotes warmth, and uplifts the spirits. An excellent herb for the elderly, it is also used in the treatment of amenorrhea, anxiety, cellulite, debility, delayed menses, depression, memory loss, menstrual cramps, stress, and vertigo. It is warm and dry, corresponding to the Sun and to the element of Fire.

Sage (*Salvia officinalis*) of the Lamiaceae (Mint) family is actually an anaphrodisiac—the opposite of an aphrodisiac. It is also antifungal, antigalactagogic, anti-inflammatory, antioxidant, antiseptic, antispasmodic, and aromatic as well as a brain tonic, circulatory stimulant, emmenagogue, estrogen promoter, nervine, and general tonic. Even just the aroma of sage helps promote mental alertness. Why mention an anaphrodisiac? Because sometimes getting it on might not be on the menu—your partner may be ill, too pregnant, away, or not available.

Sage is used in the treatment of anxiety, cystitis, depression, flatulence, hot flashes, irregular menses, memory problems, menopause, menorrhagia, migraines, night sweats, and excessive perspiration.

In folkloric tradition, sage is used to promote longevity and wisdom and to attract protection and prosperity. Avoid large doses during pregnancy and while nursing, because it can dry up a mother's milk.

Turmeric (*Curcuma longa*) is a member of the Zingerberaceae (Ginger) family. In many languages the literal translation of the common name for this plant is simply "yellow earth." The rhizome is antifungal, anti-inflammatory, antioxidant, antiseptic, and aromatic, and is also a circulatory stimulant and emmenagogue.

Turmeric, of the sunny yellow-orange ray, helps stabilize the body's microflora, thus inhibiting yeast overgrowth. It also sensitizes the body's cortisol receptor sites making it an excellent anti-inflammatory agent. It helps regulate the menses and is restorative after childbirth. It is used in the treatment of candida, eczema, flatulence, high cholesterol, trauma, and uterine tumors.

Dried or fresh turmeric root is a popular spice in Asian, and particularly Indian, cuisine. The root is eaten raw in southern India. Turmeric aids in the digestion of fats and protein.

In northern Indian traditional wedding ceremonies, turmeric is applied to the bride and groom to offer protection from "the evil eye." In folkloric tradition it is considered a symbol of prosperity and is used in cleaning for purification.

Vanilla (*Vanilla planifolia, V. pompona*) is a member of the Orchidaceae (Orchid) family. The genus name *Vanilla* derives from the Latin *vaina,* "sheath," "pod," or "little vagina," in reference to the suggestive shape of the flower. The Aztecs were the first to use vanilla; among other things, they added it to their chocolate drinks. The smell of vanilla is said to be one of the closest to mother's milk; perhaps as a result, smelling or eating vanilla can have a calming effect and help awaken childhood memories. The cured seedpod is considered aphrodisiac, aromatic, and stimulant.

Vanilla's aphrodisiac qualities perhaps result from the fact that it causes urethral irritation, which stimulates and raises awareness of the genitals. It is used infrequently in modern herbal medicine, but it can be helpful in cases of emotional trauma, hysteria, and low libido.

Vanilla bean and extract are popular flavorings for a wide variety of confections and liqueurs. Vanilla is used in love magic to scent perfumes, cosmetics, potpourri, and smoking mixtures.

EDIBLE FLOWERS

Flowers are the sex organs of plants. They add grace and beauty to any dish you make and are a colorful addition to any diet. Be sure to use only organically grown or wild edible flowers as many commercial ones are treated with chemicals. To show your beloved that he or she is adored, decorate your food with organic edible flowers such as violets, rose petals (with the white heels removed), daylilies, or hibiscus. Make food a healthful, beautiful, and flavorful mandala of your love. Other common edible flowers include apple blossoms, bachelor's buttons, bee balm, calendulas, chive flowers,

Johnny-jump-ups, lilacs, marigolds, nasturtiums, orange blossoms, pansies, petunias, plum blossoms, red clover, snapdragons, and squash blossoms.*

APHRODISIAC BEVERAGES

Sometimes a love cocktail can be more enticing than a whole meal. It's a great idea to have a supply of these around—you never know when they might come in handy!

Flower Power Sun Teas—Cold Water Infusions

The following flowers make delicious sun teas, which don't require any heat. Fill a glass pitcher with fresh flowers from the list below. Cover with pure water (use one cup of flowers per gallon of water). Allow to steep in the sun (or moonlight) for several hours. I have been known to infuse a few large crystals in the water too. Strain and imbibe the beauty of fresh infusions! The infusion will keep up to four days in the refrigerator.

- Anise hyssop leaf and flower (*Agastache foeniculum*)
- Bee balm leaf and flower (*Monarda* species)
- Lilac flower (*Syringa* species)
- Lemon balm leaf and flower (*Melissa officinalis*)
- Lemon verbena leaf (*Aloysia triphylla*)
- Peppermint leaf and flower (*Mentha piperita*)
- Rose flower (*Rosa* species)
- Rosemary leaf and flower (*Rosmarinus officinalis*)
- Spearmint leaf and flower (*Mentha spicata*)

Alcohol

Alcohol, in moderation, can be an aphrodisiac. It relaxes the mind and body, releases inhibitions, and can call passion to mind. Honey wine, also known as mead, was given to ancient Teuton brides for a month after their wedding to help them feel more responsive to sexual overtures from their new husbands. (And from this practice the word *honeymoon* evolved.) But as Shakespeare warned in *Macbeth,* "Alcohol provoketh desire, but taketh

*For more information on edible flowers see my book *Rawsome!* It lists more than 150 varieties of edible flowers.

away performance." Excessive drinking interferes with testosterone production and increases estrogen production; it decreases physical sensitivity, slows nerve functioning, and depresses the emotions. In men, prolonged excessive drinking has an adverse effect on erectile and ejaculatory functions and can even cause the male genitals to shrink. In women, it may lead to menstrual irregularity, infertility, and the inability to orgasm. It is best to avoid making the decision to sleep with someone for the first time when you are intoxicated.

While some aphrodisiac beverages are alcoholic, and in moderation a turn-on, they all become anaphrodisiac in excess. It's important, therefore, to remember that the purpose of an aphrodisiac beverage is to inspire passion and release inhibitions, not to cause loss of control.

Chartreuse, a yellow or green aphrodisiac liqueur, contains warming spices like allspice. Benedictine is another aphrodisiac liqueur, invented by monks—like Chartreuse—and also produced in monasteries. Liqueur de Damiana is a Mexican drink said to incite passion, and traditionally it is given to a bride on the morning of her wedding by her mother-in-law. Other traditional aphrodisiac alcohols include apricot brandy, champagne, cognac, palm wine, tequila, and vermouth.

Many imbibers would feel better if they avoided wines containing the preservative sulfite. Sulfite can cause allergic reactions, including breathing difficulty. It also increases the severity of hangovers.

Make your own love potion by tincturing some of the passion-inspiring herbs given in this chapter and the one following. My favorites include cinnamon, cardamom, cloves, vanilla bean, nutmeg, anise, muira puama, damiana, rose petals, vitex berries, and ginseng root. You can tincture one herb singly or in combination with other herbs. Also try adding honey to the final tincture for a delicious, sweet liqueur. (For more information about making tinctures by steeping herbs in alcohol or an alcohol substitute, see the "Herbal Tinctures" section on page 50.)

Alcohol is not the only beverage you can use to make a toast to love. Try morning smoothies or fresh juice. My favorite love tonic drink these days is the juice from young coconuts or a green smoothie. And remember, the best aphrodisiac of all is to be deeply in love. To good health and great love!

ANAPHRODISIACS

Anaphrodisiacs are the opposite of aphrodisiacs. They decrease sexual vitality and passion. In this classification are valerian, vinegar, tobacco, excessively refined sugars and carbohydrates, and cold showers. Icy foods, such as ice cream, cold sodas, and cold milk, can also cool your passions and cause congestion in the reproductive organs.

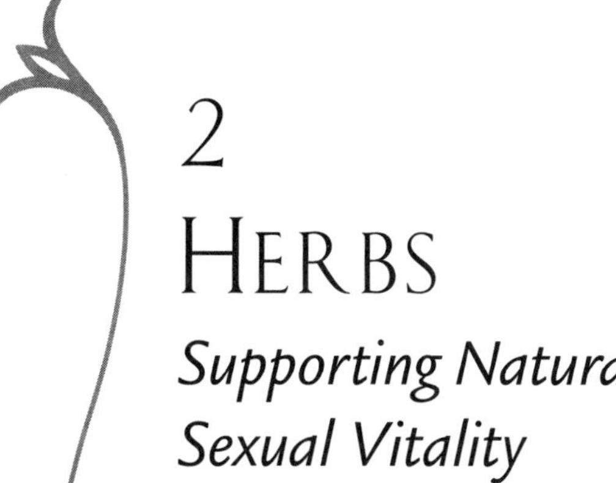

2
Herbs
Supporting Natural Sexual Vitality

HERBS OFFER A SAFE, natural way to nourish the body and boost sexual vitality. They are multifaceted, multidirectional, and multidimensional. A single herb can have many beneficial effects—some immediate, some long-term, some physical, and some emotional. Herbs can be directly healing, while they can also support the body's own healing mechanisms. For thousands of years, people around the world have used herbs to improve their health. That includes, in part, building sexual vigor and nourishing the reproductive system.

Herbs have wide-ranging actions, and they affect different people differently. They also tend to have a cumulative benefit; they work best when taken at an appropriate dosage over an appropriate length of time. So before using any herb as a health supplement, it's a good idea to educate yourself about it. Look it up in at least three herbal health books, and compare the descriptions. Consider consulting with an herbalist. Most important, if you are taking any medications—prescription or over-the-counter—consult with your health care provider before beginning a program of herbal supplements. Herbs and drugs can interact strangely, possibly leading to a serious health risk.

HERBAL PREPARATIONS

Herbs can be prepared as teas, tinctures, and capsules. All of these preparations are easy to make at home, though you can also find many premixed formulations at natural food stores and herb shops. Whether you make your own formulations or purchase commercial mixes, these time-tested botanicals are sure to spice up your love life!

Herbal Teas

Teas are soothing and warming. They can stimulate your senses, nourish your body, refresh your mind, and revitalize your energy. Having a cup of tea invites you to take time out of a busy day to sip, savor, and reflect.

To make a tea from leaves and flowers, you must prepare an *infusion.* Bring 1 cup of water to a boil in a nonaluminum pot. Remove from heat and add 1 heaping teaspoon of dried herb or 2 heaping teaspoons of fresh herb. Cover and let steep at least 10 minutes. Strain.

To make a tea from roots and barks, you must prepare a *decoction.* (One caveat: A root that is particularly high in volatile oils, such as ginger, is best infused rather than decocted.) Combine 1 heaping teaspoon of dried herb or 2 heaping teaspoons of fresh herb with 1 cup of water. Bring to a boil, reduce heat, and simmer, covered, for 20 minutes. Strain.

If you want to make a tea from a combination of herbs that must be infused and herbs that must be decocted, prepare the herbs that must be decocted first. When they have simmered for 20 minutes, remove the pot from the stovetop and strain. Then pour the hot water over the herbs that must be infused. Cover and let steep for at least 10 minutes, then strain.

Return the spent herbs to the earth by adding them to your compost pile. Give back to Mother Earth.

Herbal Tinctures

Tinctures are herbal extracts made by steeping herbs in alcohol or other liquid. Over time the liquid, known as the *menstruum,* extracts the water-soluble and alcohol-soluble elements from the herbs. As a result, the menstruum is imbued with the healing properties of the herbs. Alcohol is the most common menstruum—it must be at least 50 proof to activate the extraction process and to serve as a preservative. Most herbalists use vodka or brandy;

vodka is the purest grain alcohol, and brandy has a sweetness that balances the flavor of some of the less-palatable herbs.

Tinctures are easy to use; just put a dropperful in a bit of warm water and drink. You can buy herbal tinctures at any herb shop or natural food store; however, they're also easy to make at home, using the following method.

Chop or grind the herbs. The herbs being tinctured are known as the *mark*. Place them in a glass jar, then fill the jar with brandy or vodka so that the alcohol rises to an inch above the herbs. Screw on the cover tightly, and place in a cool, dark location. Shake daily. After a month, strain the herbs from the menstruum, first through a strainer and then through a clean, undyed cloth. Squeeze the cloth tightly to force out the last few drops of precious liquid. Put the tincture in glass bottles—dark glass is preferable, as it protects the tincture from the deactivating effects of light. Label and date the bottles, and store away from heat and light. Stored properly, these alcohol-based tinctures will keep for many years.

Tinctures can also be made using vegetable glycerin rather than alcohol. Glycerin-based tinctures, known as glycerites, are excellent for those who are alcohol intolerant as well as for children, pregnant women, and nursing mothers. Glycerin is both a solvent and a preservative with an effectiveness somewhere between that of water and alcohol. It is naturally sweet, slightly antiseptic, demulcent, and healing. Glycerites are prepared just like tinctures, but instead of alcohol they use a menstruum of one part water to two parts glycerin. A glycerite's shelf life is one to three years.

Apple cider vinegar—preferably organic—is another alternative menstruum for tincturing. It is also a digestive tonic and can be used to season food. For maximum potency, warm the vinegar before pouring it over the herbs. Do not use a metal lid to seal your container when storing a vinegar tincture; contact with vinegar causes metal to rust, which will contaminate the tincture. A vinegar-based tincture will have a shelf life of six months to two years. Look for a vinegar that is 5.7 percent acetic acid (or thereabouts) for a longer shelf life. Discard a tincture if it smells strange or contains mold.

The day of the new moon is traditionally considered the best time to start a new batch of tincture. The energy of the Moon is thought to draw out the properties of the herbs.

Herb Capsules

To make herb capsules, simply grind small amounts of dried herbs to a powder in a grinder. (Some dried herbs, such as saw palmetto berries, are very hard and will likely destroy a grinder. If that seems like it would be the case with an herb you're considering, forget about making your own capsules and purchase ready-made ones.)

You can purchase empty capsules at natural food stores and herb shops. Look for the size "00" capsules. Pull apart each capsule, scoop herbs into it, and press the two halves of the capsule together again. Store in a sealed glass jar away from heat and light. And don't forget to label the jar so that you'll remember what's in it.

A COMPENDIUM OF HERBAL LOVE TONICS

Every culture has a set of herbal favorites that nourish sexuality. Here's a compilation of herbs from around the world that have served humanity pleasurably in both ancient and modern love potions. The herbs listed below are just some of the plants known to be effective for stimulating sexual health. Also important are the culinary herbs listed in the previous chapter.

The herbs described below have many more properties than are listed here, but as this book is about sexuality, we have focused on the actions most likely to affect the reproductive system. For a more complete exploration, check out my book *The Desktop Guide to Herbal Medicine* (Laguna Beach, Calif.: Basic Health Publications, 2007).

Ashwagandha

Withania somnifera

Family Solanaceae (Nightshade)

Etymology The common name translates from the Sanskrit *ashva,* "horse," and *gandha,* "smells like," which alludes to the virility of a horse. The species name, *somnifera,* indicates that the herb is a soporific agent.

Part Used Root (primarily)

Physiological Effects Adaptogen, anabolic, anti-inflammatory, antioxidant, antispasmodic, antitumor, aphrodisiac, astringent, diuretic, hormone tonic, hypotensive, immune tonic, nervine, nutritive, rejuvenative, sedative, tonic, uterine relaxant

Medicinal Uses Ashwagandha's use has been recorded for at least three thousand years. It is excellent for those in convalescence. An ayurvedic maxim says that taking ashwagandha for fifteen days imparts strength to an emaciated body, just as rain does to a crop. Ashwagandha relaxes blood vessels and promotes an overall feeling of well-being. It enhances libido, boosts fertility, and strengthens the adrenal glands. It is often used to treat nervous exhaustion, debility, involuntary semen emission without orgasm, and sexual dysfunctions associated with stress. It also counteracts diseases associated with aging.

The herb has many other medicinal uses, including being of benefit to those with anxiety, depression, erectile dysfunction, exhaustion, infertility, low libido, lumbago, miscarriage, premature aging, and low sperm count.

Ashwagandha works as a monoamine oxidase inhibitor, thereby increasing the availability of dopamine, a neurotransmitter. It also appears to mimic the action of the neurotransmitter GABA (gamma amino butyric acid) in relaxing the body.

Constituents Thirty-five alkaloids (including ashwagandhine), steroidal lactones (withanolides), amino acids (tryptophan, alanine, ornithine), iron

Energetic Correspondences

- Flavor: sweet
- Temperature: warm
- Moisture: moist
- Polarity: yang
- Planet: Jupiter
- Element: Fire

Dosage Take 1 dropperful of tincture or 1 to 2 capsules three times daily.

CONCERNS

Avoid during pregnancy. Ashwagandha may increase the potency of barbiturates; if you are taking barbiturates, consult with your health care provider before taking ashwagandha.

Asparagus

Asparagus cochinchinensis (Chinese asparagus), *A. lucidus, A. racemosus* (Indian asparagus)

Family Liliaceae (Lily)

Etymology The word *asparagus* comes from the Greek *asparagos,* which refers to tender shoots that can be consumed. Due to its phallic shape, the plant has long been regarded as an aphrodisiac, which can be seen in its etymology; the ayurvedic name *shatavari,* for example, means "she who has one hundred husbands."

Part Used Root

Physiological Effects Aphrodisiac, brain tonic, demulcent, diuretic, female tonic, galactagogue, Kidney yin tonic, nutritive, rejuvenative, and reproductive tonic

Medicinal Uses Asparagus has been known as a supreme tonic since ancient times. The Taoist classic *Embracing the Uncarved Block,* written in AD 300 by Ko Hung, tells the story of a man named Tu Tze-wei, who drank asparagus root tea for many years and was able to have sexual relations with eighty wives and concubines, walk a distance of fifty miles a day, and attain the advanced age of 145. In general, asparagus moistens and restores the entire system.

Asparagus root increases orgasmic ability, boosts sperm count, and nourishes the ovum. It is often used to treat erectile dysfunction, and it is excellent for women who have had hysterectomies. On the emotional side, asparagus fosters deep feelings of love and compassion.

Asparagus root is used to treat cystitis, dry skin, erectile dysfunction, female organ weakness, frigidity, herpes, infertility, low libido, low sperm count, menopause, poor memory, post-hysterectomy dryness, and vaginal dryness. It can be used to encourage healing during convalescence.

Constituents Essential oil, steroidal glycoside (asparagoside), asparagine, arginine, tyrosine, flavonoids (kaempferol, quercetin, rutin), copper, iron, zinc, resin, tannin, mucilage

Energetic Correspondences

- Flavor: sweet, bitter
- Polarity: yin

- Temperature: cool
- Moisture: moist
- Planet: Venus
- Element: Water

Dosage Take 1 cup of tea or 30 to 40 drops of tincture three times daily.

CONCERNS

Safe when used appropriately. Aparagus root is not recommended in cases of chronic diarrhea or cough with excessive clear phlegm.

Burdock

Arctium lappa, A. minus

Family Asteraceae (Daisy)

Etymology The genus name, *Arctium,* derives from the Greek *arktos,* meaning "bear"—a reference to the shaggy burrs. The species name, *lappa,* is derived from a Greek word meaning "to seize," in reference to the clinginess of the seeds. The common name *burdock* is derived from the French *beurre,* "butter," and the English word *dock,* meaning "leaves"; French women would wrap their cakes of butter in leaves of burdock to transport it to the marketplace.

Parts Used Root, seed, leaf (topically)

Physiological Effects Root: adaptogen, adrenal tonic, aphrodisiac, demulcent, diuretic, galactagogue, nutritive, rejuvenative

Medicinal Uses In Chinese and Hawaiian cultures, burdock is considered an aphrodisiac. It helps you feel grounded with its deep root and in touch with your body and the earth.

As an anti-inflammatory demulcent agent, burdock root soothes and clears internal heat. It improves the elimination of metabolic wastes through the liver, lymph, large intestine, lungs, kidneys, and skin. Burdock is used to treat candida, cystitis, gonorrhea, HIV, irritability, lumbago, premenstrual syndrome, prostate inflammation, syphilis, urinary inflammation, and uterine prolapse. It makes an excellent spring detoxification or fasting tea.

Constituents Root: vitamin C, calcium, iron, magnesium, potassium, zinc, polyacetylenes, chlorogenic acid, taraxosterol, arctigen, inulin, lactone, essential oil, flavonoids, tannin, mucilage, resin

Energetic Correspondences

- Flavor: root—bitter; seed—pungent
- Temperature: cool
- Moisture: dry
- Polarity: yin
- Planet: Venus/Jupiter/Saturn/Pluto
- Element: Water

Dosage Drink 1 cup of tea or 10 to 30 drops of tincture three times daily.

CONCERNS

Avoid burdock seeds during the first trimester of pregnancy, during the later stages of measles, and in cases of open sores.

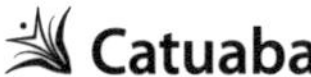 Catuaba

Erythroxylum catuaba

Family Erythroxylaceae (Coca)

Etymology The genus name, *Erythroxylum,* derives from the Greek *erythros,* "red," and *xylon,* "wood." Catuaba is an indigenous South American name for the tree.

Parts Used Bark, root

Physiological Effects Analgesic, antibacterial, antiseptic, antiviral, aphrodisiac, brain tonic, central nervous system stimulant, tonic, vasodilator, vasorelaxant

Medicinal Uses This South American herb enhances sexual desire, generally by decreasing stress. In the Amazon, where the herb originates, there is a saying that "until a father reaches sixty, the son is his; after that, the son is catuaba's," in reference to the herb's aphrodisiac qualities. Catuaba's aphrodisiac qualities benefit both women and men. The herb is used to treat agitation, anxiety, erectile dysfunction, exhaustion, low libido, and poor memory.

Catuaba is in the same family as coca, from which cocaine is derived, but it does not contain cocaine alkaloids.

Constituents Essential oils and alkaloids

Energetic Correspondences

- Flavor: pungent
- Temperature: warm
- Moisture: dry
- Polarity: yang
- Planet: Mars
- Element: fire

Dosage Drink 1 cup of tea or 10 to 20 drops of tincture three times daily.

CONCERNS

No reports of toxicity exist. However, until further research has been done, catuaba is not recommended during pregnancy.

Damiana

Turnera aphrodisiaca, T. diffusa (syn. *T. microphylla*)

Family Turneraceae (Turnera)

Etymology The genus name, *Turnera,* was given in honor of Giorgio della Turra (1607–1688), an Italian botanist. The species name, *aphrodisiaca,* is from Aphrodite, Greek goddess of love and aphrodisiacs.

Part Used Aboveground plant

Physiological Effects Antidepressant, aphrodisiac, astringent, diuretic, emmenagogue, hormone regulator, nervine, stimulant, and urinary antiseptic

Medicinal Uses The Mayans and Aztecs used damiana as a sexual stimulant and to treat respiratory disorders. It was listed in the U.S. National Formulary from 1888 to 1947. Damiana nourishes the yang, invigorates the brain and nerves, regulates the pituitary gland, and promotes physical endurance. The bitter principle, damianin, stimulates the nervous system and genitals and allows nerve messages to more readily spread through the body. Damiana is high in phosphorus, which may contribute to its energizing qualities. Damiana improves orgasmic ability, boosts nerve sensitivity, and strengthens the reproductive system.

Valued in Central America for its ability to treat erectile dysfunction and premature ejaculation, damiana also counteracts testicular atrophy and remedies sexual problems related to anxiety. There are some reports of people having unusually erotic dreams while taking damiana. The herb has been used by livestock breeders to encourage mating.

Today, damiana is used to treat anxiety, bedwetting, debility, depression, erectile dysfunction, exhaustion, hangover, hot flashes, infertility, low libido, menstrual cramps, prostatitis, urinary tract infection, and venereal disease. It has been used as a tea to help teenagers overcome the shyness and self-consciousness that sometimes accompanies puberty, and it can also be used to help adults overcome sexual "performance anxiety."

As a flower essence, damiana diminishes feelings of inadequacy and restores feelings of sensuality and energy.

Some lovers enjoy sharing a ritual smoke of damiana before making love. Combine a pinch of peppermint leaf with a pinch of skullcap leaf and two pinches of damiana leaf. Add a few shredded rose petals, then roll up in smoking paper and smoke or share in a water pipe as a prelude to lovemaking. Damiana is also sometimes burned as an incense to inspire visions.

Constituents Vitamin C, phosphorous, selenium, silicon, sulfur, flavonoids, essential oils, beta-sitosterol

Energetic Correspondences

- Flavor: bitter, pungent
- Temperature: warm
- Moisture: dry
- Polarity: yang
- Planet: Mars/Pluto
- Element: Fire/Water

Dosage Take 1 cup of tea daily or 15 drops of tincture three times daily.

CONCERNS

Damiana is generally considered safe, but avoid using it in cases of urinary tract disease, hypertension, or during pregnancy or nursing. Long-term use may interfere with the body's assimilation of iron. Large doses may be somewhat laxative.

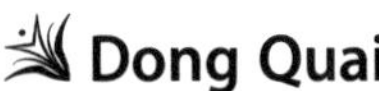 Dong Quai

Angelica polymorpha, A. sinensis

Family Apiaceae (Parsley)

Etymology The English spelling of the Chinese name appears variously as *dong quai, tang kuei,* and *tang kwei*. The Chinese name translates as "state of return," in reference to the belief that the herb helps blood return to where it belongs, rather than stagnating.

Part Used Root

Physiological Effects Antifungal, anti-inflammatory, antispasmodic, antitumor, aphrodisiac, blood tonic, chi tonic, circulatory stimulant, diuretic, emmenagogue, hepatoprotective, immune stimulant, sedative (mild), postpartum tonic, uterine relaxant, uterine stimulant, uterine tonic, yin tonic, and vasodilator

Medicinal Uses The first recorded use of dong quai appears in the *Shen Nong Ben Cao Jing* (Divine Husbandman's Classic of the Materia Medica), compiled during the Han Dynasty (AD 25–220). It is still one of the most frequently used herbs in Asia.

Dong quai is a classic women's herb, but it also benefits men. It increases a woman's sex drive, which can be particularly helpful for menopausal women. It can improve circulation and act as an energy tonic for both sexes. Dong quai is used to treat amenorrhea, anemia, candida, dry skin, dysmenorrhea, endometriosis, exhaustion, hair loss, infertility (female), insomnia, irregular menses, menopause (hot flashes, vaginal dryness, and heart palpitations), muscle spasms, pain, PMS, and traumatic injury.

On the emotional side, dong quai supports calmness and fosters compassion. In Oriental tradition, it is used to disperse congestion in the pelvic region. Though it is not estrogenic, its effects are similar in that it binds to estrogen receptor sites. Women who are going off birth control pills can use dong quai to help reestablish regular menstrual cycles. Dong quai also helps nourish dry, thin, vaginal tissues and beautifies the skin.

Constituents Vitamin B_2, niacin, folic acid, vitamin B_{12}, chromium, iron, magnesium, phosphorus, potassium, flavonoids, coumarins, polysaccharides, essential oils, beta-sitosterol, angelic acid

Energetic Correspondences

- Flavor: sweet, pungent, bitter (but extremely bitter roots are of poor quality)
- Polarity: yin
- Planet: Venus/Mars/Jupiter/Moon

- Temperature: warm
- Moisture: moist
- Element: Water

Dosage Take 1 cup of tea or 20 to 40 drops of tincture three times daily.

CONCERNS

Avoid dong quai during pregnancy, except under the supervision of a qualified health care practitioner. Avoid in cases of diarrhea, poor digestion, abdominal distention, heavy menstrual flow, high fever with a strong fast pulse, or when using blood-thinning medications such as ibuprofen. Use of dong quai can increase photosensitivity.

Eleuthero

Eleutherococcus senticosus, E gracilistylus (formerly *Acanthopanax senticosus,* and *A. spinosus*)

Family Araliaceae (Ginseng)

Etymology The name *Eleutherococcus* is from the Greek *eleutheros,* meaning "free," and *kokkos,* meaning "pip," in reference to the fruits. Formerly, this plant was called Acantho Panax from the Greek word *akanthos,* meaning "thorn." In the 1970s the herb was known as Siberian Ginseng, as part of a marketing effort to associate a lesser-known product with a popular one.

Although eleuthero has many similar properties to American and Asian ginsengs, it is not a true ginseng but rather a second cousin. However, it is the subject of much research. It is also less expensive, easier to grow, and more sustainable than ginseng.

Parts Used Root, root bark

Physiological Effects The root, root bark, and, to a lesser degree, the leaves are used as an adaptogen, antioxidant, antispasmodic, aphrodisiac, immune tonic, metabolic regulator, rejuvenative, tonic (adrenal, cardiac, chi, immune, nerve, and yang tonic), and vasodilator. Eleuthero is also considered an antifungal, anti-inflammatory, antitumor, blood tonic, circulatory stimulant, diuretic, emmenagogue, hypotensive, sedative (mild), postpartum tonic, uterine relaxant, uterine stimulant, uterine tonic, and yin tonic.

Medicinal Uses Eleuthero has been used for centuries by the tribal communities of Siberia and by the Chinese for more than four thousand years. An ancient Chinese proverb says, "I would rather take a handful of eleuthero than a cartload of gold and jewels." Legend says that reindeer, a symbol of strength and endurance, consume this plant in the frigid regions of China, Russia, and Japan.

Since 1962 Russian cosmonauts have been given rations of eleuthero to help them acclimate to the stresses of being weightless and living in space. Athletes, deep-sea divers, rescue workers, and explorers also use it for nourishing support during times of stress. In the past forty years there have been more than a thousand studies on eleuthero that demonstrate it to share many of the same therapeutic properties as *Panax* ginsengs.

Considered an adaptogen that helps people acclimate to stressful situations, eleuthero is an excellent treatment for a weakened nervous system or adrenal gland insufficiency. It relieves fatigue, improves stamina, and helps remedy erectile dysfunction.

Eleuthero is used in alcoholism, AIDS, athletic recovery, depression, edema, erectile dysfunction, chronic fatigue syndrome, convalescence, fatigue, hepatitis, hypertension, infertility, lumbago, low sperm count, and stress. In Asia it is sometimes included as an ingredient in liqueurs and wines that are sold as sexually tonifying beverages, such as Wu Jia Pi wine.

Constituents Beta-carotene, vitamins B_1, B_2, C, and E, niacin, calcium, chromium, copper, iron, zinc, phenylpropanoids, lignans, coumarins, sterols (beta-sitosterol), glycosides (eleutherosides—considered one of the "active ingredients"), polysaccarharides

Energetic Correspondences

- Flavor: sweet, pungent, bitter (but extremely bitter roots are of poor quality)
- Temperature: warm
- Moisture: dry
- Polarity: yang, more neutral than *Panax* varieties
- Planet: dominion of Mars and Jupiter
- Element: Fire

Dosage Take 1 cup of tea or 20 to 40 drops of tincture three times daily.

CONCERNS

Eleuthero is safe when used appropriately. In rare cases, eleuthero may contribute to diarrhea, elevation of blood pressure, and mild blood platelet antiaggregation properties. Taking eleuthero too close to bedtime may interfere with sleep.

Epimedium

Epimedium spp., including *E. aceranthus, E. acuminatum, E. brevicornum, E. grandiflorum, E. koreanum, E. macranthum, E. pubescens, E. sagittatum*

Family Berberidaceae (Barberry)

Etymology The genus name, *Epimedium,* derives from the Greek *epi,* "upon," and *media,* in reference to the ancient country of Media, southwest of the Caspian Sea. The Mandarin name *yín yáng hùo* translates as "licentious goat wort," a.k.a. horny goat weed, in reference to the fact that goats that graze upon this herb have increased seminal emissions and are more sexually active.

Part Used Aboveground plant

Physiological Effects Antiviral, aphrodisiac, circulatory stimulant, endocrine tonic, hormone regulator, hypotensive, immune stimulant, Kidney yang tonic, nervous system tonic, restorative, tonic, and vasodilator

Medicinal Uses Epimedium stimulates the sensory nerves, thereby increasing sexual desire and strength. It stimulates the pituitary gland and thus the gonads and increases sperm production and motility as well as testosterone production. It strengthens the adrenal system, dilates capillaries, improves circulation, and is a traditional remedy for erectile dysfunction.

Epimedium warms the kidneys, tonifies yang, and removes excess moisture from the body. It also strengthens bones, improves metabolism, and exhibits a mild androgenic effect.

Epimedium is used to treat depression, drug and chemical withdrawal symptoms, erectile dysfunction, exhaustion, forgetfulness, herpes, infertility, low libido, lumbago, memory loss, menopause, numbness, osteoporosis, pain, polyuria, poor circulation, premature ejaculation, and prostatitis.

Constituents Vitamin E, manganese, flavonoids (quercetin, luteolin, kaempferol), linolenic acid, palmitic acid, polysaccharides, alkaloid, sterols, tannin

Energetic Correspondences

- Flavor: pungent, sweet
- Temperature: warm
- Moisture: dry
- Polarity: yang
- Planet: Jupiter
- Element: Fire

Dosage Drink ½ cup of tea or 15 to 30 drops of tincture three times daily.

CONCERNS

Epimedium is not recommended for those who have an excessive sex drive, experience wet dreams, or are overly hot or irritable. Excess use can cause vertigo, vomiting, dry mouth, decreased thyroid activity, or nosebleed. Use for short periods of time only.

Fenugreek

Trigonella foenum-graecum

Family Fabaceae (Legume)

Etymology The genus name, *Trigonella,* derives from the Greek *trigonon,* meaning "triangle," in reference to the three-sided corolla of the flower. The species name, *foenum-graecum,* is Latin for "Greek hay," a nod to the fact that fenugreek was once used to scent inferior grades of hay.

Parts Used Seed; in ayurvedic medicine, the entire plant

Physiological Effects Aphrodisiac, aromatic, diuretic, emmenagogue, galactagogue, nutritive, phytoestrogenic, restorative, stimulant, and yang tonic

Medicinal Uses Fenugreek has long been used in Egyptian, ayurvedic, and Chinese medicine. In the Middle East, the seeds were eaten by harem women to sweeten the breath, increase libido, and enhance sexual allure. In Oriental tradition, they are used to warm and nourish the Kidneys and glands.

Fenugreek is used in the treatment of erectile dysfunction, debility, Kidney chi deficiency, menopause, menstrual cramps, premature ejaculation, and vaginal dryness. It is sometimes used as an ingredient in breast growth enhancement formulas.

Constituents Beta-carotene, B-complex vitamins (especially niacin and choline), vitamin C, vitamin E, calcium, iron, lysine, tryptophan, glutamic acid, aspartic acid, lecithin, carbohydrates (galactomannans), steroidal saponins (diosgenin, yamogenin), alkaloids (trigonelline, carpaine, gentianine), glycosides, flavonoids (apigenin, quercetin, luteolin), coumarin, mucilage, protein, fatty acids (linoleic, linolenic, oleic)

Energetic Correspondences

- Flavor: bitter
- Temperature: warm
- Moisture: moist
- Polarity: yang
- Planet: Mercury
- Element: Metal

Dosage Take 1 or 2 capsules, 1 or 2 dropperfuls of tincture, or 1 cup of tea three times daily.

CONCERNS

Avoid fenugreek seed during pregnancy as it can be a uterine stimulant. Although fenugreek can be used to lower blood sugar levels, diabetics should use it for this purpose only with guidance from a qualified health care practitioner.

Ginkgo

Ginkgo biloba

Family Ginkgoaceae (Ginkgo)

Etymology The genus name, *Ginkgo,* derives from the Japanese *ginky,* meaning "silver apricot." The species name, *biloba,* derives from the Latin *bi* ("double") and *loba* ("lobes") in reference to its two-lobed leaves.

Parts Used Leaf (harvested when starting to yellow, then dried)

Physiological Effects Antibacterial, anticoagulant, antifungal, anti-inflammatory, antioxidant, brain tonic, circulatory stimulant, decongestant, Kidney tonic, neuroprotective, rejuvenative, vasodilator

Medicinal Uses Ginkgo is the oldest tree species on the planet—common even when dinosaurs roamed the earth—and it is tolerant to disease, insects, and pollution.

Ginkgo leaf relaxes blood vessels, improving circulation and the delivery of nutrients (like oxygen and glucose) throughout the body, including the genitals and brain. Concentrated ginkgo leaf increases the synthesis of dopamine, norepinephrine, and other neurotransmitters. It also helps reverse erectile dysfunction without altering blood pressure, unlike some pharmaceuticals that are used to treat this condition. Ginkgo prevents blood platelet aggregation and may boost sperm production.

Ginkgo leaf is used in the treatment of anxiety, depression, erectile dysfunction, fatigue, hemorrhoids, leukorrhea, memory loss, shortness of breath, and vision loss.

Constituents Beta-carotene, vitamin C, superoxide dismutase, flavonoids (ginkgolide, quercetin, rutin, kaempferol, and proanthocyanidins)

Energetic Correspondences

- Flavor: sweet, bitter
- Temperature: leaf—neutral; seed—warm
- Moisture: dry
- Polarity: yin
- Planet: Sun/Mercury/Venus/Mars
- Element: Metal

Dosage Drink 1 cup of tea or 20 to 40 drops of tincture three times daily.

CONCERNS

Side effects from ginkgo leaf are rare. However, large amounts have been reported to cause gastrointestinal disturbance, irritability, restlessness, and headache. Ginkgo leaf can negatively affect the blood's ability to clot, so avoid ginkgo for at least a week before surgery, in cases of hemophilia, or in concurrence with anticoagulant drugs such as Coumadin, aspirin, or monoamine oxidase inhibitors.

Ginseng

Panax ginseng (Asian ginseng), *P. quinquefolium* (American ginseng)

Family Araliaceae (Ginseng)

Etymology The genus name, *Panax,* derives from the Greek *panakos,* meaning "panacea." The species and common name, *ginseng,* derives from the Mandarin name for the plant, *ren shen,* which translates roughly as "essence of the earth in the form of a man," a reference to the humanlike shape of some ginseng roots. The American species name, *quinquefolium,* refers to its five-part leaves.

Part Used Root

Physiological Effects Adaptogen, antioxidant, aphrodisiac, chi tonic, endocrine tonic, hepatoprotective, phytoandrogenic, rejuvenative, restorative, stimulant, and tonic

Medicinal Uses In the sacred Hindu Vedas, ginseng is described as capable of bestowing "the power of the bull." In case you're wondering what that means, read on. In the 1700s French missionaries discovered that a plant growing near the Great Lakes and being used by Native peoples in love potions and as a tonic was a New World relative of the Asian species. Daniel Boone was a ginseng harvester.

American ginseng has properties similar to Asian ginseng but is considered milder and as a tonic is prescribed more frequently for younger people.

Ginseng of either kind helps the body better utilize oxygen, relieving fatigue and calming anxiety. It also strengthens adrenal glands, improves general blood flow and cerebral circulation, supports endocrine function, increases testosterone levels in both men and women, boosts sperm counts, endows virility, and supports testicle and ovarian growth in young men and women, respectively. It improves muscle tone and even aids in the production of DNA.

Ginseng improves stamina, reaction time, and concentration, which make it useful for such pursuits as studying, taking tests, long-distance driving, making love, and meditating. It also speeds recovery time from sickness, surgery, childbirth, athletic performance, and other stressors to the body.

Ginseng is used in the treatment of adrenal deficiency, anemia, chronic fatigue, depression, drug addiction and withdrawal symptoms, erectile dysfunction, fatigue, infertility (male and female), insomnia, low libido, low sperm count, memory loss, menopause, night sweats, organ prolapse, and post-traumatic stress (physical and emotional).

American ginseng is white; the root is simply harvested and cleaned. Asian ginseng, on the other hand, is often steamed with herbs and wine, which gives it a reddish color and a more warming quality. Thus American ginseng is more often used during the warmer times of the year, while Asian ginseng is best used during cooler seasons.

Ginseng's effects are cumulative, and most benefit occurs after a period of use, although some users will notice immediate effects. Some athletes use it for a week prior to an event. Although the root is the primary medicinal component of the plant, the leaves of both varieties can be used to treat hangover and fever.

WHEN TO TAKE GINSENG

For best effect, take ginseng between meals rather than with food. It is best not to take ginseng at night, as it could impair sleep.

Constituents B vitamins, acetylcholine, copper, germanium, manganese, phosphorous, selenium, saponins (ginsenosides, also known as panaxosides), phytosterols (beta-sitosterol, stigmasterol, campesterol), essential oils

Energetic Correspondences

- Flavor: sweet, slightly bitter
- Temperature: *P. ginseng*—warm; *P. quinquefolium*—slightly warm
- Moisture: *P. ginseng*—dry; *P. quinquefolium*—moist
- Polarity: yang
- Planet: Sun
- Element: Fire

Dosage Take 1 to 2 capsules, cups of tea, or dropperfuls of tincture between meals. Most effective when taken over a period of time. American ginseng is at risk of becoming endangered in the wild; use only cultivated—never wildcrafted—supplies.

CONCERNS

Avoid ginseng in cases of heat and inflammation, such as fever, flu, pneumonia, hypertension, or constipation. Since ginseng can be energizing, avoid taking it within four hours of bedtime. The herb is not recommended for children for prolonged periods as it may cause early sexual maturation. Avoid during pregnancy and while nursing. Do not take ginseng in conjunction with cardiac glycosides except under the guidance of a qualified health care professional.

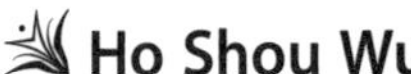

Polygonum multiflorum

Family Polygonaceae (Rhubarb)

Etymology The genus name, *Polygonum,* is Latin for "many knees," in reference to the many joints on the stems. The species name, *multiflorum,* is Latin for "multiflowered." The Mandarin common name *he shou wu,* which is also the English common name, means "black-haired Mr. He," a reference to a story about a fifty-six-year-old, gray-haired Mr. He who ate ho shou wu root for a year, then fathered a son and grew a full head of black hair. Also known as fo ti.

Part Used Root (raw or cooked)

Physiological Effects Antibacterial, antidepressant, anti-inflammatory, antioxidant, antispasmodic, antiviral, aphrodisiac, astringent, blood tonic, cardiotonic, chi tonic, demulcent, diuretic, Liver tonic (when raw), Kidney tonic, rejuvenative, restorative, sedative, yin tonic

Medicinal Uses Ho shou wu root is available either raw and dried or cooked in a black soybean broth. It is one of China's most common blood tonics. It strengthens the bones and muscles, moistens the intestines, builds bone marrow, and calms the spirit. This classic Chinese herb improves circulation, boosts libido, and relieves anxiety. In Oriental tradition, it helps in cases of Liver or Kidney deficiency.

Cooked ho shou wu root is used to treat anemia, atherosclerosis, blurred vision, exhaustion, hair loss, infertility, high cholesterol, hot flashes, hypertension, infertility, knee weakness, low sperm count, lumbago, premature ejaculation, scrofula, insomnia, menopausal complaints, numbness, premature aging, premature gray hair, premature menopause, schizophrenia, spermatorrhea, spleen weakness, and vaginal discharge.

Constituents Magnesium, phosphorous, potassium, unsaturated fatty acids, lecithin, anthraquinones, allantoin, tannins

Energetic Correspondences

- Flavor: sour, bitter, sweet
- Temperature: warm
- Moisture: moist
- Polarity: yin
- Planet: Mars/Saturn
- Element: Water

Dosage Drink ¼ cup of tea four times daily, or take 15 to 30 drops of tincture three times daily.

CONCERNS

Avoid ho shou wu during bouts of diarrhea and excessive phlegm. The raw root is more laxative than the cooked variety. If using the cooked root and suffering from weak digestion, combine it with a digestive tonic herb such as ginger or dried orange peel. There have been rare reports of dermatitis or numbness in the extremities after ingestion of large doses.

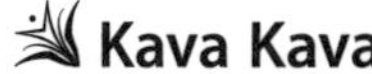 Kava Kava

Piper methysticum

Family Piperaceae (Pepper)

Etymology The genus name, *Piper,* derives from the Greek name for pepper, *peperi.* The species name, *methysticum,* is thought to be Latin for "intoxicating." The common name, *kava,* is Tongan for "bitter."

Parts Used Root, upper rhizome

Physiological Effects Anaphrodisiac (if used excessively), anesthetic, antifungal, antibacterial, aphrodisiac, diuretic, euphoric, hypnotic, muscle relaxant, nervine, psychoactive, sedative, soporific, and stimulant

Medicinal Uses Kava calms the heart and respiration, relaxes the muscles without blocking nerve signals, and calms physical tension without numbing mental processes. Users claim it promotes increased sound sensitivity, more fluent speech, and feelings of euphoria. Part of its mood-elevating ability might be due to its activation of mesolimbic dopaminergic neurons. Kava kava is also said to increase tolerance of pain; Native people in the South Pacific often took kava kava before being tattooed, and women in labor sometimes drink kava kava juice as a calmative and to facilitate birth.

Kava kava is used in the treatment of anger, anxiety, attention deficit disorder, cramps, cystitis, depression, dysuria, fear, gonorrhea, headache (tension), hot flashes, hyperactivity, incontinence (nocturnal), insomnia, irritable bladder, menstrual cramps, nervousness, pain, restlessness, stress, urinary tract infection, uterine inflammation, withdrawal symptoms (from alcohol, nicotine, or tranquilizers), and vaginitis.

In the South Pacific, kava kava is used in ceremonies to celebrate marriages, births, deaths, and other life passages. It is often used to honor a guest or to enhance communication, such as in settling a dispute, counseling a couple, or sealing a business agreement.

Kava kava is thought to have been cultivated for at least three thousand years in the South Pacific. It is said that the noble classes used kava for pleasure, the priests for ceremony, and the working classes for relaxation. When European missionaries began to have strong influence in the area, many thousands of kava plants were ripped out of the ground. Where this occurred, rates of alcoholism increased.

Kava kava helps warm the emotions, and small amounts can produce a pleasant euphoric sensation. It is also used for divination and to produce inspiration. Taking kava kava before bed can help induce pleasant sleep and vivid dreams.

Constituents Flavonoids, sesquiterpene, lactones (methysticin, yangonin, kavahin, dihydrokavain)

Energetic Correspondences

- Flavor: pungent, bitter
- Temperature: hot
- Moisture: dry
- Polarity: yin
- Planet: Saturn/Uranus/Venus/Pluto
- Element: Water

Dosage Drink ¼ cup of tea, take 1 to 2 capsules, or take 15 to 30 drops of tincture three times daily; add some milk or coconut milk to the tea, because the active compounds in kava kava are fat soluble and will be assimilated better by the body when delivered with a small amount of fat.

CONCERNS

Avoid kava kava during pregnancy and while nursing, and do not give to young children. Avoid in cases of Parkinson's disease and severe depression. Do not take in conjunction with alcohol, sedatives, tranquilizers, or antidepressants as it can potentiate their effects. Remain aware of kava kava's soporific effects; try to avoid driving, operating heavy machinery, or other activities that require fast reaction times after taking kava kava. On the plus side, kava kava, unlike many sedatives, is not habit forming. Daily use of kava shouldn't exceed three months, though occasional use on an ongoing basis is fine for those in good health.

Kava kava may cause the tongue, mouth, and other body parts to feel temporarily numb and rubbery; this is normal. However, excess amounts can cause disturbed vision, dilated pupils, and difficulty walking. Large doses taken for extended periods can have a cumulative effect on the liver, causing kawaism, a condition marked by a yellowish tinge to the skin, a scaly rash, apathy, anorexia, and bloodshot eyes.

In Europe there have been some reports of severe liver damage resulting from use of kava kava, prompting a number of nations to ban sales of it. The problem appears to be caused by a compound called pipermethystine that is found in the stem peelings and leaves of the kava plant but not in the roots. Traditional kava preparations are extracted from the roots only, and the peelings and leaves are discarded. However, some European pharmaceutical companies bought up the kava waste products when demand for kava extract soared in the early 2000s. The cases of liver damage appear to have involved people who took standardized extract capsules, which may have contained kava stem peelings and roots as well as chemical solvents. For this reason, avoid kava products made from the leaves or stems of the plant. The traditional tea prepared from the root appears to be quite safe.

Licorice

Glycyrrhiza glabra (European licorice), *G. inflata, G. lepidota* (American licorice), *G. uralensis* (Chinese licorice)

Family Fabaceae (Pea)

Etymology The genus name, *Glycyrrhiza,* derives from the Greek *glyky ryhiza,* "sweet root," as does the common name, *licorice.* The species name, *glabra,* is Latin for "smooth," in reference to the smooth seedpods.

Part Used Root (stolon)

Physiological Effects Adrenal tonic, antifungal, anti-inflammatory, antioxidant, antiseptic, antispasmodic, antitumor, antiviral, aphrodisiac, chi tonic, demulcent, emollient, galactagogue, hepatoprotective, immune tonic, nutritive, phytoestrogenic, rejuvenative, sedative, and tonic

Medicinal Uses Licorice is one of the most commonly used herbs in traditional Chinese medicine. It enters all twelve meridians and harmonizes the effects of other herbs, helping to prolong their effects. Its constituent glycyrrhizin (which is similar to the human hormone cortisol) inhibits the production of the inflammatory prostaglandin E2. Licorice soothes irritated mucous membranes, restores pituitary activity, and helps normalize the function of glands and organs. It also helps induce feelings of calmness, peace, and harmony.

It is used to treat adrenal weakness, AIDS, alcoholism, bladder infection, candida, chronic fatigue, debility, depression, dysuria, eczema, emotional instability, fatigue, hair loss, infertility, irregular ovulation, irritability, menstrual cramps, prostatitis, and stress. It is also used as a lubricating enema or douche. In magical traditions licorice is a love charm and promotes fidelity.

Constituents B-complex vitamins, choline, phosphorus, potassium, glycosides (glycyrrhizin, also known as glycyrrhic acid), saponins, phytoestrogens, coumarins, flavonoids (isoflavones, liquiritin, isoliquiritin), amines (asparagine, betaine), essential oil, coumarins, protein, fat

Energetic Correspondences

- Flavor: sweet, slightly bitter
- Temperature: neutral
- Moisture: moist
- Polarity: yin
- Planet: Venus
- Element: Water

Dosage Take ½ cup of tea or 30 to 60 drops of tincture three times daily.

CONCERNS

Avoid licorice in cases of edema, nausea, vomiting, and rapid heartbeat. Licorice is not recommended during pregnancy or in combination with steroid or digoxin medications. Excessive or prolonged use can cause sodium retention and potassium depletion, elevated blood pressure, as well as vomiting, headaches, and/or vertigo. Continuous use is not recommended in excess of six weeks, except under the guidance of a qualified health care practitioner. Chinese licorice (*G. uralensis*) is said to be less likely to cause side effects than the European variety (*G. glabra*). All these precautions notwithstanding, licorice is often added in very small amounts to other herbal formulas to harmonize them and prevent undesirable side effects.

Maca

Lepidium meyenii, L. peruvianum

Family Brassicaceae (Mustard)

Etymology The genus name, *Lepidium,* derives from the Greek *lepis,* "scale," perhaps in reference to the heavy root. The common name, *maca,* is a Quechua word for the plant.

Part Used Root

Physiological Effects Adaptogen, antioxidant, aphrodisiac, immune tonic, nutritive, rejuvenative, tonic

Medicinal Uses Maca increases strength and stamina and helps the body deal with stress.

Alkaloids in maca are believed to affect the hypothalamus-pituitary axis, which has a positive effect on the adrenals, thyroid, and pancreas. Maca increases the production of estrogen, testosterone, and progesterone and improves the quantity and motility of sperm. It is also used as a tonic for recovering alcoholics, helping to decrease cravings.

Maca root enhances libido and improves fertility in both men and women. It can be used to treat erectile dysfunction and vaginal dryness. Maca is used in the treatment of adrenal exhaustion, anemia, chronic fatigue, erectile dysfunction, infertility, irregular menses, low sperm count, memory loss, menopausal symptoms (hot flashes, night sweats, mood swings), osteoporosis, premature aging, and vaginal dryness. It is also used to support convalescence.

Maca roots can be eaten much like sweet potatoes. They have a flavor like that of butterscotch and are often added to smoothies and "superfood" confections. The Inca cultivated maca more than two thousand years ago. Legend has it that Incan warriors would consume it before battle as a strengthening tonic. During the Spanish colonialization of Peru, maca was used as currency. There are chronicles of Spanish conquistadors finding that their horses and pigs became infertile at the high altitude (a common phenomenon). Incan farmers recommended that the Spaniards feed the animals maca as they had found that it increased reproduction in their own llamas and alpacas.

Constituents Maca contains important essential fatty acids, including omega-3 and omega-5, as well as vitamin B_1, vitamin B_2, vitamin B_{12}, vitamin C, vitamin E, calcium, iodine, iron, phosphorus, zinc, amino acids (histidine, glycine, tyrosine, lysine, phenylalanine, valine, methionine), carbohydrates, saponins, alkaloids, phytosterols (sitosterol, stigmasterol, campesterol, and ergosterol).

Energetic Correspondences

- Flavor: sweet
- Temperature: warm
- Moisture: moist
- Polarity: yin
- Planet: Venus/Jupiter
- Element: Metal

Dosage Take 5 to 20 grams of the dried root daily, or 30 to 40 drops of tincture three times daily.

CONCERNS

Maca root is generally regarded as safe, though high doses may contribute to insomnia.

Marijuana

Cannabis sativa

Family Cannabaceae (Cannabis)

Etymology The genus name, *Cannabis,* is thought to derive from the Hebrew *kanehbosm,* meaning "aromatic reed," and/or from the Greek name for this plant, *kannabis,* which means "two dog." The genus name, *sativa,* derives from the Latin *satus,* "planting," and denotes the plant's long history of cultivation. In fact, Carl Sagan, author of *Cosmos,* believed *Cannabis sativa* to be this planet's most ancient cultivar.

Parts Used Bud (flowering top of female plant), resin, leaf

Physiological Effects Antidepressant, antispasmodic, aphrodisiac (but can also be anaphrodisiac, depending on dosage and circumstance), cerebral sedative, euphoric, hallucinogen, hypnotic, vasodilator

Medicinal Uses Marijuana's effects can vary in different people but most noted are the dilation of blood vessels and alveoli sacs in the lungs, resulting in deeper respiration and an increase in heart rate. Low doses tend to promote a sense of relaxation. The bud increases levels of phenylethylamine (as does chocolate), a neurotransmitter that makes us feel more in love.

Cannabis can encourage great sex by allowing one to become less inhibited, more creative, and more responsive to pleasure. Some people, with the right partner, can experience mind-blowing sexual union. It is highly individual in its effects, however, and may inhibit desire in some people, even reducing testosterone levels after prolonged use. Cannabis is used in the treatment of AIDS, anorexia, menstrual cramps, and nervousness in the elderly, as well as for chronic pain. It increases the sensations of the parasympathetic nervous system. The leaves need to be cooked or heated before they become psychoactive.

Though marijuana is most often smoked to achieve therapeutic effect, it can also be consumed as food, tinctured, encapsulated, put in a vaporizer, or made into a sublingual spray. The buds, young leaves, and seeds are all edible. In India marijuana is used to prepare *bhang,* an herbal milkshake that is traditionally served at wedding banquets to produce great joy. A myth from Nepal tells that Shiva, the world's creator and destroyer, lived with his goddess wife Parvati in the Himalayas. Yet Shiva wandered, amusing himself with nymphs and other goddesses. This displeased Parvati, so she sought a way to keep her husband close to home. She took the resin from a female hemp plant, and when Shiva returned home she offered him its smoke. He was filled with joy and arousal, and they experienced divine bliss together. After this he remained with his wife and proclaimed that the doors to paradise were now open to his devotees.

Constituents Cannabinoids (tetrahydrocannabinol), flavonoids, essential oils, alkaloids (cannabisativine, muscarinem trigonelline), calcium

Energetic Correspondences

- Flavor: sweet, pungent
- Temperature: warm
- Moisture: drying, though the seed is moistening when consumed as a food
- Polarity: yin
- Planet: Saturn/Mars/Neptune
- Element: Fire/Water

CONCERNS

Smoking marijuana may affect some people adversely, possibly inducing paranoia, personality deviations, short-term memory loss, and perceptual distortions. Because of these possible effects, and marijuana's sedative properties, avoid driving, operating heavy machinery, or other activities that require fast reaction times after using marijuana. It can also promote weird visions, which can be frightening. Smoking in general can be hard on the lungs, and though cannabis has been used to treat asthma and bronchitis, smoking it to excess can aggravate those conditions. Marijuana can also inhibit testosterone production, cause hypoglycemic states, and lower HDL production. Dryness in the mouth and eyes is a common side effect.

Though marijuana has been used medicinally for centuries, it is currently illegal to grow or possess it in many countries, including the United States. Products made from seeds, however, are legal and available in the U.S.

Muira Puama

Ptychopetalum olacoides, P. uncinatum

Family Olaceae (Olive)

Etymology The origins of this herb's common and Latin names are uncertain.

Parts Used Inner bark, root

Physiological Effects Adaptogen, androgenic, antidepressant, antioxidant, aphrodisiac, nervous system stimulant, and tonic

Medicinal Uses Muira puama has been a premier remedy for centuries in South America, especially as an aphrodisiac. Muira puama is famous in Brazil for its effectiveness in treating erectile dysfunction and improving orgasmic ability. It can be used to enhance both the physical and psychological enjoyment of sex. It improves erectile dysfunction, fatigue, fertility, hair loss, low sperm count, and low libido. It also prolongs virility, lessens inhibitions, and relieves depression and other emotions caused by sexual trauma. It is believed to increase testosterone production.

Natives of South America apply the cooled tea to their genitals as a sexual stimulant.

Constituents Fatty acids (behenic acid), alkaloids (muirapuamine), coumarin, phytosterols (beta-sitosterol), essential oils (beta-carophyllene, alpha-humulene), triterpenes (lupeol), tannin

Energetic Correspondences

- Flavor: sweet, pungent
- Temperature: warm
- Moisture: dry
- Polarity: yang
- Planet: Mars
- Element: Fire

Dosage Drink ½ cup of tea or 10 to 30 drops of tincture three times daily.

CONCERNS

Muira puama is generally regarded as safe. Some people may find that it causes insomnia if taken before bedtime.

Nettle

Urtica dioica, U. urens

Family Urticaceae (Nettle)

Etymology The genus name, *Urtica,* is Latin, meaning "I burn." The species name, *dioica,* is Latin for "two dwellings" or "two houses," in reference to the plant being dioecious, or bearing male and female flowers on different plants. The common name, *nettles,* is thought to derive from the Anglo-Saxon *noedl,* meaning "needle," in reference to either the use of nettles as a textile fiber or their sharp prickles.

Part Used Aboveground plant

Physiological Effects Adrenal tonic, antioxidant, blood tonic, circulatory stimulant, decongestant, diuretic, endocrine tonic (seed), galactagogue, Kidney tonic, nutritive, parturient, rejuvenative (seed), thyroid tonic (seed), tonic (leaf, root, seed), styptic, uterine tonic

Medicinal Uses Nettles build the blood and strengthen the kidneys. Nettle leaf curbs the appetite and alkalizes the body, enabling it to eliminate toxins. Nettle tea is energizing, making it a motivating ally in attempts to stay on a healthy diet. Nettle is used in the treatment of acne, amenorrhea (due to blood or kidney deficiency), anemia, candida, cellulite, cystitis, eczema, hemorrhoids, infertility (men and women), menorrhagia, nephritis, night sweats, obesity, and premature gray hair.

Nettle, especially its seeds, have been used as a remedy for impotence for thousands of years. Second-century herbalist Galen (AD 131–200) wrote that nettle seeds "taken in a draught of mulled wine arouse desire," while traditional Arab cultures used nettle seeds soaked in honey as a cure for impotence. And since ancient times, fresh nettles have been used for the practice of flagellation, or, more properly termed, *urtication,* in which the genitals are whipped with fresh stinging nettles to increase blood flow to the area—a painful sort of herbal Viagra that is not for the unadventurous! (*If you get your partner to agree to this experiment, you must kiss and make it better for them!*)

The nettle plant's individual parts have some targeted uses. Nettle leaf and root in particular are known to tone and firm tissues, muscles, arteries, and skin. Taken internally, they decrease uric acid buildup and increase circulation to the skin's surface. The leaf can be used to prevent hair loss, while the root is used in the treatment of prostatitis. Nettle root also deactivates aromatase, the enzyme that helps convert testosterone into estradiol, thus keeping testosterone levels high. It improves both BPH and prostatitis. Though the root does not contain androgen, it does help existing androgens from becoming inactivated. Nettle seed is also used in the treatment of erectile dysfunction, and it can be used to prevent hair loss.

As a flower essence, nettle is recommended in times of anger or emotional coldness that can lead to spitefulness and cruelty. It encourages fearlessness in people who feel isolated or "stung" by others, helping them regain the ability to connect with others by expressing their anger. It also helps users to release stress and reestablish harmony and unity within themselves.

Nettles can be described as a superfood, being even more nutritive than spinach. Before they can be consumed, however, the sting must be deactivated. Cooking the nettles will do this, as will juicing or pureeing them, or drying and powdering them. Our favorite tonic here at home is a glass of fresh nettle juice daily. We are able to harvest it from March until October. If you harvest your own nettles, cut off the bottom ends to keep the young tops fresh, and juice the tops into Green Smoothies. Should your hands get stung while collecting the nettles, know that the sting is an excellent remedy against sore joints.

Constituents Protein, beta-carotene, xanthophylls, vitamin B, vitamin C, vitamin E, vitamin K, flavonoids (quercitin, rutin, kaempferol, rhamnetin), calcium, chromium, iron, silica, betaine, mucilage, tannin, chromium, silica, chlorophyll, amines (histamine, acetylcholine, serotonin, 5-hydroxyaliphatic acid), hydroxycoumarins, mucilage, saponins (lignin, sitosterol), glycosides, tannin

Energetic Correspondences

- Flavor: salty, slightly bitter
- Temperature: cool, seed is warming
- Moisture: dry
- Polarity: yang
- Planet: Mars
- Element: Fire

Dosage Drink 1 cup of tea or 20 to 40 drops of tincture, or take 3 to 4 capsules three times daily. We drink fresh nettle juice almost daily, except in winter. (The rest of the time we enjoy tea.)

CONCERNS

Stick with the *urens* and *dioica* species of nettle unless you have consulted with local herb authorities on the safety of local varieties.

Nettle is not known as stinging nettle for nothing; avoid touching or eating the fresh plant unless it is very young and/or you are very brave. Touching the fresh plant can cause a burning rash. Wearing gloves when collecting can help prevent this, but the hairs in large plants may still pierce through. A nettle sting can be soothed with a poultice of yellow dock or plantain or even the juice of the nettle plant itself (but good luck obtaining this without getting many more stings). However, you can learn to love the sting. I admit to collecting nettles barehanded with a pair of scissors and a paper bag. The arthritis I was developing twenty years ago has now become a thing of the past—and I attribute its disappearance to nettle stings.

Eating raw nettles can cause digestive disturbances, mouth and lip irritation, and urinary problems; however, these side effects are rare when the plant is pureed before ingestion and practically nonexistent when the plant is dried.

When used appropriately nettle is considered safe, even over an extended period of time, although those with overly cold, deficient conditions should not use nettle for prolonged periods. Only the aboveground portions of young plants should be consumed as older plants can be irritating to the kidneys and may cause digestive disturbances.

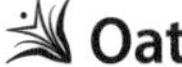 Oat

Avena fatua (wild oat), *A. sativa* (cultivated oat)

Family Poaceae (Grass)

Etymology The genus name, *Avena,* is Latin for "nourishing." The common name, *oat,* derives from the Old English term for the grain.

Parts Used Seed (unripe), stem (also known as oatstraw)

Physiological Effects Antidepressant, antispasmodic, aphrodisiac, blood tonic, brain tonic, chi tonic, demulcent, diuretic, endocrine tonic, mood elevator, nervine, nervous system tonic, nutritive, rejuvenative, reproductive tonic, restorative, and uterine tonic

Medicinal Uses The spikelets (unripe milky seeds) of oat have a relaxing effect; they nourish the nervous system and help the body handle stress. Oatstraw is rich in magnesium and polysaccharides that promote energy. It is an excellent herb to use during convalescence. It also benefits the libido, liberating testosterone, and makes tactile sensations more pleasurable. Oatstraw promotes vaginal lubrication and makes it possible for women to experience multiple orgasms. It can be used to treat cases of erectile dysfunction and premature ejaculation.

With its high silicon content, oat helps nourish the skin, nails, teeth, bones, and hair. It also builds the blood, relaxes the nerves, and strengthens the nervous system, making tactile sensations more pleasurable. It even supports the elasticity of blood vessels. Oat seeds and stems are used in the treatment of addiction, alcoholism, anxiety, convalescence, debility, depression, emotional distress, erectile dysfunction, exhaustion, hemorrhoids, incontinence, infertility (male and female), low libido, menopause, nervous breakdown, nervousness, osteoporosis, post-traumatic stress, and withdrawal symptoms (from tobacco, drugs, or alcohol). It is also used to facilitate recovery from childbirth.

As a flower essence, oat is helpful for those who are filled with uncertainty and dissatisfaction and who are unable to find their life's direction.

Constituents Beta-carotene, B and E vitamins, calcium, iron, magnesium, manganese, potassium, selenium, silicon, zinc, histamine, lysine, methionine, lipids, saponins, flavonoids, gluten, alkaloids (trigonelline, avenine), phytosterols (beta-sitosterol)

Energetic Correspondences

- Flavor: sweet
- Temperature: warm
- Moisture: moist
- Polarity: yin
- Planet: Mercury/Mars/Jupiter/Moon/Pluto/Venus
- Element: Earth

Dosage Drink 1 cup of tea or 20 to 40 drops of tincture three times daily.

CONCERNS

Oat is safe when used appropriately. Those with gluten allergies may need to begin with small dosages and increase cautiously, or use the oat straw, which is gluten-free, rather than seed.

Pine

Pinus spp., including *P. nigra* (black pine), *P. contorta* (lodgepole pine), *P. pinaster, P. pinea, P. strobus* (white pine), *P. sylvestris* (Scots pine), *P. tabuliformis* (Chinese red pine)

Family Pinaceae (Pine)

Etymology The genus name, *Pinea,* from which the common name, *pine,* derives, is the Latin name for the nuts derived from this tree. Pollen, the part used in tantric medicine, is Latin for "flour."

Parts Used Pollen, essential oil, flower

Physiological Effects Antioxidant (bark), antiseptic, antiviral, rubefacient, stimulant, tonic

Medicinal Uses Every spring the male catkins of the pine release pollen; each catkin can produce six million grains that then inseminate the pine cones. Pine pollen is the sperm of the potent pines and has been used for more than a thousand years in Asian medicine as a longevity and libido tonic. It is high in amino acids and hormonal compounds that increase androsterone and testosterone in the body.

The essential oil of pine is said to normalize male hormones; it can be prepared as a steam inhalation or as a massage or bath oil.

As a flower essence, pine is helpful for those who are filled with guilt and self-blame and for those who are never satisfied with their success. It helps bring about true understanding and forgiveness and releases responsibility. Pine increases psychic awareness as well as insight and helps users learn from past mistakes.

Constituents Pine pollen contains significant amounts of arginine, cystine, glycine, leucine, lysine, methionne, phenylananine, tryptophan, and tyrosine, and smaller amounts of serine and valine. Black pine pollen contains the raw material to make androsterones, androstenedione, testosterone, and DHT.

Energetic Correspondences

- Flavor: bitter
- Temperature: warm
- Moisture: dry
- Polarity: yang
- Planet: Mars/Pluto
- Element: Metal, Earth

Dosage Take 1 dropperful of tincture three times daily. We enjoy raw pine pollen and flax crackers.

CONCERNS

Pine is generally regarded as very safe. Some people may experience contact dermatitis from the wood, resin, or sawdust. Those with known pine pollen allergies should avoid this product.

Raspberry

Rubus spp.

Family Rosaceae (Rose)

Etymology The genus name, *Rubus,* is Latin for "blackberry" or "bramble."

Part Used Leaf

Physiological Effects Adrenal tonic, anti-abortifacient, antiseptic, antispasmodic, astringent, hormone tonic, Liver tonic, Kidney tonic, nutritive, oxytoxic, parturient, phytoestrogenic, postpartum tonic, prostate tonic, stimulant, uterine tonic, yin tonic

RASPBERRY FRUIT

Raspberries have many therapeutic effects on the body, including antacid, antioxidant, antiviral, aphrodisiac (when unripe), blood tonic, laxative (mild), parturient, and refrigerant properties.

Medicinal Uses There are many, many species in the *Rubus* genus, but most herbalists agree that all red raspberry plants share common uses, detailed here.

Raspberry leaf is considered a supreme tonic for pregnant women because it can tonify the uterus, nourish the mother and the growing baby, prevent miscarriage and false labor, and facilitate birth and placental delivery. When used after birthing it can decrease uterine swelling and minimize postpartum hemorrhaging as well as increase colostrum in the mother's milk. Raspberry leaf also reduces inflammation and excess dampness. Its nourishing mineral content and ability to support the reproductive and nervous systems can even be of benefit in encouraging healing from sexual trauma and abuse. And though it is often regarded as an herb for women, raspberry leaf is also nourishing for men.

Raspberry leaf is used in the treatment of anemia, dysmenorrhea, hemorrhage, herpes, incontinence, infertility, muscle cramps, miscarriage (threat of), menorrhagia, morning sickness, overactive bladder, ovulation difficulty, prolapse of the uterus or anus, thrush, and weak vision.

Raspberry leaf tea can be used as a douche to treat leukorrhea or organ prolapse. As a flower essence, raspberry helps release resentment, bitterness, and old emotional wounds.

Constituents Vitamin B_1, vitamin E, calcium chloride, iron citrate, magnesium, manganese, potassium, phosphorous, potassium, selenium, sulfur, flavonoids, pectin, alkaloid (fragarine), organic acids (citric, malic, gallic, ellagic), furanones, tannins

Energetic Correspondences

- Flavor: bitter
- Temperature: neutral
- Moisture: dry
- Polarity: yin
- Planet: Venus/Mars/Jupiter
- Element: Water

Dosage Drink 1 cup of tea three times daily.

CONCERNS

There are no known toxic levels of raspberry leaf. Once nursing is established, excess consumption of raspberry leaf should be avoided as its astringent properties could lessen the amount of breast milk.

Rehmannia

Rehmannia glutinosa

Family Scrophulariaceae (Foxglove)

Etymology Rehmannia is named after the German physician Joseph Rehmann (1753–1831). The literal translation of the Mandarin name for this herb, *di huang,* is "yellow earth" or "cooked yellow earth," due to the yellowish orange color of the roots. The species name, *glutinosa,* is Latin for "very sticky," in reference to the properties of this plant.

Part Used Root

Physiological Effects Blood tonic (when cooked), cardiotonic, demulcent, diuretic, hypertensive, hypoglycemic, Kidney tonic (when cooked), Liver tonic (when raw), rejuvenative, yin tonic

Medicinal Uses Traditional Oriental medicine draws a distinction between the properties of the root when it is raw and when it is cooked. The raw root is used to quiet inflammation and heat. The cooked root is more of a building tonic to correct deficiency; it is used to strengthen the bones, marrow, and tendons, to nourish the eyes and ears, and as a tonic after birthing.

The cooked root is used in the treatment of anemia, dysmenorrhea, fatigue, irregular menses, lumbago, menorrhagia, muscle weakness, night sweats, postpartum bleeding, and spermatorrhea.

Constituents Phytosterols (beta-sitosterol, stigmasterol), glycosides, saponins, sugars (mannitol, galactose, glucose, raffinose), rehmannin, tannin

Energetic Correspondences

- Flavor: sweet, sour, bitter
- Temperature: cool
- Moisture: moist
- Polarity: raw root—yin; cooked root—yang
- Planet: Jupiter
- Element: Water

Dosage Take 1 to 3 capsules three times daily. Root slices can also be added to medicinal soups.

CONCERNS

Avoid excessive use of rehmannia in cases of loose stools or a very coated tongue.

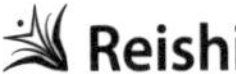 Reishi

Ganoderma lucidum

Family Polyporaceae (Polypor)

Etymology The genus name, *Ganoderma,* derives from the Latin *gan,* meaning "shiny," and *derm,* meaning "skin." The species name, *lucidum,* is Latin for "shining." Both refer to the mushroom's naturally glossy appearance.

Part Used Fruiting body

Physiological Effects Adaptogen, antioxidant, antiviral, cardiotonic, expectorant, rejuvenative

Medicinal Uses Reishi mushroom is considered a longevity herb in Asian medicine and has been in use in that tradition for more than four thousand years. In the Taoist tradition reishi is said to enhance spiritual receptivity, and it is used by monks to calm the spirit and the mind. It is considered a symbol of feminine sexuality. Reishi is used in the treatment of AIDS, cancer, depression, fatigue, hemorrhoids, HIV, hypertension, hypotension, insomnia, and nephritis.

Constituents Vitamin B_2, vitamin C, adenosine, ganoderic acid S, ganoderic acid R, ganesterone, lipids, ash, protein, glucans, polysaccharides, phytosterols, coumarin

Energetic Correspondences

- Flavor: bitter
- Temperature: cool
- Moisture: dry
- Polarity: yin
- Planet: Saturn
- Element: Earth

Dosage Drink 1 cup of tea, or take 1 to 2 capsules or 20 to 40 drops of tincture three times daily.

CONCERNS

Reishi has a very low potential for toxicity. However, long-term use may cause dry mouth, dizziness, and digestive distress. Because reishi can inhibit blood clotting, it should be avoided at least one week before surgery, before childbirth, and in conjunction with blood-thinning medications. When pregnant or while nursing, use it only under the guidance of a qualified health care practitioner.

Rhodiola

Rhodiola rosea (syn. *Sedum roseum, Sedum rhodiola*)

Family Crassulaceae (Stonecrop)

Etymology The former genus name, *Sedum,* may be from the Latin *sedere,* meaning "ground hugging," or perhaps from *sedare,* meaning "calming." The species name, *rosea,* derives from the Latin *rosa,* "rose," in reference to the plant's rose-scented roots and flowers.

Part Used Root

Physiological Effects Adaptogen, antioxidant, nootropic, stimulant, and tonic

Medicinal Uses Rhodiola enhances T-cell immunity and can improve the function of neurotransmitters, including serotonin and dopamine, by inhibiting their destruction by enzymes; it has been found to increase serotonin levels in the brain by up to 30 percent. Rhodiola also increases mental and physical performance; it can shorten recovery time between athletic endeavors, such as workouts, and can improve memory and work productivity. In Siberia it is traditionally given to couples prior to marriage to help them bring forth healthy children.

Rhodiola is used in the treatment of depression, erectile dysfunction, fatigue, hysteria, insomnia, nervous system disorders, pain, premature ejaculation, and stress.

Constituents Organic acids, kaempherol, flavonoids (rhodiolin, rhodionin, rodiosin, tricin), rosavin, monoterpenes (rosaridin, rosiridol), phenolic acids (hydroxycinnamic acid, gallic acid), beta-sitosterol

Energetic Correspondences

- Flavor: sweet, sour
- Temperature: cool
- Polarity: yin
- Planet: Venus/Mars/Jupiter/Neptune/Pluto
- Element: Water

Dosage Take 1 to 2 capsules or 20 to 30 drops of tincture three times daily.

CONCERNS

Rhodiola is generally regarded as safe.

Sarsaparilla

Smilax aristolochiifolia (syn. *S. medica*), *S. aspera, S. officinalis, S. ornata, S. papyracea, S. regelii* (Jamaican sarsaparilla)

Family Smilacaceae (Smilax)

Etymology The genus name, *Smilax,* is the classical Greek name for this plant. The common name *sarsaparilla* derives from the Spanish *zarza,* meaning "bramble," and *parrilla,* meaning "little vine."

Part Used Rhizome

Physiological Effects Alterative, antibacterial, anti-inflammatory, antiseptic, antitumor, antiviral, aphrodisiac, astringent, carminative, cholagogue, demulcent, depurative, diaphoretic, diuretic, emetic, febrifuge, hepatoprotective, rejuvenative, stimulant, stomachic, sudorific, tonic

Medicinal Uses Sarsaparilla is rich in phytosterols, which provide the raw material for the body to produce hormones. It also contains the trace minerals selenium and zinc. It strengthens the adrenal system and sexual organs, making men more virile and women more passionate. It is a traditional Mexican remedy for low libido and erectile dysfunction.

When it was first brought from Mexico to Spain in the 1500s, sarsparilla was exalted as a treatment for venereal diseases such as gonorrhea and syphilis; perhaps this is the reason it was so very popular with pirates and cowboys. It was an official herb in the United States Pharmacopoeia for the treatment of venereal disease from 1820 to 1910.

Sarsaparilla soothes the mucous membranes, increases all of the body's metabolic processes, and facilitates the excretion of uric acid and cleansing of the genitourinary system. It is used in the treatment of acne, AIDS, anemia, arthritis, boils, depression (menopausal), eczema, endometriosis, erectile dysfunction, fatigue, hot flashes, infertility, leukorrhea, menstrual cramps, ovarian cysts, pelvic inflammatory disease, premenstrual syndrome, psoriasis, skin dryness, syphilis, and urinary tract infection. In folkloric tradition it is used to attract love and prosperity.

Constituents Iron, sulfur, zinc, steroidal saponins (sarsapogenin, smilagen, sitosterol, stigmasterol, pollinastanol), glycosides, resin, fat, sugar

Energetic Correspondences

- Flavor: sweet, pungent
- Temperature: neutral
- Moisture: moist
- Polarity: yang
- Planet: Mars/Jupiter
- Element: Fire

Dosage Drink ½ cup of tea or 10 to 20 drops of tincture three times daily.

CONCERNS

Sarsaparilla is safe when used appropriately.
Avoid during pregnancy.

Saw Palmetto

Serenoa repens (syn. *S. serrulata*)

Family Arecaceae (Palm)

Etymology The genus name, *Serenoa,* was given in honor of American botanist Sereno Watson (1826–1892). The species name, *repens,* is Latin for "creeping."

Part Used Berry

Physiological Effects Alterative, anabolic (muscle-building), antiandrogenic, anti-inflammatory, antiseptic, antispasmodic, aphrodisiac, diuretic, galactagogue, hormonal regulator, nutritive, rejuvenative, reproductive tonic, restorative, sedative (in small amounts), stimulant, thyroid tonic, urinary antiseptic, uterine tonic, yang tonic, yin tonic

Medicinal Uses Saw palmetto is best known for its ability to inhibit the conversion of testosterone to dihydrotestosterone (DHT), a substance that can contribute to swelling of the prostate. It also helps rebuild atrophying genitals, including thinning of the vaginal walls in women. It reduces the occurrence of nocturnal urination and can be used to treat erectile dysfunction, premature ejaculation, and "honeymoon cystitis" (irritation occurring from excessive sex). It improves orgasmic ability and boosts libido.

Saw palmetto was an official herb in the United States Pharmacopoeia from 1905 to 1926 and in the National Formulary from 1926 to 1950. It strengthens the reproductive organs, prevents atrophy of the genitals and bladder tissue, enhances sexual arousal, and reduces inflammation.

Saw palmetto is used in the treatment of acne, dysuria, epididymitis, erectile dysfunction, genital atrophy, hirsutism, HIV, incontinence, irregular menses, low libido, low sperm count, nocturia (excessive nighttime urination), polyuria (frequent urination), premature ejaculation, prostatitis, orchitis, sexual debility, urinary infection, urinary hesitancy, and wasting diseases. It also can be used to encourage convalescence, enhance breast size (many women vouch for it!), and even initiate sexual maturation when it has been slow to start.

Saw palmetto berries also can be mixed with cocoa butter and used as a bolus to treat uterine or vaginal problems.

Constituents Carotene, calcium, phosphorous, potassium, essential oil, fatty acids (caproic, capric, lauric, oleic, palmitic, stearic, myristic), tannin, phytosterols (beta-sitosterol, campesterol, stigmasterol), polysaccharides, dextrose, resins

Energetic Correspondences

- Flavor: pungent, sweet
- Temperature: warm
- Moisture: dry
- Polarity: yang
- Planet: Mars/Pluto
- Element: Fire

Dosage Take 20 to 30 drops of tincture three times daily.

CONCERNS

Saw palmetto is considered safe when used appropriately. There have been rare reports of saw palmetto causing stomach distress.

Avoid during pregnancy and while nursing, at least until further research has been done to ascertain its safety during these times.

Schizandra

Schisandra chinensis (syn. *Kadsura chinensis*), *S. sphenanthera*

Family Schisandraceae (Magnolia Vine)

Etymology The genus name, *Schisandra,* derives from the Greek *schisis,* meaning "crevice," and *andros,* meaning "man," in reference to the cleft on the stamen of some varieties.

Part Used Berry

Physiological Effects Adaptogen, antibacterial, antidepressant, antioxidant, aphrodisiac, astringent, brain tonic, cholagogue, emmenagogue, hepatoprotective, immune tonic, Kidney tonic, nervous system tonic, rejuvenative, reproductive tonic, restorative, sedative (mild), yang tonic, yin tonic restorative

Medicinal Uses Schizandra was widely used by the royalty of ancient China as a youth preserver, beautifier, and reproductive tonic. Schizandra increases staying power in men. It also helps one overcome trauma associated with sexual abuse. It is a supreme adaptogen; Russian pilots of the 1940s used it to help them tolerate the low-oxygen conditions of high altitudes, while to this day hunters in Siberia consume schizandra berries for energy and to help their bodies function in the harsh conditions.

Schizandra improves coordination, intellect, and sensory perception. According to Oriental medicine, it also protects the Heart, Lungs, and Liver; nourishes Kidney chi; and purifies the blood. Chinese medicine calls for eating a few berries one hundred days in a row as a tonic to improve coordination and concentration. It is used to nourish the "water of the genitals," or the fluids that help sensitize and moisturize the genitals. Long-term use helps beautify the skin.

Schizandra is used in the treatment of anxiety, chronic fatigue, depression, eczema, exhaustion, headache, hepatitis, HIV, hives, infertility, insomnia, irritability, low libido, low sperm count, lung weakness (shortness of breath), memory loss, night sweats, nocturnal emissions, polyuria, premature aging, premature ejaculation, post-traumatic stress disorder, spermatorrhea, stress, excessive sweating, and wasting diseases. It also can facilitate athletic recovery and improve sexual stamina.

Constituents Vitamin C, vitamin E, manganese, phosphorous, silicon, sesquicarene, lignans (schizandrin, gomisin), essential oils, phytosterols (stigmasterol, beta-sitosterol), mucilage, citric acid, malic acid, tartaric acid

Energetic Correspondences

- Flavor: sweet, sour, salty, pungent, bitter
- Temperature: warm
- Moisture: dry
- Polarity: yang
- Planet: Mars/Jupiter
- Element: Fire

Dosage Take ½ cup of tea or 20 to 30 drops of tincture three times daily.

CONCERNS

Avoid schizandra in cases of excess heat (such as fever), overly acidic conditions, cough, epilepsy, intracranial pressure, or in the early stages of rash. Schizandra is not recommended during pregnancy or for children under the age of two, except under the guidance of a qualified health care practitioner.

Tribulus

Tribulus cistoides, T. terrestris

Family Zygophylaceae (Caltrop)

Etymology *Tribulis terrestris* means "terrible earth," which is exactly what you might think when you step barefooted on one of its spiky seeds.

Part Used Fruit

Physiological Effects Aphrodisiac, diuretic, galactagogue, Kidney tonic, nervine, parturient, rejuvenative, restorative, sedative, tonic

Medicinal Uses Tribulus has been used in India since ancient times as a remedy for low libido in men and women. It can boost sperm count and remedy erectile dysfunction. It increases testosterone production by activating luteinizing hormone secretions from the pituitary gland. It also increases semen production, sperm moltility, sex drive, and performance.

In women it increases levels of follicle-stimulating hormone. It also improves the metabolism of fats, thus improving the circulation of chi and blood throughout the body.

Tribulis is also used in ayurvedic medicine to enhance mental clarity. It is often suggested for athletes as an agent to increase muscle and burn fat, though more research is needed to substantiate these claims. It is known to relieve pain, improve the flow of Liver chi, clear the lungs, stimulate circulation, and soothe the mucous membranes of the urinary tract.

Tribulis is used in the treatment of amenorrhea, anemia, cystitis (chronic), eczema, edema, erectile dysfunction, gonorrhea, hemorrhoids, high cholesterol, hives, hypertension, incontinence, infertility, kidney stones, leucorrhea, low libido, low sperm count, lumbago, nocturnal emissions, premature ejaculation, polyuria, postpartum bleeding, spermatorrhea, and venereal disease. It also can be used to ease labor that has been difficult. And to think it is considered a noxious weed in many parts of the United States!

Constituents Beta-carotene, protein, iron, vitamin C, linoleic acid, kaempferol, sapogenins (chlorogenin, diosgenin, gitogenin), essential oil, alkaloids (harmine), tribuloside, tannin

Energetic Correspondences

- Flavor: sweet, bitter
- Temperature: warm
- Moisture: dry
- Polarity: yang
- Planet: Mars
- Element: Fire

Dosage Take 1 cup of tea, 20 to 40 drops of tincture, or 1 to 2 capsules three times daily.

CONCERNS

Avoid during pregnancy, except under the guidance of a qualified health care practitioner. Avoid in cases of dehydration or blood or chi deficiency. There have been a few rare reports of stomach upset from using tribulus, which diminishes if the herb is taken with food.

Vitex

Vitex agnus-castus

Family Verbenaceae (Vervain)

Etymology The genus name, *Vitex,* derives from the Latin *vitilis,* which means "made by plaiting," in reference to the use of the flexible branches in making braided fences. The species name derives from ancient Greek; *agnus* means "lamb," and *castus* means "chaste" or "spotless." The common names, monk's pepper and chaste tree, refer to the berries' ability to reduce sexual desire.

Part Used Berry

Physiological Effects Anaphrodisiac for men, antiandrogenic, aphrodisiac for women, aromatic, diuretic, emmenagogue, galactagogue, ophthalmic, phytoprogesteronic, reproductive tonic

Medicinal Uses Vitex increases the production of progesterone, luteinizing hormones, and prolactin, and inhibits the release of follicle-stimulating hormone. It helps to reregulate the menstrual cycle for women coming off birth control pills and to normalize irregular cycles, shortening a long cycle or lengthening a short one. It also helps normalize the functions of the pituitary gland.

Vitex is used in the treatment of amenorrhea, cysts (in the breasts, ovaries, and uterus), depression (related to menopause), dysmenorrhea, endometriosis, fibroids (in the breasts, ovaries, or uterus), infertility, herpes (related to menses), menorrhagia, migraines (related to menstrual cycle), polymenorrhea, premenstrual acne, premenstrual syndrome, and threatened miscarriage. It can also be beneficial after hysterectomy.

In order to improve hormonal problems with vitex, the herb should be taken for at least six months.

Constituents Essential oils (cineol, limonene, pinene, sabinene), flavonoids (casticin, isovitexin, orientin), alkaloids (vitticine), iridoglycosides (agnuside, aucubin, eurostoside)

Energetic Correspondences

- Flavor: sweet, bitter, pungent
- Temperature: neutral
- Planet: Venus/Mars/Moon/Pluto

- Moisture: moist
- Element: Metal
- Polarity: yin

Dosage Drink 1 cup of tea or 20 to 40 drops of tincture three times daily.

CONCERNS

Discontinue if diarrhea, nausea, or abnormal menstrual changes occur. Large doses can cause formication, a strange symptom in which one feels as if ants were crawling on one's skin. Avoid during pregnancy except under the supervision of a health care professional. Vitex can decrease the effectiveness of birth control pills. Rare individuals may experience contact dermatitis. Vitex has the reputation of decreasing sex drive in some people.

Yohimbe

Pausinystalia yohimbe (formerly *Corynanthe yohimbe*)

Family Rubiaceae (Madder)

Etymology The name yohimbe is thought to have been borrowed from a Bantu language of southern Cameroon.

Part Used Bark

Physiological Effects Analgesic, antidiuretic, aphrodisiac, cardiac stimulant, cerebral stimulant, hallucinogen (mild), hypertensive, Kidney yang tonic, nerve stimulant, serotonin inhibitor, stimulant, vasodilator

Medicinal Uses Yohimbe has been used medicinally in Africa for hundreds of years, especially by the Bantu people. It increases blood flow to the genitals, compresses the veins, and prevents blood from flowing back out of the genital area. It also affects the ganglion nerve center at the base of the spine, stimulates erection, and excites the "sex center" of the human brain in the hypothalamus. It increases levels of norepinephrine, which causes a temporary boost in energy.

Yohimbe is used by veterinarians to encourage unenthusiastic bulls and stallions to mate. In humans, it has been found to restore erectile function in many cases of psychogenic (psychological) impotence. It is also sometimes recommended as an herb for weight loss (though there are safer herbs for this purpose), and it increases adrenaline production. It is used in the treatment of depression, dysmenorrhea, erectile dysfunction, and low libido.

The powdered bark is sometimes rubbed on the body as an aphrodisiac.

Constituents Indole alkaloids (yohimbine, yohimbiline, ajmaline, pseudoyohimbine, corynantheine), tannins

Energetic Correspondences

- Flavor: pungent, bitter
- Temperature: warm
- Moisture: dry
- Polarity: yang
- Planet: Mars
- Element: Fire

Dosage Take 1 cup of tea or 40 drops of tincture; take only as needed.

CONCERNS

Yohimbe is best used under the guidance of a qualified health care practitioner. It should be ingested no more than twice a week and used only in small doses as large doses can cause depression and reduced sex drive. Do not use for more than three days in a row. Yohimbe can elevate blood pressure and cause insomnia, mania, tremors, nausea, and vomiting. Avoid using in conjunction with pharmaceuticals, particularly MAO inhibitors and medications for treating diabetes, high blood pressure, and heart problems. Avoid in cases of anxiety, bipolar conditions, diabetes, heart disease, hypertension, kidney disease, liver disease, peripheral vascular disease, prostate inflammation, and schizophrenia. It's also best to avoid tyramine-rich foods (bananas, cheese, chocolate, sauerkraut, red wine) for twelve hours before using yohimbe as the combination can elevate blood pressure. Pregnant women, the elderly, and children should not ingest yohimbe.

Let herbs feed, heal, and fill your needs!

LOVE POTIONS FROM FRIENDLY HERBALISTS

The following recipes and potions were devised and graciously donated by several of my herbalist friends. They're delicious and designed to brighten every encounter with your loved one. Try them and see!

Several of the recipes call for herbal tinctures, which you can either buy premade or make for yourself by following the instructions on page 50.

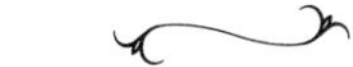

Damiana Rose Cordial

This formula is a tonic for the nervous and reproductive systems. Try drizzling it over fruit pieces or baked pears, adding it to orange juice, tea, or carbonated water, or sipping it from little cordial glasses. A little bit goes a long way. Try your belly button as a cordial cup!

1 cup damiana leaf
2 cups brandy
1½ cups spring water
1 cup honey
1 tablespoon rose water
1 tablespoon vanilla

1. Place the damiana in a clean glass jar and pour the brandy over it. Stir well, then cover. Let soak for five days.
2. Strain the liquid from the leaves. Reserve the leaves, and store the liquid in a clean bottle.
3. Place the alcohol-drenched leaves in a clean glass jar. Pour the spring water over them. Stir well, then cover. Let soak for three days.
4. Strain the liquid from the leaves and reserve it. Compost the leaves.
5. Place the water in a saucepan. Warm it over low heat, then add the honey. Stir and heat just until the honey is melted and mixed into the water. Remove from heat.
6. When the honey water has cooled, combine it with the brandy extract. Add the rose water and vanilla. Pour into a glass jar, cover, and shake well. Let sit for one to four weeks before using.

Diana De Luca, author of *Botanica Erotica: Arousing Body, Mind and Spirit* (Healing Arts Press, 1998)

Aphrodisiac Formula for Women

This recipe combines some of nature's best.

2 cups damiana herb
2 teaspoons schizandra berry
1½ teaspoons rosemary leaves
1½ teaspoons organic rose flower
1 teaspoon clove bud
3 cups water

1. Combine all the herbs.
2. Place 3 tablespoons of the herb mixture into a canning jar. Add 3 cups of boiling water. Cover and let sit overnight.
3. Strain the infused water from the spent herbs. Drink 1 cup of the tea before each meal during the day.
4. Continue this daily program for one to two months.

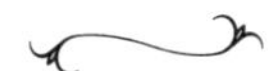

Aphrodisiac Formula for Men

A potent herbal blend for men!

3 parts Syrian rue seed
3 parts muira puama inner bark
2 parts nettle seed
2 parts milky oat seed
1½ parts polygala roots
Vodka

1. Combine all the herbs in a quart canning jar. Cover with vodka, so that the vodka rises one inch over the top of the herbs.
2. Let steep for one month, shaking every day.
3. Strain the infused vodka from the spent herbs through fine cheesecloth. Bottle in amber glass dropper bottles. Take 1½ dropperfuls in a bit of warm water three or four times daily on an empty stomach; continue for one to two months.

The above two formulas are from Matthew Becker, clinical herbalist for Pharmaca Integrative Pharmacy.

Herbal Salve

A "must have" in every home medicine chest. Can be used on sore muscles, cuts, and bruises or even applied to dry or overindulged genitals.

2 cups good-quality vegetable oil (such as olive, almond, coconut, sesame, or avocado)

8 ounces fresh or dried chopped blossoms of chamomile, calendula, or Saint John's wort

2 ounces beeswax, cocoa butter, or shea butter (if you're using coconut oil, skip this ingredient)

1. Add the oil to a heavy-bottomed, nonaluminum pot.
2. Stir in fresh or dried herbs.
3. Warm over low heat for 30 to 60 minutes. If you're using fresh herbs, keep uncovered so that moisture can evaporate. If you're using dried herbs, cover.
4. Line a clean container with cheesecloth or muslin, and pour the oil and flowers onto it. Let the oil drip from the flowers through cheesecloth or muslin to filter. When the flowers have stopped dripping, measure the amount of oil.
5. Reheat the filtered oil in a clean pot until it is warm enough to melt the beeswax, cocoa butter, or shea butter. Then add the beeswax, cocoa butter, or shea butter. (If you're using coconut oil as your base, you do not need to add any additional thickener.) Stir until the ingredients are thoroughly combined.
6. While the oil is warm, pour it carefully into salve containers.
7. When the salve has hardened, secure the lid and seal tightly.
8. Store in a cool, dark location and use within one year.

From Cascade Anderson Geller. As a voice for the green world, Cascade shares her experiences with plants and discusses the interconnection of plants and people—in the clinical herbal setting, the home, and, most importantly, outdoors in forest, field, and garden.

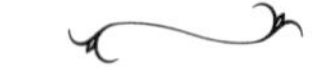

Coconut-Avocado Love Elixir

This spicy dish will really get the blood flowing.

1½ cups coconut water
Meat of 1 coconut and 1 avocado
1 inch fresh gingerroot
Juice of 2 limes
½ cup spinach
1½ cups water
1 large clove garlic
2 tablespoons unpasteurized miso
Pinch of cayenne pepper
½ cup basil
1 tomato, chopped
Spearmint leaves, pine nuts, and sunflower sprouts for garnish

1. Combine all ingredients except the tomato and garnish ingredients in a blender and puree.
2. Place the chopped tomato in a bowl and pour the puree over it.
3. Garnish with spearmint leaves, pine nuts, and sunflower sprouts. Serves 4.

From Peter Ragnar, author of *Wisdom of the Mystic Mountain Warrior*. See www.roaringlionpublishing.com for books, DVDs, and course offerings.

The Love Shake

This is way beyond your average smoothie!

2 tablespoons organic chocolate powder
2 cups almond milk
4 dried figs (preferably organic Turkish), soaked
1 frozen banana
A touch of vanilla extract
2 tablespoons maca powder
Frozen organic raspberries (optional)
2 dropperfuls fresh damiana tincture (optional)
2 dropperfuls ginger tincture (optional)
½ to 1 teaspoon red ginseng powdered extract

Combine all ingredients in a blender and blend.

Christopher Hobbs, L.Ac., A.H.G., coauthor of Peterson's *A Field Guide to Western Medicinal Plants and Herbs* (Houghton Mifflin, 2002) and author of *Natural Therapy for Your Liver* (Avery, 2002). See www.christopherhobbs.com.

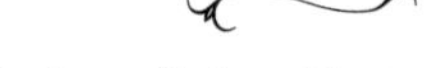

Aphrodisiac Date Parfait

After this, you may become the final dessert.

2-pound package of pitted dates
Brandy (I prefer apricot brandy.)
Vanilla ice cream
Whipped cream
Jasmine essential oil
Nuts (optional)

1. Chop the dates.
2. Stir the brandy into the chopped dates until they are gooey. Refrigerate until chilled.
3. In a parfait glass, layer the date mixture with vanilla ice cream. Top with whipped cream to which 1 drop of jasmine essential oil per 8 servings has been added. Sprinkle with nuts, if desired. Chill again until ready to serve.

Diana De Luca, author of *Botanica Erotica: Arousing Body, Mind, and Spirit* (Healing Arts Press, 1998)

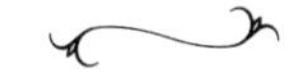

Easy Massage Oil

This massage oil encourages passion. It can also be dripped moderately over desserts to add flavor.

1 drop jasmine absolute
1 drop sandalwood essential oil
1 drop ylang ylang essential oil
1 drop neroli essential oil
1 drop spikenard essential oil
1 ounce vegetable oil (I prefer hazelnut, sunflower, or olive.)

Combine the absolute and essential oils in a small container and shake vigorously. Then add the vegetable oil and shake again until it is truly blended.

Jeanne Rose, founder of New Age Creations, the first body-care company in the United States to use aromatherapy, author of *Herbal Body Book* (Frog, Ltd., 2000) and *Herbs and Aromatherapy for the Reproductive System* (Frog, Ltd., 1994), and director of the home-study courses "Herbal Studies Course" and "Aromatherapy Studies Course." See www.jeannerose.net.

Male Sexual Vitality Tonic

This formula is an adaptogenic sexual tonic. It can enhance sexual health and performance in healthy men, while it is also useful in cases of sexual weakness or exhaustion. It is especially indicated for male sexual impotence.

5 parts *Panax* ginseng root tincture
4 parts saw palmetto berry tincture
2 parts cardamom seed tincture
5 parts Jamaican sarsaparilla root tincture
4 parts "milky" oat seed tincture

Combine all ingredients. Take 40 drops in a bit of water or juice two or three times a day.

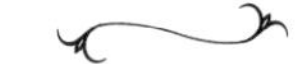

Herbal Ed's Sexy Smoothie

After drinking this smoothie, I feel completely energized, and sexual vitality and stamina are definitely enhanced. All ingredients are approximate, so feel free to experiment.

2½ cups almond milk
1 cup blueberries, strawberries, or other berries
2 tablespoons maca root powder
1 tablespoon raw flaxseeds
1 tablespoon raw pumpkin seeds

Combine the ingredients in a blender and blend.

The above two recipes are from "Herbal Ed" Smith, founder of Herb Pharm. See www.herb-pharm.com and www.herbaled.org.

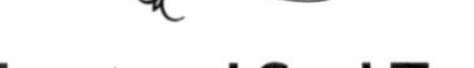

Heart and Soul Tonic

Maintaining good love requires more than mere engagement on the sexual level. It is equally important for the heart and the soul to be involved. In this tonic, hawthorn is for the heart, damiana is for the sexual excitement, and sacred basil is for the soul. Chambord is added because it tastes so good!

- 2 ounces hawthorn brandy (berries steeped in brandy for six weeks)
- 8 ounces sacred basil infusion (sacred basil leaf steeped in boiling water for four hours)
- 2 ounces damiana brandy (damiana leaf and flower steeped in brandy for six weeks)
- A splash of Chambord

Combine all ingredients. Store in the refrigerator, where it will keep for several weeks.

Pam Montgomery, author of *Partner Earth: A Spiritual Ecology* (Destiny Books, 1997) and *Plant Spirit Healing* (Bear & Company, 2008), director of Partner Earth Education Center and Green Nations Gatherings.

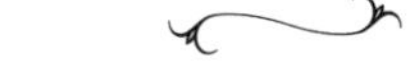

Asparagus-Epimedium Tea

Epimedium is also known as horny goat weed. Meditate on that name while sharing this tea with your beloved over a large shrimp cocktail.

- 1 quart water
- 1 heaping teaspoon Chinese asparagus root
- 3 heaping teaspoons epimedium leaf

1. Drop the asparagus root into the water. Bring to a boil, cover, and simmer for 20 minutes.
2. Remove from heat. Add the epimedium leaf. Cover and let steep for 20 minutes.
3. Strain and share.

Lesley Tierra, author of *The Herbs of Life* (Crossing Press, 1992), *Healing with Chinese Herbs* (Crossing Press, 1997), and *A Kid's Herb Book* (Robert D. Reed Publishers, 2000), and coauthor of *Chinese Traditional Herbal Medicine* (Lotus Press, 1998). See www.planetherbs.com.

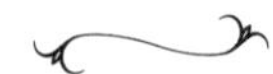

A Romantic Love Potion

An herbal beverage to enjoy by the glass.

1 quart red wine (or red raspberry or pomegranate juice)
1 teaspoon vanilla extract
1 tablespoon damiana tincture
½ teaspoon nutmeg powder
2 tablespoons rose water
1 teaspoon ginseng tincture
3 drops cardamom essential oil
2 tablespoons honey (optional)

Combine all the ingredients. Let sit for a couple of days to allow the flavors to blend and mellow.

Kathi Keville, author of *Herbs for Health and Healing* (Rodale Press, 1996), coauthor of *Aromatherapy: A Complete Guide to the Healing Art* (Crossing Press, 1995), and director of the American Herb Association. See www.ahaherbs.com.

Kava Kava Brew

Prepare your brew at least twenty-four hours before your love fest.

Use ½ to 1 ounce of dried kava kava root per person.

1. Chop the roots and place in a glass jar or enamel pan.
2. Pour 2 cups of boiling water per person over the cut roots.
3. Cover and let steep, away from heat, until you're ready to drink it.
4. Serve chilled or warmed, with honey and milk and a little cinnamon or nutmeg if you like. Hint: When your nose starts to tingle, drink another half glass of kava kava, no more. Then concentrate on love.

Susun S. Weed, author of *Wise Woman Herbal for the Childbearing Year* (Ash Tree Publishing, 1985), *New Menopausal Years the Wise Woman Way* (Ash Tree Publishing, 2001), and *Breast Cancer? Breast Health!* (Ash Tree Publishing, 1997). She is the director of Wise Woman Center in Woodstock, New York. See www.susunweed.com.

CHINESE PATENT FORMULAS

Making tea is not everyone's cup of tea. If you prefer pills, look for herbal formula combinations in natural food stores, or try an Asian market where patent formulas are available. Patent medicines are ready-made herbal formulas that are usually found in pill form. Chinese patent formulas are often used in combination with other therapies, such as acupuncture. There are several Chinese patent formulas, some based on ancient recipes, that can do wonders for sexual vigor. Keep in mind, however, that Chinese formulas are medicines, designed to treat specific conditions and constitutions; using a formula that isn't right for you can make you ill or exacerbate an existing condition. For these reasons, it's a good idea to consult a practitioner of traditional Chinese medicine before you take them.

CONG RONG BU SHEN WAN tonifies Kidney yin and yang and nourishes *jing,* or life essence. It is often recommended in cases of weak lower back, erectile dysfunction, and premature ejaculation.

NAN XING BU SHEN WAN warms and tonifies the Kidneys. It can be used to remedy coldness in the extremities, lower back pain, urinary incontinence, and sexual weakness.

REHMANNIA SIX PILLS are recommended in cases of Kidney yin deficiency. The formula calms the heart, builds the blood, and remedies low libido and/or erectile dysfunction resulting from illness.

TIAN WANG BU XIN WAN is recommended in cases of emotional instability, premature ejaculation, and sexual anxiety.

TZEPAU SANPIEN PILLS strengthen the Kidneys and thus improve sexual function. They remedy erectile dysfunction, weakness, and dizziness.

YAO JIAN SHEN PIAN is often recommended in cases of Kidney yang depletion, weak lower back, and fatigue, especially when due to sexual excess.

YOU GUI WAN, also known as YUDAI WAN, can be used to treat incontinence, weakness following illness, and Kidney yang depletion. It is often recommended in cases of erectile dysfunction, leukorrhea, premature ejaculation, and lower back pain.

ZAN YI DAN nourishes Kidney yang and is recommended in cases of apathy, weak lower back, erectile dysfunction, and infertility.

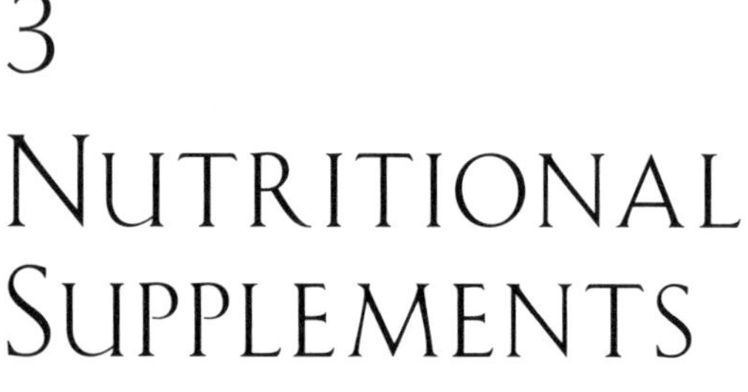

3 Nutritional Supplements

Balancing and Rebuilding Sexual Health

YOUR PRIMARY SOURCE OF nutrition should always be a healthy diet. A balanced, varied range of organic, unprocessed food served up for breakfast, lunch, dinner, and all the snacks in between should supply adequate vitamins, minerals, and nutrients for a healthy body, a sound mind, and an ardent sexual appetite. If we all ate this way, we would pay less for supplements.

There are situations, however, in which diet alone is not adequate to supply the nutrients an individual needs, and supplements become necessary: when a person is recovering from an illness or childbirth, for example. Even during an illness, supplements can be an opportunity to avoid using a pharmaceutical drug. You can buy supplements yourself, and they are often more effective than pharmaceutical prescriptions; they always have fewer side effects.

There are several nutrients that have a direct effect on sexual vitality and may be added as supplements to the diet when necessary. If you intend to take these supplements in pill form, instead of as food, look for pills that are free of artificial dyes and preservatives. As with just about everything, supplements in excess can be detrimental to your health. Your health care provider or a nutrition advisor will be able to give you guidelines for establishing a safe, healthy supplement program.

VITAMINS

Vitamins are familiar to many of us, but did you know what a profound effect these nutrional powerhouses can have on your sexuality?

Beta-carotene (vitamin A)

Action: The body converts beta-carotene to vitamin A, which is necessary for the production of sex hormones. It strengthens mucous membranes, prevents atrophy of the genitals, and can help increase sperm levels.

Therapeutic use: Supplementation with beta-carotene can counteract vaginal dryness and thinning of the vaginal walls in postmenopausal women and can improve sperm count in men.

Recommended dosage: 25,000–50,000 IU of beta-carotene daily

Natural sources: Apricots, beet greens, broccoli, cabbage, cantaloupes, carrots, dandelion greens, grapefruit, green leafy vegetables, green peppers, kale, lamb's-quarter, mangoes, mustard greens, nori, oranges, papaya, parsley, persimmons, peppers, pumpkin, romaine lettuce, spinach, sweet potatoes, Swiss chard, tomatoes, watermelon, winter squash, yam, and yellow squash

B-complex vitamins

Action: Taken as a whole, the B-complex vitamins support the production of hormones in both men and women.

Therapeutic use: Both men and women who suffer from inadequate hormone levels may benefit from supplementation with B-complex vitamins.

Recommended dosage: 50–300 mg daily

Natural sources: Brown rice, Brussels sprouts, green leafy vegetables, nutritional yeast, nuts (all), and whole grains

CHOLINE

Action: Choline, one of the B-complex vitamins, aids in the production of the neurotransmitter acetylcholine, which relays nerve messages between the brain and the sexual organs and can intensify orgasms. Choline can help improve mood and memory and enhance the brain's perception of pleasure.

Therapeutic use: Those who have trouble achieving orgasm or who feel particularly tense or anxious about sex may benefit from supplementation with choline.

Recommended dosage: 25–500 mg daily

Natural sources: Avocados, beans (especially garbanzo beans, lentils, split peas, and soybeans), cabbage, cauliflower, corn, fish (particularly salmon), green beans, nutritional yeast, nuts (all), oats, peanuts, potatoes, rice, seeds (all), soybeans, and wheat germ

NIACIN (VITAMIN B_3)

Action: Niacin is also known as vitamin B_3. It stimulates histamine release, which increases mucous-membrane secretions, enables orgasm, and causes that "flush" or glow that occurs on the face, neck, and chest when arousal is high. Niacin also improves circulation and tactile sensations.

Therapeutic use: Niacin can be used to correct erectile dysfunction and help women achieve more orgasms.

Recommended dosage: 25–300 mg daily. For a "niacin rush," which can make a sexual encounter feel hot and intense, take 100 mg about fifteen minutes before getting started.

Natural sources: Avocados, barley, beans, bee pollen, broccoli, fish (particularly anchovies, haddock, halibut, mackerel, salmon, and swordfish), mushrooms, nutritional yeast, oysters, peanuts, potatoes, raspberries, rice, sesame and sunflower seeds, soybeans, squash, strawberries, tempeh, tomatoes, tuna, watermelons, and whole grains

---

CAUTION

Large doses of niacin can contribute to acid indigestion and make you feel hot and prickly for about ten minutes.

PANTOTHENIC ACID (VITAMIN B_5)

Action: Pantothenic acid is needed for hormonal function and energy production.

Therapeutic use: People with hormonal deficiencies may benefit from supplementation with B_5, but note that it is part of the vitamin B complex and should therefore be taken in combination with other B vitamins.

Recommended dosage: 25–500 mg daily

Natural sources: Asparagus, avocados, beans (especially lentils and soybeans), bee pollen, broccoli, buckwheat, cabbage, chicken, chicken liver, clams, corn, crabs, eggs, fish (particularly anchovies, flounder, haddock, herring, mackerel, salmon, sardines, and trout), flaxseeds, green leafy vegetables, nutritional yeast, nuts (cashews, hazelnuts, peanuts, and pecans), papaya, peas, pineapples, potatoes, royal jelly, sesame seeds, shiitake mushrooms, sunflower seeds, watermelons, wheat germ, whole grains, yams, and yogurt

PYRIDOXINE (VITAMIN B_6)

Action: Pyridoxine, another B-complex vitamin, plays a vital role in hormonal balance and in the production of testosterone and ejaculatory fluid. It also helps convert the amino acid histidine into histamine. A B_6 deficiency is often associated with low libido.

Therapeutic use: Supplementation with B_6 can facilitate orgasmic ability in women and boost libido.

Recommended dosage: 25–300 mg daily

Natural sources: Apples, asparagus, avocados, bananas, barley, beans (particularly garbanzo beans, lentils, lima beans, navy beans, and soybeans), bee pollen, blueberries, brown rice, buckwheat, cabbage, cantaloupe, carrots, cheese, corn, crabs, eggs, fish (particularly cod, halibut, herring, mackerel, salmon, sardines, trout, and tuna), flax, green leafy vegetables, hazelnuts, kale, lettuce, mangoes, molasses, nuts (particularly Brazil nuts, chestnuts, peanuts, and walnuts), nutritional yeast, onions, oranges, peas, potatoes, prunes, sesame and sunflower seeds, spinach, squash, sweet potatoes, tomatoes, and watermelons

Vitamin C

Action: Vitamin C strengthens the body, clears heat, nourishes the adrenal glands, and supports collagen activity so that the skin remains elastic and supple. It is also an excellent antioxidant. Look for a vitamin C supplement that also includes bioflavonoids, which have a chemical activity similar to that of estrogen.

Therapeutic use: Supplementation with vitamin C can reduce excessive bleeding during menstruation, normalize menstrual cycles, relieve hot flashes, increase vaginal lubrication, and counteract phimosis.

Recommended dosage: 1,000 mg of vitamin C with 500 mg of bioflavonoids daily

Natural sources: Acerola berries, amla fruit, avocados, Brussels sprouts, cabbage, cauliflower, collard greens, cantaloupe, grapefruit, kale, mangoes, oranges, papaya, red peppers, rose hips, spinach, strawberries, and tomatoes

Vitamin D

Action: Ultraviolet rays on the skin stimulate the manufacture of vitamin D in the body. Vitamin D stimulates calcium absorption and supports bone and tooth growth, blood clotting, and nervous system function.

Therapeutic use: Vitamin D is being proclaimed a steroid hormone that impacts the prostate gland. Vitamin D enhances virility and endurance and may be helpful in preventing breast cancer.

Recommended dosage: Dosage guidelines for vitamin D have recently increased from no more than 1000 IU once daily to up to 3000 IU daily being acceptable.

Natural sources: Foods are generally low in vitamin D, but small amounts can be found in alfalfa, basil, chickweed, bee pollen, fenugreek, green leafy vegetables, horsetail, mullein, nettle, papaya, parsley, shiitake mushrooms, sunflower seeds and greens, sweet potatoes, watercress, and wheatgrass. Getting more full-spectrum light helps too.

Vitamin E

Action: Vitamin E, a natural antioxidant, is sometimes referred to as "the sex vitamin." It stimulates vasodilation and improves blood flow to all parts of the body, including the sexual organs, thereby aiding in erection and orgasm. Vitamin E supports the production of sex hormones, increases stamina, boosts fertility, and nourishes the pituitary gland. It also eases the symptoms of hot flashes, limits or slows the thinning of vaginal walls, reverses or improves cases of vaginal dryness, helps improve sperm count, and counteracts loss of libido.

Therapeutic use: Women who suffer from hot flashes, thin vaginal walls, vaginal dryness, or difficulty achieving orgasm may benefit from supplementation with vitamin E, as may men who suffer from erectile dysfunction and low sperm count. Vitamin E can also be helpful for both men and women with low libido, hormone deficiencies, and fertility problems.

Recommended dosage: 100–1,200 IU daily

Natural sources: Almonds, asparagus, beet greens, blackberries, Brazil nuts, brown rice, dandelion greens, dark green leafy vegetables, eggs, hazelnuts, kale, leeks, lettuce, liver, lobster, oats, parsley, peanuts, purslane, quinoa, salmon, spinach, sprouted grains, sunflower seeds, sweet potatoes, tomatoes, turmeric, tuna, vegetable oils, and whole grains

ESSENTIAL FATTY ACIDS

Essential fatty acids (EFAs) improve skin and hair, lower blood pressure and cholesterol levels, and reduce the risk of blood clots. They are found in high concentrations in the brain and are used by all cells, including those involved in the production of hormones.

Action: EFAs are needed for proper hormone function; they also help promote soft skin and vaginal moisture. Low levels of EFAs can cause women to experience more cramping and men to lack sufficient ejaculate.

Therapeutic use: Supplementation with EFAs may counteract vaginal dryness and cramping and improve ejaculate production.

Recommended dosage: If you're taking an EFA supplement, follow the dosage guidelines on the package label.

Natural sources: Cod liver oil, corn oil, fish (particularly eel, mackerel, and salmon), flaxseeds, hemp seeds, purslane, sesame seeds, sunflower seeds, and walnuts

Omega-3 Fatty Acids (Alpha-Linolenic Acids)

Omega-3 and omega-6 fatty acids are the only types of fatty acids that the body cannot synthesize. Omega-3 fatty acids are found in cell membranes and are necessary for the production of anti-inflammatory prostaglandins.

Natural sources: Beans, blue-green algae, cabbage, chia seed, flaxseed, green leafy vegetables, hemp seeds, pine nuts, pumpkin seeds, purslane, sesame seeds, soy foods (fermented are easiest to assimilate), spinach, sprouts, squash, and walnuts

Omega-6 Fatty Acids (Linoleic Acids)

Like omega-3 fatty acids, omega-6 fatty acids cannot be synthesized in the body. A deficiency of linoleic acid can contribute to eczema, hair loss, liver degeneration, susceptibility to infections, infertility in men, and miscarriage in women.

Natural sources: Beans, black currant oil, borage seed oil, corn, evening primrose oil, pumpkin seeds, sesame seeds, vegetable oils, and whole grains

Gamma-linolenic acid

Action: Gamma-linolenic acid (GLA) is an essential fatty acid that invigorates the sexual organs, improves moods, and normalizes hormonal output.

Therapeutic use: GLA has been found useful in treating low libido, erectile dysfunction, inability to orgasm, and premature ejaculation.

Recommended dosage: If you're taking a GLA supplement, follow the dosage guidelines on the package label.

Natural sources: Barley, black currant seed oil, borage seed oil, evening primrose oil, hemp seeds, oats, and spirulina

MINERALS

Minerals provide our bodies with vital building blocks, so it is important to be aware of our intake of them.

Calcium

Action: Calcium is vital for the health of bones and teeth. It also calms the emotions and supports good sleep.

Therapeutic use: Ingested in adequate amounts throughout adolescence and the menstrual years, calcium can prevent many of the concerns associated with menopause, most notably osteoporosis. It also may relieve cramping associated with dysmenorrhea and some symptoms of premenstrual syndrome.

Recommended dosage: 1,000–1,500 mg daily

Natural sources: Almonds, beans (black, garbanzo, pinto, soy, and white), blackstrap molasses, Brazil nuts, broccoli, carob powder, clams, collards, dairy products, dandelion greens, eggs, figs, flounder, green leafy vegetables, hazelnuts, kombu, lentils, miso, oats, oysters, peanuts, salmon, sardines, scallops, seaweeds, sesame seeds, shrimp, sunflower seeds, tofu, and turnip greens

Iron

Action: Iron transports oxygen throughout the body; low levels can manifest as lack of energy and low libido. Iron is needed for production of hemoglobin. Vitamin C aids the absorption of iron; therefore, a vitamin C deficiency can lead to an iron deficiency.

Therapeutic use: Supplementation with iron may benefit those with low energy or libido, as well as those who have been diagnosed as iron deficient.

Recommended dosage: 10–25 mg daily for men; 18–30 mg for women. Take only if needed.

Natural sources: Almonds, apricots, beans, blackberries, blackstrap molasses, burdock root, carrots, dandelion greens, fish, green leafy vegetables, grapes, green peppers, Jerusalem artichokes, kidney, millet, miso, nettles, nori, oatmeal, oysters, parsley, persimmons, prunes, pumpkin seeds, raisins, seaweeds (dulse, hiziki, kelp, and kombu), sesame seeds, shellfish, spinach, squash, sunflower seeds, turkey (dark meat), venison, watercress, and sprouted grain such as wheat

---

CAUTION

Excessive levels of commercial iron supplements can cause constipation and may increase the risk of heart attack. Try a daily glass of prune juice or eat figs as they are mildly laxative and high in iron.

Magnesium

Action: Magnesium is needed for the production of sex hormones and may be helpful in treating prostate problems. It helps prevent many of the health concerns associated with menopause and is also a muscle relaxant that plays an important role in skeletal, muscle, and nerve function. We sometimes say, "If you have spasms, take magnesium." I know it doesn't rhyme, but it gets the message across.

Therapeutic use: Supplement with magnesium in cases of muscle spasms, cramps, and premenstrual syndrome, especially when PMS is accompanied by mood swings.

Recommended dosage: 500–750 mg daily

Natural sources: Almonds, apricots, artichokes, avocados, bananas, barley, beans, beet greens, blackstrap molasses, Brazil nuts, brown rice, buckwheat, carrots, cashews, celery, chard, chocolate, corn, crabs, dandelion greens, dates, dulse, figs, fish (particularly flounder, halibut, salmon, sole, and tuna), green leafy vegetables, kelp, millet, oatmeal, oranges, peas, peaches, peanuts, pecans, peppers, pine nuts, potatoes, prunes, quinoa, rye, seaweeds, seeds (especially pumpkin, sesame, and sunflower), shrimp, spinach, soybeans, squash, tofu, tomatoes, walnuts, watermelon, whole grains, and wild rice

Selenium

Action: The antioxidant selenium is concentrated in the testes and believed necessary for sperm production. It works synergistically with vitamin E and prevents the formation of free radicals. Selenium is best obtained from food or in the form of selenomethionine, a compound derived from selenium-rich sea vegetables.

Therapeutic use: Selenium supplements may be helpful in cases of muscle weakness, lack of mental alertness, and depression.

Recommended dosage: 50–400 micrograms daily

Natural sources: Alfalfa, asparagus, barley, beets, black-eyed peas, blackstrap molasses, Brazil nuts, broccoli, brown rice, cabbage, carrots, cashews, catnip, cayenne, celery, chamomile, chickweed, fennel seed, fenugreek seed, fish, garlic, ginseng, green leafy vegetables, hawthorn berries, honey, hops, horsetail, kelp, lentils, lobster, meat, milk, mushrooms, nutritional yeast, oatstraw, onions, oysters, parsley, raspberry leaf, rose hips, salmon, scallops, seaweeds, shrimp, soybeans, spinach, sprouts, squash, sunflower seeds, tomatoes, tuna, whole grains, yarrow, yellow dock, and yogurt

Zinc

Action: Zinc stimulates the thymus gland to manufacture thymosin, which aids in the production of sex hormones and neurotransmitters. Zinc is needed for normal genital development, vaginal lubrication, and sperm count and motility. Be aware that zinc levels decline with age and that coffee, alcohol, and smoking deplete the body of zinc. Zinc improves one's sense of taste, sight, and smell.

Therapeutic use: Supplement with zinc to counteract low libido, prostatitis, erectile dysfunction, vaginal dryness, and low sperm count.

Recommended dosage: 22.5–50 mg daily

Natural sources: Almonds, beans, bee pollen, Brazil nuts, brown rice, buckwheat, cashews, corn, crabs, eggs, garlic, green, leafy vegetables, herring, kelp, lobster, maple syrup, milk, mushrooms, mussels, nutritional yeast, oatmeal, oysters, peanuts, peas, potatoes, poultry, pumpkin seeds, rice bran, rye, sesame seeds, sunflower seeds, tuna, walnuts, and whole grains

OTHER SUPPLEMENTS

Arginine

Action: Arginine, an amino acid, is a precursor to nitric oxide, a compound that is responsible for vasodilation and thus plays a role in the flow of blood to the genitals and increasing arousal. Arginine appears to stimulate the release of growth hormone from the pituitary gland. It is a component of seminal fluid and accelerates tissue repair. It also relaxes smooth muscle contractions in the arteries of the penis, resulting in stronger erections.

Therapeutic use: Arginine can improve libido in both sexes and strengthen erections in men. Applied topically in a cream, it can be used to increase arousal and intensify orgasms.

Recommended dosage: 1,000–2,000 mg twice daily, taken with food

---

CAUTION

Those carrying the herpes virus or suffering from diabetes should avoid taking arginine as a supplement, except under the supervision of a health care professional. Avoid during pregnancy and while nursing.

Natural sources: Apples, apricots, berries, cacao, coconut, eggplants, nuts, oats, pineapple, tomatoes, seeds (all), strawberries, and wheat (best sprouted)

Dimethylglycine

Action: Dimethylglycine (DMG) can boost energy, support endurance, improve libido, and benefit the entire urogenital system. It balances neurotransmitters including dopamine and serotonin.

Therapeutic use: Dimethylglycine can be used to treat vaginal dryness, cryptorchidism, and low libido.

Recommended dosage: 250 mg daily

Natural sources: Nutritional yeast, pumpkin seeds, rice bran, sunflower seeds, and whole grains. It is also found in small amounts in brown rice and liver.

Superoxide Dismutase

Action: Superoxide dismutase is an antioxidant enzyme that increases libido, supports sexual stamina, and prevents premature aging.

Therapeutic use: Supplementation with superoxide dismutase can counteract low libido.

Recommended dosage: 100 IU daily.

Natural sources: Barley grass, broccoli, Brussels sprouts, green, leafy vegetables, nutritional yeast, and wheatgrass

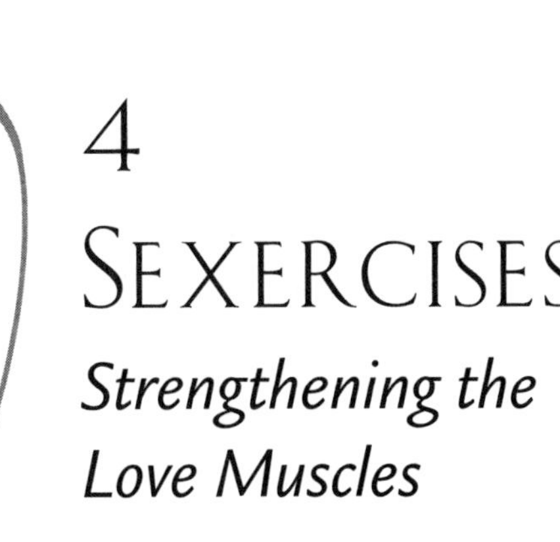

4 SEXERCISES

Strengthening the Love Muscles

WE'VE ALL HEARD THE RAP. To stay healthy, we must exercise. To reduce stress, we must exercise. To lose weight, we must exercise. Somehow most of us still find ourselves unable to fit three twenty-minute exercise sessions into our schedule each week. But would it make a difference if I told you that you'd have the best sex of your life if you started exercising?

It's true. Regular exercise is one of the most efficient and inexpensive methods for promoting the "urge to merge." Psychologically, exercise relieves depression, reduces stress, relaxes the mind and body, and opens the heart. Physically, it encourages strength, stamina, flexibility, and sensitivity. Chemically, it boosts the production of endorphins, adrenaline, and testosterone, all of which contribute to arousal. As a result, exercise also boosts libido and intensifies orgasms.

Exercising for twenty minutes three times a week can effect an astonishing change in your health, psyche, and sex life. The hardest part is just getting started. Once you do, you'll find that exercise is almost addictive—when you miss sessions, you'll feel restless and unsettled.

Making a commitment to exercise doesn't mean that you have to pay membership fees at a health club or start running marathons. Anything that increases your heart rate qualifies as exercise, and that includes cleaning the house, going for a walk, playing tag with your kids, dancing, gardening, and any other everyday activity that is undertaken with energy and enthusiasm. Taking walks together can be time for romance and exercise. Tai chi, qi gong, and martial arts can be aligning and empowering. Making love itself is good exercise—you can burn about a hundred calories per session!

Be aware, however, that anything done to excess can drain energy and libido. Therefore, while it's important to get adequate exercise, it's also important not to overdo it.

EXERCISES FOR SEXUAL VITALITY

There are many exercises designed specifically for boosting sexual vitality, either for an individual or between two people in a relationship. Some of these exercises focus on the strength and flexibility of the muscles used in making love; others work to increase the flow of sexual energy through the body; still others harmonize the energies between two people in a relationship. You'll find that regular practice of these exercises increases your orgasmic ability, improves your stamina as a lover, enhances your sensitivity to your lover's needs, and endows you with strong sexual confidence.

Kegel Exercises

The Kegel pelvic exercises have been known for thousands of years to practitioners of tantra as *mool bandha,* or "root locks." These exercises strengthen and tone muscles in your pelvic region. They are named after Dr. Arnold Kegel, who popularized them in North America in the 1950s as a treatment for stress-related incontinence. For both men and women, Kegels release tension, improve circulation, and strengthen muscles in the pelvic area. For women, they can be used to strengthen muscles weakened by childbirth and to increase the occurrence and intensity of orgasms. For men, they give greater staying power and also massage the prostate, contributing to prostate health. Kegels can also help men differentiate between orgasm and ejaculation.

To practice Kegels, you must tighten and then release the pubococcygeus muscles, which control the anal sphincter as well as the flow of urine. To find these muscles, stop midstream the next time you are urinating. Can you feel the muscles in the pelvic area that allow you to halt the flow of urine? Now release them, allowing your urine to flow again.

That tightening followed by release amounts to one Kegel contraction.

When you practice Kegels, inhale while tightening and exhale while releasing. Hold each contraction for one to five seconds, and be sure to relax fully between contractions. Do the exercises three times daily, starting with twenty-one contractions at each session and working your way up to one hundred. Kegels are a very subtle exercise; if you practiced them in a room full of people, no one would ever notice. Kegels are, therefore, a great way to make good use of time when you're stuck in traffic, waiting in line, riding in a crowded elevator, or sitting on a large ball writing a sex help book.

A variation of Kegels for men is to hang a damp washcloth over the erect penis while performing Kegels. The washcloth serves as a weight, and will be carried up and down with each Kegel. When the washcloth becomes easy to manage, use a hand towel instead.

Once you've undertaken Kegel exercises seriously, you'll notice dramatic improvement in your orgasmic ability within a few weeks. Doing Kegels is also one of the best ways to prevent incontinence later in life.

The Deer

The Deer, also known as Stoking the Golden Stove, is one of the most important Taoist exercises for promoting long life and sexual vitality. The Deer moves blockages of energy, stimulates hormonal production, and relieves a wide range of reproductive disorders. This exercise can also help prevent prostate problems, hemorrhoids, and erectile dysfunction. There are male and female versions.

For women, sit up straight on a bed, chair, or the floor, and place the heel of your foot gently against your clitoris. Rub your hands together to warm them, and then massage around each breast (excluding the nipples) in a slow, circular motion thirty-six times. Massage inward to make your breasts grow larger and outward to make them smaller. If your breasts are overly large, tender, or prone to lumps, massage away from the heart. After the breast massage, lower your hands to your sides and do thirty-six deep Kegels.

For men, the Deer is performed standing or while sitting on a chair or a bed. Rub your hands together to warm them. Hold your scrotum with one hand. With the palm of the other hand, massage right below the navel in a circular motion eighty-one times. Then switch hands and directions and massage again. Follow with thirty-six Kegels.

The Deer should be practiced twice daily, in the morning when you wake up and at night before you go to bed. It is essential to focus on the exercise, rather than thinking about what you're going to wear or have for lunch. Be mindfully present during your practice.

The Mounted Archer

This Taoist exercise, also known as the Horseman, strengthens the Kidneys, improves blood quality and circulation, calms the mind, and improves digestion.

Stand with your legs shoulder width apart and cross your arms in front of your chest. Keeping your heels on the floor, bend your knees, lower your upper body, and lean forward as if you were riding a horse. Pull one arm back as if you were drawing back a bowstring. Inhale, then resume the crossed-arm position. Repeat eight times, alternating arms. Practice daily.

Male Tonifying Exercise

In the Taoist tradition the simple act of urinating can build sexual energy and strengthen Kidney chi in men. But it's important to do it right. Stand on tiptoe, tighten the buttocks, keep the waist and back straight, hold in the stomach, and clench the teeth. Urinate forcibly, all the while exhaling slowly. This practice also helps treat erectile dysfunction and premature ejaculation.

The Wild Duck

The Wild Duck is a beneficial Taoist exercise for women. It can help with menstrual concerns, low libido, and leukorrhea. It tonifies the lower abdomen, including the Kidneys, Liver, Spleen, and reproductive center.

Stand on the balls of your feet and stretch upward, simultaneously inhaling and raising your arms. Then drop your heels to the floor, and as you slowly lower your arms, bend at the waist until your head is between your knees, all the while gently exhaling. Stand and repeat.

When you've done the standing stretch five times, sit down on the floor or another firm surface. Extend your legs in front of you and place your hands on your thighs. Slowly exhale, bending toward your legs and stretching your arms, attempting to touch your feet with your hands. When you've stretched as far as you can, begin to inhale and slowly return to your original position, keeping your arms extended.

Practice the Wild Duck daily for maximum benefit.

These next exercises benefit both women and men.

Squatting

Squatting as a general practice—for stretching, resting, watching something—is a wonderful tonic for the reproductive system. It opens the pelvis, moves blockages, releases tension, and improves the circulation of chi in the lower body. Just squat, breathe, and relax. I also believe that sitting cross-legged (even if it is on the couch while watching a movie) helps open the pelvic area, allowing for better circulation of chi throughout our bodies. Tight belts and clothes that encircle the waist tightly impede this flow of energy between the upper and lower chakras.

Hip Circles

Like squatting, regularly doing hip circles will move blockages and improve chi circulation in the pelvic area. Hip circles also help you to feel grounded in your pelvis rather than too much "in your head."

Stand with your feet shoulder width apart. Bend your knees as if you were about to sit, keeping your spine straight and your hands on your hips. Rotate your hips in a circle, starting first to the right and then to the left, as if you were dancing. Do thirty-six circles in each direction.

Pelvic Lifts

Pelvic lifts strengthen the lower back and buttocks. They also increase circulation and energy in the pelvic region.

Lie on your back and bend your knees enough to place your feet flat on the floor about hip width apart. Place your arms at your sides. Tightly squeeze the muscles of your buttocks while contracting the abdominal muscles and pressing the small of your back to the floor. While exhaling, push your hips toward the ceiling, drawing your buttocks off the floor. Keep your abdominal and buttocks muscles held tightly. Hold for a few seconds at the high point, then lower yourself slowly to the floor, rolling your spine down vertebra by vertebra from the middle back until your buttocks reach the floor. Rest for thirty seconds, then repeat. Start with five lifts and work up to twenty.

Kidney Rub

The kidney rub can be a fun exercise to perform with a partner. As explained on pages 6–7, Oriental medical tradition holds that the Kidneys govern sexual energy. A kidney massage, therefore, will strongly benefit libido and sexual vitality. The kidneys respond best to stimulation on the back. To perform a kidney massage, rub up and down over the bare lower back thirty-six times every morning and evening. The massage will warm and energize this vital area.

The Butterfly

This is an excellent exercise to open and relax the pelvis, which can make you more flexible and open to a wide variety of love positions.

Sit on the floor with your knees bent and the soles your feet touching each other. Gently bring your knees up and down, like the wings of a butterfly perched on a flower, and try to touch the floor with your knees several times.

Cat Stretch

Cats take stretching to a new dimension, and we could learn a thing or two from them. This exercise helps relieve tension in the back, allowing chi to move more freely. Get down on your hands and knees with your arms and thighs vertical. While exhaling, slowly lower your head and arch your back, making a convex curve. Then inhale, stretching your head up and arching your spine down, making a concave curve. Repeat seven times.

Stretching for Partners

These stretching exercises also help to open the pelvis. Better still, they're a lovely way to play together!

Sit across from each other with your legs flat on the floor and spread wide, feet touching at the soles. Reach across and grasp hands. Swing back and forth so that one partner brings his or her head to the ground in front while the other leans back, and then vice versa. Use your arms to balance yourselves and create a smooth transition.

The second exercise has the partners sitting in the same position and grasping hands. Now swing back and forth in a circular fashion, first clockwise and then counterclockwise. By opening the pelvis, you awaken your sexual energy.

Shake, Shake, Shake!

Whenever you're feeling stressed or tight, turn on some upbeat music and spend three minutes shaking every part of your body. Don't think about what you're doing; just do what feels good, letting your body take over. This wild and free movement releases tensions stored in the body. When you're done, sit cross-legged and quiet on the floor, or lay down and feel the energy flow throughout your body.

Dance, Dance, Dance!

Dancing charges your chakras, loosens you up, and makes you flexible for love. It aligns your vertebrae better than many chiropractic adjustments, improves circulation, and helps you let go of constricted body patterns that keep you "uptight." Dancing with a partner can be its own kind of foreplay. If you are not a dancer, just pretend you are underwater and swim!

Here's a poem I wrote in the dark while driving home from Santa Fe in 1981 with my husband, Tom:

Dancing is like flying
It's really free.
Making love to music gets into me.
Tossing my head
Like a defiant child
Nothing lets me be so wild.
I feel I'm electric
I know I'm divine
Dancing takes me
Way beyond time.
I get lighter than light
And higher than air.
Being one with the music
It takes me all there.

Yoga

I highly recommend yoga, both for its overall health benefits and for its particular benefits for sexual vitality. Yoga harmonizes the nervous and glandular systems. Yoga postures that are especially beneficial for sexual energy

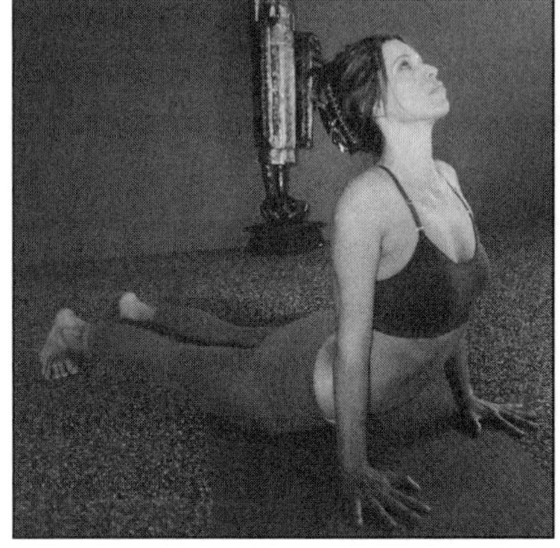

Cobra

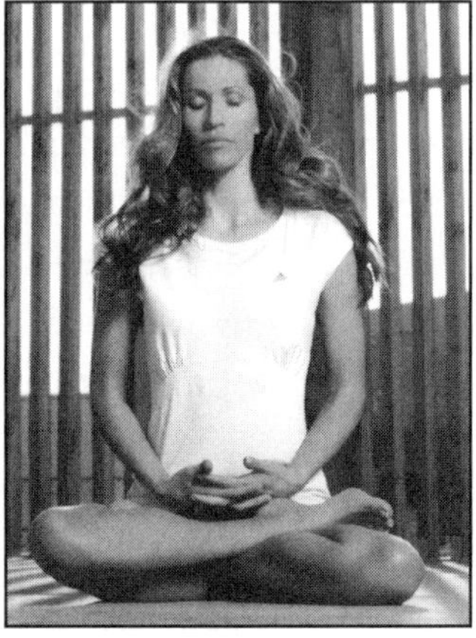

Lotus

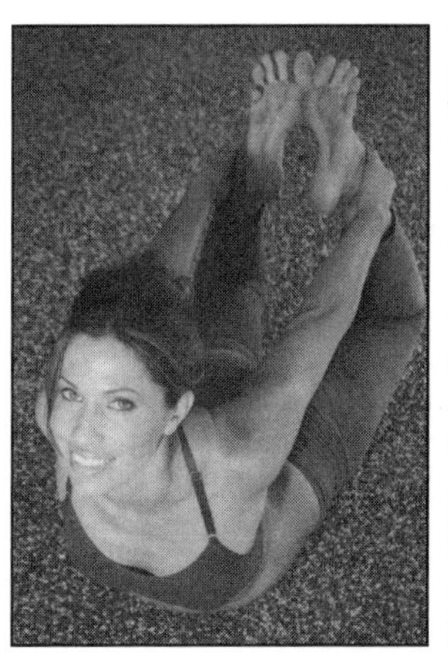

Bow

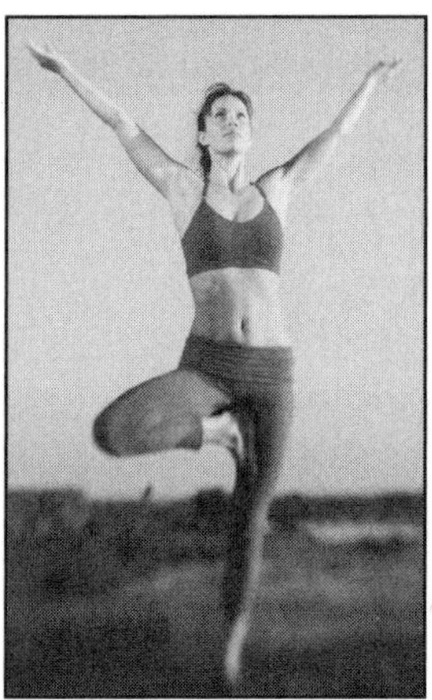

Tree

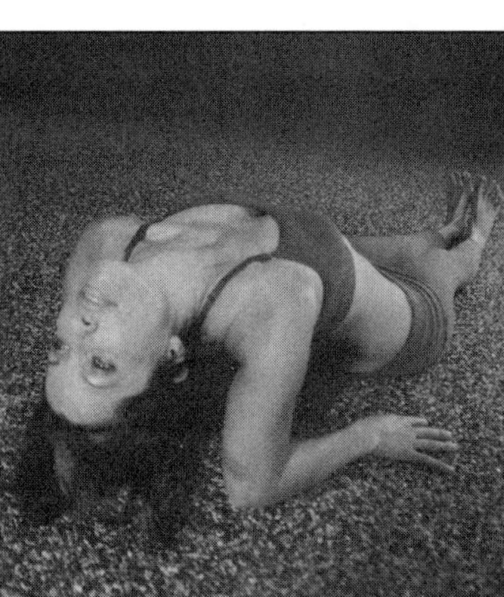

Fish

and vitality include Cobra, Bow, Fish, Lotus, and Tree. Partners can benefit tremendously from taking a yoga class together. There are even newer forms of yoga, called Partner Yoga and Contact Yoga, that call for interactive yoga between partners.

Deep Breathing

Breathing deeply increases our awareness of the present moment, promotes health, invites serenity, and massages the internal organs. During sex, deep breathing allows a man to make love longer without ejaculating and a woman to be more open to orgasm.

A deep breath is capable of containing seven pints of air; most people, however, inhale only a pint of air with each breath. That's unfortunate, because shallow breathing quickens the heart rate and increases stress levels.

Daily practice of deep-breathing exercises makes deep breathing a habit. Inhale slowly and deeply for a count of five, drawing breath all the way down into the belly and allowing both the belly and chest to expand. As you inhale, do the contraction phase of Kegels (described on page 118). Hold for a count of five (unless you have high blood pressure, in which case you should begin to exhale immediately). Inhale an extra sniff of air, then exhale slowly to a count of five, relaxing the shoulders, pulling the belly inward, and releasing the Kegel contraction. Repeat seven times.

Synchronized Breathing

Breathing in harmony while making love can help lovers connect in a deep and powerful way. Partners can synchronize their breathing to harmonize together, or alternate to exchange energy, so that one is breathing in while the other is breathing out.

There are a couple of exercises that can help lovers learn to synchronize their breathing. In the first, the partners sit cross-legged with their backs touching and elbows interlaced. Though you may feel a gentle stretch in the shoulders while sitting like this, avoid pulling on your partner's arms. Breathe deeply together, feeling the breath of your partner fill his or her lungs.

In the second exercise, partners sit cross-legged on the floor facing each other. Press the palms of your hands against your partner's palms. Keep your wrists, elbows, and shoulders relaxed. Slow your breathing and try to synchronize it, always keeping eye contact. Allow the breath of life to dance between you!

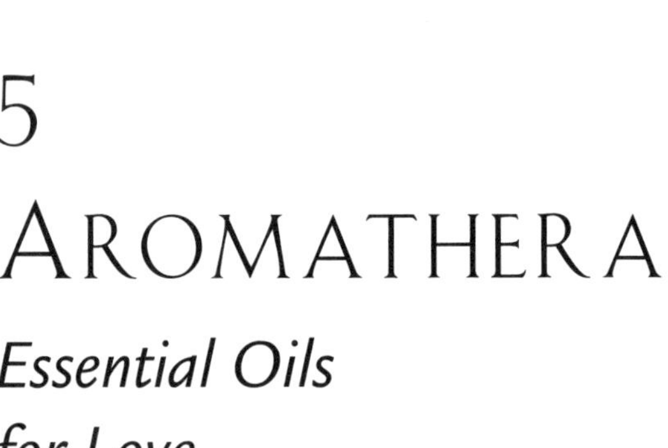

5
Aromatherapy
Essential Oils for Love

AROMATHERAPY RELIES ON THE essential oils of plants for physical and emotional healing. Essential oils are aromatic, volatile, chemically rich substances that plants produce to support all of their life processes, including growth and reproduction. Plant oils attract pollinators, repel predators, and protect plants from disease. Doesn't it make sense that these precious oils could also do the same things for you?

A single plant contains just a tiny amount of essential oil, but that small dose has potent and wide-ranging effects. Scent can lift or depress the spirits, calm or excite the mind, inspire passion or promote good sleep, and much more. Essential oils are sharply aromatic; more importantly, they have a direct chemical effect on the olfactory system and the brain. When the molecules that make up essential oils are inhaled through the nose, they travel up the nasal passages to the brain. These molecules are so small that they bypass the blood-brain barrier (a wall of tissue that prevents substances in the blood from crossing over into brain tissue) and enter the brain itself. Once in the brain, essential oils have a direct impact on the limbic system, the part of the brain associated with emotion, memory, and learning, and so evoke a powerful emotional response. They can also stimulate the production of neurotransmitters.

Essential oils can be directly inhaled or applied to the skin, where the small size of the molecules again contributes to the oil's healing effect. The molecules penetrate the skin and enter the bloodstream, which carries them throughout the body. Many essential oils have antiviral and immunostimulating properties. Some are antibacterial, and unlike many of the synthetic antibacterial agents in use today, bacteria do not seem to develop a resistance to them.

And keep in mind that bringing a bottle of an essential oil can be a lovely social icebreaker. You can say, "*Want a hit of tuberose*?" while offering an open bottle. Suggest at least two deep inhalations, one through each nostril, and you're sure to make friends easily.

While an essential oil is the purest abstraction of these powerful plant oils, there are other ways to obtain them. An absolute is a plant oil that has been extracted with a solvent. It is not a pure essential oil and should never be taken internally. Other methods of extraction include hydrosols and carbon dioxide extractions.

ESSENTIAL OILS TO INSPIRE PASSION

Fragrance is a gateway to the brain. The sense of smell is underused in the realm of romance. Pleasantly fragranced oils, lotions, and other potions can encourage us to engage in healing-touch therapy—like massage or acupressure—or even foreplay. Equally important are the direct healing, soothing, energizing, stimulating, and aphrodisiac effects that aromatic essential oils can have on the human psyche. Whether mixed with oil in preparation for a massage, diffused to scent the air, dabbed on the neck and navel as a delicate perfume, or spritzed onto the sheets and mattress to refresh the bed, essential oils have the power to turn our thoughts to passion.

The essential oils described here are handpicked from a vast array of choices and chosen for their powerful effects on human sexuality. Some are potent aphrodisiacs, others are wonderful tonics for the reproductive system, and still others promote emotional openness. When you want to encourage passion in the bedroom, these are the essential oils to turn to.

When you're working with essential oils, keep in mind that quality is imperative. Be sure to use pure essential oils and not synthetic fragrances. Be suspicious of companies whose essential oils are all the same price; some essential oils are harder to extract than others, or are unusual or rare. These differences should be reflected in the price. Essential oils should be packaged in dark-colored glass bottles. The label on the bottle should give both the common name and the botanical name of the plant whose essential oil is contained in the bottle.

Store essential oils away from light, heat, plastic, and metal and beyond the reach of children. Be careful when using them, as some oils can stain clothing or damage the finish on furniture. Keep essential oils away from broken skin and mucous membranes such as those of the eyes, mouth, and genitals. Some essential oils can induce uterine contractions, so pregnant women should avoid them unless they are under the supervision of a qualified aromatherapist or health care professional.

Most essential oils are very potent and should be diluted in a carrier oil. I like to use almond, grapeseed, and apricot kernel oils because they are light and don't have a strong odor. When I want to create a more warming blend, I use a heavier oil, such as hazelnut or sesame.

The scent of an essential oil application should be subtle, not overpowering. Dizziness, nausea, and rashes can all be signs that you are overdoing it or that you are sensitive to a particular oil. If an essential oil mixture begins to irritate your skin, wash it off and apply pure vegetable oil directly to the irritation.

Cardamom

Elettaria cardamomum

Family Zingiberaceae (Ginger)

Energetics Sweet, pungent, warming

Therapeutic Effects Cardamom fosters joy and clarity, and in ayurvedic medicine it is considered to be an aphrodisiac. It helps improve poor concentration, worry, and overthinking. It is uplifting and encourages our hunger for life as well as a desire for contentment. It is also a stimulant and a breath freshener.

CAUTION

Do not use cardamom undiluted.

Champa

Michelia champaca

Family Magnoliaceae (Magnolia)

Energetics Sweet, bitter, warm

Therapeutic Use Champa has a floral, sensuous scent. It aids in the release of anger and can help bring couples closer together. It alleviates frigidity and is considered to be an aphrodisiac.

Cinnamon

Cinnamomum cassia, c. verum

Family Lauraceae (Laurel)

Energetics Sweet, warm

Therapeutic Use Cinnamon essential oil invigorates the senses, calms the nerves, and improves circulation. It also increases desire and creativity. It is often used to treat erectile dysfunction and frigidity. One study found that the smell of cinnamon buns increased blood flow to the penis. Pumpkin pie spice also had this effect.

CAUTION

Do not use cinnamon undiluted.

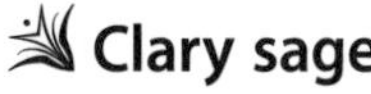

Clary sage

Salvia sclarea

Family Lamiaceae (Mint)

Energetics Sweet, bitter, pungent, warm

Therapeutic Use Clary sage arouses the emotions and helps one feel more grounded in the body. It is antidepressant, aphrodisiac, and a mild euphoric. It is often used in the treatment of amenorrhea, anxiety, emotional confusion, indecision, premenstrual tension, menopause, and postnatal depression.

Clove

Syzygium aromaticum

Family Myrtaceae (Myrtle)

Energetics Sweet, pungent, warm

Therapeutic Use Clove combats exhaustion and nervousness and is considered to be an aphrodisiac. It also has anesthetic properties and can be used to prevent premature ejaculation.

CAUTION

Do not use clove undiluted.

Coriander

Coriandrum sativum

Family Apiaceae (Parsley)

Energetics Pungent, warm

Therapeutic Use Long used in love potions, coriander is mentioned in the tales of *The Arabian Nights* as an aphrodisiac. The first-century Greek physician Dioscorides recommended adding coriander seeds to wine to increase semen output. During medieval times it was thought to encourage women to part with their virtue. Coriander seed is a gentle stimulant that helps relieve depression and stress. Coriander is said to promote harmony in relationships and to improve a bad mood.

Fennel

Foeniculum vulgare

Family Apiaceae (Parsley)

Energetics Sweet, warm

Therapeutic Use Folklore recommends fennel essential oil for promoting courage, self-esteem, and strength. Because it has phytoestrogenic activity, it is considered a tonic for the female reproductive system; it can be used to treat cramps and amenorrhea and to improve the flow of breast milk in nursing mothers. In Mediterranean tradition, eating fennel is used to curb the appetite and promote slenderness.

Geranium

Pelargonium graveolens, P. odorantissimum

Family Geraniaceae (Geranium)

Energetics Sweet, penetrating, cool

Therapeutic Use Geranium essential oil calms anxiety, reduces stress, alleviates fatigue, and stimulates sensuality. It helps one feel at ease, improves relationships, and aids in resolving passive-aggressive issues. Geranium essential oil has phytoestrogenic properties and can be used to treat PMS, excessive menses, menopause, and infertility and as a tonic for the reproductive system. It is a thyroid stimulant, antidepressant, antiseptic, aphrodisiac, cell regenerator, and hormonal balancer for both men and women.

Ginger

Zingiber officinale

Family Zingiberaceae (Ginger)

Energetics Pungent, sweet, warm

Therapeutic Use Ginger's stimulating fragrance has aphrodisiac properties and helps to open the heart. It improves circulation, alleviates depression, and can be used to treat erectile dysfunction.

CAUTION

Do not use ginger undiluted.

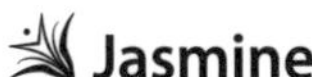

Jasmine

Jasminum officinale

Family Oleaceae (Olive)

Energetics Sweet, warm, stimulating

Therapeutic Use Essence of jasmine is available as an absolute, not an essential oil, but it still has potent healing powers. The fragrance of the absolute is rich and sensual. It relieves stress, helps move emotional blocks, calms fears and anxiety, and is mildly euphoric. Jasmine is sacred to Kama, the Hindu god of love (the Eastern version of Cupid), who uses it to anoint the tips of his arrows. Try using a mister of Jasmine floral water.

Neroli

Citrus bigaradia, C. aurantium

Family Rutaceae (Rue)

Energetics Sweet, cool

Therapeutic Use Neroli essential oil, which is extracted from orange blossoms, has antidepressant properties and eases anxiety, stress, and grief. Neroli helps relieve first-encounter apprehensions when one is spending time with a new partner. It helps the body and mind to feel more connected and is used to calm premenstrual tension and cramps.

Nutmeg

Myristica fragrans

Family Myristicaceae (Nutmeg)

Energetics Stimulating, pungent, warm

Therapeutic Use The scent of nutmeg essential oil invigorates the brain and calms and strengthens the nerves. It has long been considered an aphrodisiac and is helpful for resolving erectile dysfunction and irregular menses. Nutmeg's principle component, myristicin, served as a starting point for Ecstasy, the "love drug."

CAUTION

Do not use nutmeg undiluted.

Patchouli

Pogostemon cablin

Family Lamiaceae (Mint)

Energetics Sweet, warm

Therapeutic Use Patchouli calms anxiety, lifts spirits, stimulates the nervous system, overcomes frigidity, improves clarity, and attracts sexual love. It has antifungal, antidepressant, antiseptic, aphrodisiac, and regenerative properties. It is often used to treat yeast and other vaginal infections and to balance libido levels. It is used for those that are too mentally active to tune in to their senses.

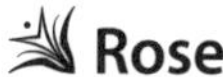

Rose

Rosa spp.

Family Rosaceae (Rose)

Energetics Sweet, cool

Therapeutic Use Rose is both sensual and romantic; it is the supreme heart opener. Rose is considered sacred to Aphrodite, the goddess of love (also known as Eve and Venus), and is a favorite of Mother Mary. Its rich fragrance is deeply floral. Essence of rose is available as both an absolute and an essential oil; the oil is much more expensive. (Before you balk at the price, consider that it takes about 180 pounds of rose blossoms to make just one ounce of essential oil.)

The open rose is a symbol for the opening of the heart and vulva. Rose calms anger and relieves exhaustion.

Rose oil is considered an antidepressant, aphrodisiac, cerebral tonic, kidney tonic, rejuvenative, restorative, and sedative. Rose is helpful for those who feel distanced from their emotional center; it promotes a sense of happiness, relieves anger and jealousy, deflates relationship conflicts, and helps heal grief caused by emotional trauma. To rekindle the spark of love, apply rose oil to the body while making love. In addition to being an aphrodisiac, rose strengthens the uterus, regulates menses, and relieves cramps. It can be used to treat uterine disorders, menorrhagia, menopause, erectile dysfunction, frigidity, and low sperm count.

To have dreams of love, prepare a dilution of rose oil, using the proportions given for massage oil on page 139. Place a drop of rose-scented oil on your forehead before sleep for a beautiful *knight.*

Organic distilled rose oil is the safest for the culinary arts. When buying rose water, be sure that the packaging specifies that the rose water is distilled; otherwise, you may end up with a synthetic product. Add rose water to desserts such as fruit smoothies, nut desserts, hot chocolate, or raw cacao smoothies.

Sandalwood

Santalum album

Family Santalaceae (Sandalwood)

Energetics Sweet, bitter, warm

Therapeutic Use Sandalwood has a chemistry similar to that of the male hormone androsterone. Its scent is earthy and reminiscent of the odors of the reproductive organs. It is regarded as spiritually uplifting, ecstatic, and erotic. It helps build sexual confidence and has been used to treat anxiety that can contribute to erectile dysfunction and frigidity. In tantric practices, sandalwood is used to awaken the kundalini energy. It has antifungal, antidepressant, antiseptic, aphrodisiac, and relaxing properties, and it is often recommended as a treatment for genitourinary infections, such as cystitis. It has a calming effect upon the nervous system.

CAUTION

Sandalwood is at risk of becoming endangered in the wild; use essential oil that was extracted from cultivated—never wildcrafted—supplies. However *S. spicatum* is a species of sandalwood that is being maintained and sustainably harvested by Aboriginal tribes in Australia; products derived from this species are friendlier to the planet.

Tuberose

Polianthes tuberosa

Family Amaryllidaceae (Amaryllis)

Energetics Sweet, cool

Therapeutic Use Tuberose is often used in perfumes for its sweet, floral scent. It is available only as an absolute. Tuberose is both an antidepressant and an aphrodisiac; it also strengthens and evokes the emotions.

Vanilla

Vanilla planifolia, V. tahitensis

Family Orchidaceae (Orchid)

Energetics Sweet, warm

Therapeutic Use Vanilla calms the mind, appeases anger, and soothes irritability. The smell of vanilla may stimulate the release of the neurotransmitter serotonin, causing feelings of arousal and satisfaction. It is an aphrodisiac and a mild menstrual stimulant. Vanilla is available as an absolute or oleoresin.

Vetivert

Vetiveria zizanioides

Family Poaceae (Grass)

Energetics Sweet, bitter, warm

Therapeutic Use The essential oil of vetivert calms, comforts, grounds, uplifts, and sedates. Vetivert—also known as vetiver—has antiseptic, aphrodisiac, and rejuvenative properties. It stimulates circulation and can also help women through postpartum depression and menopause. It helps relax an overactive mind.

Ylang ylang

Cananga odorata

Family Annonaceae (Custard Apple)

Energetics Sweet, bitter, cool

Therapeutic Use In the Malayan language *ylang ylang* means, "flower of flowers." The essential oil, extracted from the flower of the ylang ylang tree, is a euphoric used to calm anger, anxiety, and fear. It can also be used to relax a nervous partner prior to sex. Ylang ylang is antidepressant, antiseptic, and aphrodisiac. It stimulates the senses, improves self-esteem, fosters a sense of peacefulness, and helps overcome frigidity. It is often recommended for treating PMS, hormonal imbalance, and erectile dysfunction and is known to stimulate orgasmic ability. In Indonesia ylang ylang flowers are scattered on the beds of newlyweds to promote desire and bless the union with children.

AROMATHERAPY LOVE POTIONS

There are hundreds of ways to incorporate aromatherapy into your life, especially your love life. It doesn't have to be complicated. For an aphrodisiac effect, aromatherapy can be as simple as smelling the flowers. You might also dab a drop of essential oil on the nape of your neck as perfume, or anoint your bed with a few drops of a passion-inspiring fragrance. If you're interested in pursuing the therapeutic use of essential oil to resolve a physical or emotional dysfunction, consult with a qualified aromatherapist.

As I sit at my desk writing, I often take deep whiffs from the selection of essential oil bottles that grace a shelf nearby, rather than indulging in copious amounts of coffee, which many writers are known to overuse. Following are a few of my favorite ways to inspire "scentual" delight with essential oils. For more information on aromatherapy uses, safety, and preparations, read *Aromatherapy: A Complete Guide to the Healing Art* by Kathi Keville and Mindy Green (Berkeley, Calif.: Crossing Press, 2009).

Bath

Stir 5 to 8 drops of an essential oil into your bathwater after filling the tub. Mix it in before you get in the tub so that it is well diluted.

Bath Salts

Combine ⅛ teaspoon (about 12 drops) of essential oil with ½ cup of sea salt, Epsom salt, or baking soda (or a combination thereof). Add this mixture to the bathwater before you get in the tub. You can mix up big batches of bath salts ahead of time, using just ½ cup at a time in the tub. A scalloped seashell is delightful as a bath salt scoop.

Bedding

When changing the sheets, anoint the mattress with a few drops of a clear-colored essential oil such as cardamom, coriander, or ylang ylang.

Body Powder

Combine ½ to 1 teaspoon (50–100 drops) of essential oil with 1 ounce of orrisroot powder. Add ½ pound of dried, powdered herbs. (I like to use lavender.)

Chakra Anointment

According to Mindy Green, author of *Natural Perfumes* (Interweave Press, 1999) and *Calendula* (Keats Publishing, 1998) and coauthor of *Aromatherapy: A Complete Guide to the Healing Art,* a classic tantric ritual involves anointing a woman's chakras with sacred fragrances. Before intercourse, a woman is worshipped as Shakti, the embodiment of the feminine creative force. She is anointed with five fragrances on different areas of her body, arousing her five senses and lifting her spirits so that she can manifest as a goddess.

The fragrances and sites of anointment are:

- Jasmine—hands
- Patchouli—neck and cheeks
- Amber or ambrette seed—breasts and genitals
- Spikenard—hair
- Sandalwood—thighs

Each oil should be diluted before application to the body: Add 5 drops of essential oil to a half ounce of body lotion or oil.

Diffusers

There are various kinds of aromatherapy diffusers, all of which can fill your home with the beautiful fragrance of essential oils. Some are powered by candles, others by electricity. They range in price depending on their materials and design.

Facial Spray

Combine 1 teaspoon of vodka, ¼ teaspoon (25 drops) of essential oil, and 4 ounces of distilled water or aloe vera juice in a bottle with a gentle sprayer attached. (If you use aloe vera juice, keep this spray refrigerated.) Spray onto your face after washing and before bed. (Remove your glasses first, and keep eyes and mouth closed.) The spray may also be applied throughout the day for a moisturizing and pleasantly cooling effect. See if your beloved enjoys a cool blast too. This spray is lovely to have by the bed to spritz overheated bodies. Try blasting the neck, chest, or back, especially on a hot day. This spray can also be used to scent the air, the sheets, and your clothes closet.

Footbath

Add 10 drops of essential oil to 2 gallons of very warm water. Drop in those tired feet and enjoy! Offer your beloved a foot massage while his or her feet are soaking in the fragrant waters.

Foot Powder

Add 8 drops of essential oil to ½ cup of arrowroot powder, baking soda, white clay powder, or cornstarch (or a combination thereof).

Hair Brush

After washing the hairbrushes in your home, apply one or two drops of essential oil to the brush of any family member who might enjoy having their hair provide a gentle cloud of *scentual* fragrance.

Hair Rinse

Add 2 drops of essential oil and 2 tablespoons of apple cider vinegar to a cup of herbal tea of your choice. Apply after shampooing for sensuously fragrant hair.

Inhalations

Essential oils can be used like smelling salts. Hold a bottle of essential oil an inch or two from your nose and take ten deep, slow breaths, inhaling through your nostrils and exhaling through your mouth.

Steam inhalations can be especially helpful for breaking up congestion and clearing sinus passages; they're also a wonderful facial treatment. To prepare a steam inhalation, bring 2 cups of water to boil in a large pot and remove it from the heat. Stir in 4 drops of essential oil. Tent a towel over both your head and the aromatic pot. Breathe in the steam, with eyes closed, for at least ten minutes, coming up for air when it becomes too hot.

Massage Oil

Mix 25 drops of essential oil with 2 ounces of a carrier oil like olive, almond, or sesame oil. To allow the skin to benefit from the therapeutic use of the oils, don't bathe for at least an hour after the massage.

Perfume

Apply a single drop of your favorite essential oil to your temples, the nape of your neck, your throat, behind your ears, your pubis, and the insides of your wrists. To perfume your hair, dab 1 or 2 drops of essential oil onto your hairbrush as described above.

Sauna

Add 10 to 15 drops of essential oil to 16 ounces of water. Throw a bit at a time onto the hot rocks in the sauna.

CAUTION

Never use the oils undiluted in the sauna; the heat in combination with the oils can cause an explosion. That would only detract from your evening of passion.

Scented Shampoo and Conditioner

Add 20 drops of essential oil to 4 ounces of good-quality unscented shampoo or conditioner.

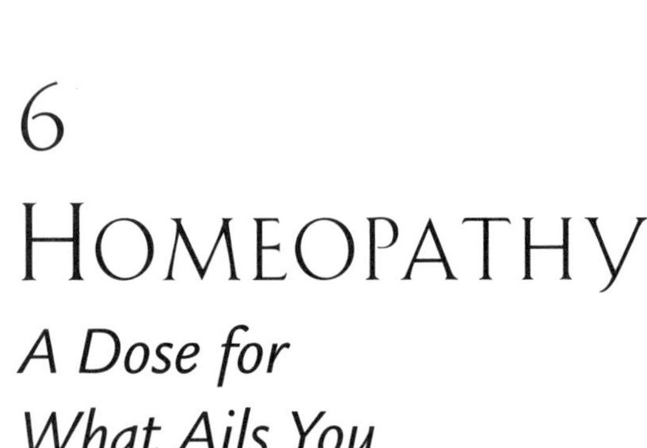

6 HOMEOPATHY

A Dose for What Ails You

HOMEOPATHY IS BASED ON the law of similars, or the philosophy that "like cures like." It was developed from the work of Dr. Samuel Hahnemann (1755–1843), who sought an alternative to the barbaric medical practices of his time and wanted to offer a safer, more effective form of treatment.

Do not confuse homeopathic remedies with herbal remedies. A homeopathic remedy is a tremendously diluted solution of a substance that would, in the body of a healthy person, produce symptoms similar to those of a particular illness. The solution contains an infinitesimal amount of the substance; you might say it contains a pattern or replica of the substance. Exposure to the pattern, however, triggers a powerful healing response from the body. In other words, by stimulating the body's own healing response, a homeopathic remedy encourages the body to heal itself.

Homeopathic remedies can effect amazingly fast-acting and profound cures. The degree of success, however, depends on selecting the right remedy for a person's constitution. Some basic guidelines for choosing and using homeopathic remedies follow, but you may also benefit from consultation with a professional homeopath to gain insight into the best remedies for your constitution. Note that homeopathy often calls for very small doses of substances that in large doses could be toxic.

USING HOMEOPATHIC REMEDIES

Homeopathic remedies come in the form of small pellets, alcohol solutions, and water solutions. The usual dosage is 4 pellets, or as many liquid drops as the package label recommends, taken under the tongue four times daily. Rather than swallowing the pellets whole, allow them to dissolve slowly under your tongue to be better absorbed into your bloodstream.

For best results, do not eat or drink for ten minutes before and after taking a homeopathic remedy.

HOMEOPATHY FOR SEXUAL VITALITY

Homeopathy offers useful methods for balancing body, mind, and spirit and can therefore be a powerful ally in the healing of sexual dysfunctions that have both physical and mental roots. Homeopathy helps the healing energy of the body realign itself and, in so doing, improves health issues of all kinds, including those that affect sexual vitality.

Note that homeopathic remedies have different effects on different people, depending on the temperament of the individual. The effects described here are of a general nature and may not encapsulate your experience with a particular remedy.

AGNUS CASTUS

Source: Chaste tree (*Vitex agnus-castus*)

Therapeutic use: AGNUS CASTUS alleviates depression that is accompanied by a sense of foreboding. It improves orgasmic ability and is recommended for use when sexual organs have "cooled their fire"—for example, in cases of erectile dysfunction, especially in older men, and a distaste for intercourse in women. AGNUS CASTUS is also recommended for women who have light menses or who are sterile.

BERBERIS

Source: Root of barberry (*Berberis vulgaris*)

Therapeutic use: BERBERIS is recommended for those who have a suppressed sex drive. It is particularly helpful for those who have pale and sunken cheeks, dry mucous membranes, a feeling of constriction in the genitals, and rapidly changing symptoms.

CALADIUM SEGUINUM

Source: American arum (*Caladium seguinum*)

Therapeutic use: CALADIUM SEGUINUM is recommended in cases where leakage of sexual fluids occurs without any excitement. It also helps those who suffer from cold sweating around the genitals.

CALCAREA CARBONICA

Source: Carbonate of lime

Therapeutic use: CALCAREA CARBONICA is recommended for those who experience an excessive sex drive, premature ejaculation, or sharp menstrual cramps.

CANTHARIS

Source: Spanish fly (*Lytta vesicatoria, Cantharis vesicatoria*)

Therapeutic use: CANTHARIS is recommended in cases of weak ejaculation, loss of normal erection, temporary erectile dysfunction, and frigidity. It is also helpful for those who have excessive sex drive, especially in cases where excess has led to irritation of the genitals. It is sometimes indicated for those with violent tendencies.

CARBO VEGETABILIS

Source: Vegetable charcoal

Therapeutic use: CARBO VEGETABILIS suppresses libido and can be used to prevent premature ejaculation. It is often recommended for those who feel exhausted and have low vitality and for those who have not "felt like themselves" since an accident or illness.

CINCHONA OFFICINALIS

Source: Peruvian bark

Therapeutic use: CINCHONA OFFICINALIS is a remedy for intense, hypersensitive individuals who have a hard time sharing their feelings. It helps individuals with lascivious fantasies balance their sexual desire.

CONIUM

Source: Poison hemlock (*Conium maculatum*)

Therapeutic use: CONIUM can be used to treat erectile dysfunction as well as painful premature ejaculation. It is particularly helpful for those who feel emotionally paralyzed due to excess or lack of sex.

GELSEMIUM

Source: Root of yellow jasmine (*Gelsemium sempervirens*)

Therapeutic use: GELSEMIUM can help curb the frequency of wet dreams and the leakage of semen when passing a stool. It is indicated for those who have facial pallor with dark circles around the eyes and a feeble mind. It can also help relieve fears, phobias, and overexcitement that impair a person's ability to function and enjoy life.

GRAPHITES

Source: Black lead

Therapeutic use: GRAPHITES is indicated for those who experience extreme sexual excitement. It can help women who have scanty menses, sore nipples, and a distaste for intercourse, as well as men who have high levels of sexual desire but are debilitated, having premature or no ejaculation. GRAPHITES can prevent or limit flatulence for those who tend to become gassy when they are sexually excited.

IGNATIA

Source: Saint Ignatius bean (*Ignatia amara*)

Therapeutic use: IGNATIA opens emotional doors and aids recovery from grief. It is recommended for those who are irritable and cry easily, and it can aid the recovery or normalization of libido after grief or trauma. Use if grief causes menses to cease.

LYCOPODIUM

Source: Club moss (*Lycopodium clavatum*)

Therapeutic use: LYCOPODIUM is recommended for the person who fears solitude, responsibility, and intimacy, and who is prone to oversensitivity and angry outbursts. It can be used to treat cases of enlarged prostate, urination difficulties, cold penis, incomplete ejaculation, tenderness in the ovaries, painful intercourse, and liver and digestive problems. It might be recommended for a person who tends to fall asleep during intercourse. It is especially helpful for resolving erectile dysfunction when the dysfunction is psychological in nature.

NATRUM MURIATICUM

Source: Salt, chloride of sodium

Therapeutic use: NATRUM MURIATICUM is recommended for those who are irritable, feel like crying, and lack desire and energy for sex. It can be used to prevent or limit loss of pubic hair, vaginal dryness, and genital odor (when it is atypically strong or unpleasant).

PHOSPHORUS

Source: Phosphorus

Therapeutic use: PHOSPHORUS is best suited for those with a fiery personality, who are full of light and life. It calms nervous tension and anxiety and can help those who are easily confused, lack perspective, and burn out easily. It also helps regulate excessive sexual desire and can prevent or limit premature ejaculation.

SABAL SERRULATA

Source: Saw palmetto (*Serenoa repens*)

Therapeutic use: SABAL SERRULATA improves tissue strength in the genitals, builds sexual vitality, and decreases fears of sexual intimacy.

SELENIUM

Source: Selenium

Therapeutic use: SELENIUM is helpful for men who have great sexual desire but suffer from exhaustion, erectile dysfunction, insomnia, memory loss, or melancholy. It is the most effective remedy for premature ejaculation accompanied by weakness in the back.

SEPIA

Source: Inky juice of the cuttlefish (*Sepia officinalis*)

Therapeutic use: SEPIA is recommended particularly for dark-haired, dark-eyed women who are unhappy and overburdened, and for men who have low sex drive, mental fatigue, and frequent erections. It can help those of both sexes who feel exhausted after intercourse. It also can ease symptoms of burning in the urethra. It is indicated for those with hormonal imbalances, such as premenstrual syndrome, cramps, heavy menses, and hot flashes as well as prolapsed uterus and pain during intercourse.

STAPHYSAGRIA

Source: Stavesacre, also known as palmated larkspur (*Delphinium staphysagria*)

Therapeutic use: STAPHYSAGRIA is recommended for those who are oversensitive, easily excited, and prone to sudden outbursts of passion and violence. It helps individuals come to terms with repressed feelings of shame and anger and can be of great help in cases where incest issues impair healthy sexual enjoyment. It also can help relieve cross-dressers from feelings of shame. It is indicated for women who experience physical pain with a new sex partner.

YOHIMBE

Source: Bark of yohimbe (*Pausinystalia yohimbe*)

Therapeutic use: YOHIMBE helps increase sensation in the sexual organs. It can help improve and prolong erections that are otherwise impaired by atherosclerosis and diabetes.

ZINCUM METALLICUM

Source: Zinc

Therapeutic use: ZINCUM METALLICUM is recommended for those who fidget and touch their genitals excessively, have excessive sex drive, and experience chronic wet dreams. It also can prevent or limit hair loss and is used to treat depression.

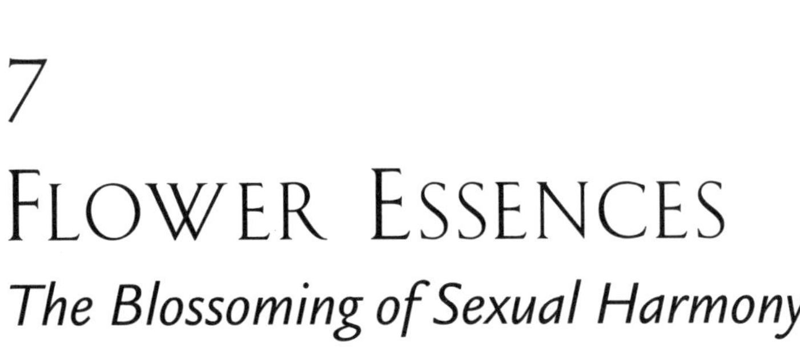

7
FLOWER ESSENCES
The Blossoming of Sexual Harmony

FLOWER ESSENCES ARE POTENTIATED plant preparations that carry the vibrational energy patterns of specific flowers. As an energy medicine, they strengthen the relationship between body, mind, and spirit. They do not have a strong aroma or flavor but, rather, just a hint of the flower that was used in preparing them.

While healing with flowers is an ancient tradition, the system of producing and prescribing flower essences that's in use today was first developed by Dr. Edward Bach, a British physician and bacteriologist. As Bach discovered, flower essences are strong allies in healing emotional patterns that block true joy and intimacy. They can help release some of the emotional barriers that keep us from sexual bliss.

OBTAINING AND USING FLOWER ESSENCES

Do not confuse flower essences with herbal or homeopathic remedies. Flower essences are made by soaking flowers in spring water for several hours in the sun. The water is then collected and bottled.

Flower essences are available at most health food stores and herb shops. You can find the original thirty-eight Bach Flower Remedies as well as newer remedies made by various manufacturers. You can also make your own. Just fill a clear glass bowl with about 12 ounces of spring water. Collect organically grown flower blossoms at their ripest in the early hours of the morning. Use a leaf as a "napkin" to pinch them off so that you don't touch them directly. Gently drop the flowers into the water and let them soak for three to four hours in direct sunlight. Then remove the flowers, again using a leaf so that you don't touch them. Add an equal amount of brandy to the water. Now you have made a "mother tincture."

To make a stock bottle, from which you'll obtain doses of the flower essence, place 2 to 4 drops of mother tincture in a clean, 1-ounce glass dropper bottle using a nonmetallic (preferably glass) funnel. Then fill the bottle almost to the top with spring water. Add 1 teaspoon of brandy as a preservative. Store away from extreme heat, extreme cold, and electromagnetic devices.

Before measuring out a dosage of flower essence, shake the bottle. The usual dosage is 3 drops under the tongue or in a small glass of water three or four times daily. You can also add flower essences to bathwater, massage oils, and body lotions. Try applying them to the sensitive skin on the insides of your wrists and to the "third eye" at the center of your forehead.

CHOOSING THE RIGHT FLOWER ESSENCE

Flower essences work well individually and in combinations of up to six different essences. You'll find that the healing effects range from subtle to dramatic. Most people find that flower essences, used over time, bring clarity, a sense of well-being, and an improved self-image.

Aspen

One of Dr. Bach's original thirty-eight remedies, Aspen eases anxiety, apprehension, and phobias pertaining to sex.

Banana

This tropical essence helps you find balance between the left and right sides of the brain. It can help resolve sexual insecurity in men and decrease machismo.

Basil

Basil lends strength to those who tend to seek sexual relationships outside of their main partnership and aids couples that want to get to the root of a conflict. It encourages a sense of completeness and can help resolve conflicts about sexual abuse.

Black-eyed Susan

This flower essence helps "shine the light" on buried sexual issues, such as rape or incest, and encourages the transformation of pain.

Clematis

One of the Bach Flower Remedies, Clematis helps those who feel unconnected to the physical body regain a sense of connection.

Crab Apple

Crab Apple helps overcome feelings of "dirtiness" or shame about sexuality. It is another of the original Bach Flower Remedies.

Easter Lily

Easter Lily helps integrate spirituality and sexuality. It can bring perspective to those who repeatedly choose unsuitable partners and help those who have experienced sexual abuse overcome feelings of uncleanliness about sex.

Elm

This essence eases anxiety about sexual performance and helps resolve feelings of inadequacy. It is one of the original Bach Flower Essences.

Fuchsia

Use Fuchsia when you want to let go of sexual and emotional repressions.

Hibiscus

Hibiscus fosters responsiveness and warmth. It is especially helpful for women who have been sexually traumatized.

Holly

Holly is an original Bach Flower Essence. It opens the emotional heart and helps overcome chronic suspicion. It eases feelings of jealousy, insecurity, and neediness.

Mariposa Lily

Mariposa Lily alleviates lingering trauma resulting from sexual abuse during childhood. It can help overcome feelings of not being loved and not having been adequately mothered. It can move you closer to the feminine aspect of creation.

Mimulus

Mimulus, a Bach remedy, helps overcome shyness. It eases general fear and anxiety.

Rescue Remedy

Rescue Remedy is a combination of five flower essences developed by Dr. Edward Bach. It is also sold under the name Five-Flower Essence. It helps relieve shock after physical and emotional trauma, including arguments and heartbreak. Take 2 drops under the tongue as often as needed. This is one of those "Don't leave home without it" remedies that often comes in handy for any of life's challenges.

Nasturtium

This essence is indicated for those who are "too into their heads" to have an interest in sex; it helps them come out of their shells. It also can be used to increase vitality.

Scarlet Monkeyflower

When you're going through therapy, Scarlet Monkeyflower can help give you the courage to express your emotions. It also helps restore sexual harmony after anger.

Sticky Monkeyflower

Sticky Monkeyflower helps balance feelings about sexual issues. It can help dispel fears of intimacy and release emotional pain resulting from past relationships.

Walnut

Walnut helps to protect you from outside influences, shoring up those who are oversensitive. It is one of the thirty-eight Bach Flower Remedies.

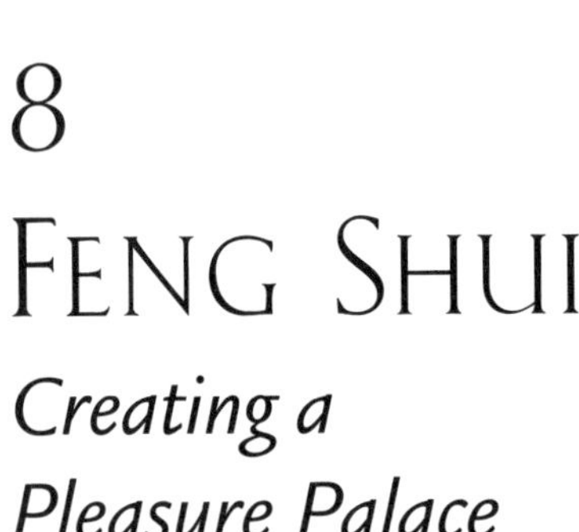

8

Feng Shui

Creating a Pleasure Palace

FENG SHUI, TRANSLATED FROM the Chinese as "wind and water," is the Oriental art of placement. Feng shui has been used for more than five thousand years to harmonize the chi that flows around and through our environment, just as chi flows through the body (see page 6). Because your living environment does affect your psyche, it is important to create and maintain your living space consciously. For example, it is much easier to feel calm when you are in an uncluttered environment. Learning about feng shui is one of the most immediate steps you can take to attract and enhance love in your life. Feng shui is more than a fad. It is a five-thousand-year-old practice that inspires focus and intention to make all of our dreams come true.

THE BAGUA

The *bagua* is a grid that divides a space into nine sectors, each associated with a particular aspect of life: career, relationship, family, prosperity, health, helpful people/travel, children and creativity, new knowledge, and reputation (see illustration). The career sector is at the entrance to the space, and determines where the other sectors fall. The bagua can be applied to an entire house or to a single room. Proper arrangement of living quarters in a particular sector strengthens the energy that corresponds to that sector; when the energy in all nine sectors is strong and balanced, the people who live in the home have strong and balanced chi.

Feng shui also prescribes the auspicious arrangement of elements within a particular room. With proper feng shui, the bedroom becomes the bedrock of passion and marital harmony; the kitchen, a realm of healing nourishment; the living room, an oasis of relaxation; and the bathroom, a temple in which to purify the body.

In our continuing quest for great sex, love, and health, we will focus here on the bedroom and the relationship sector. No matter how small or simple your space, you can create positive feng shui to encourage greater joy

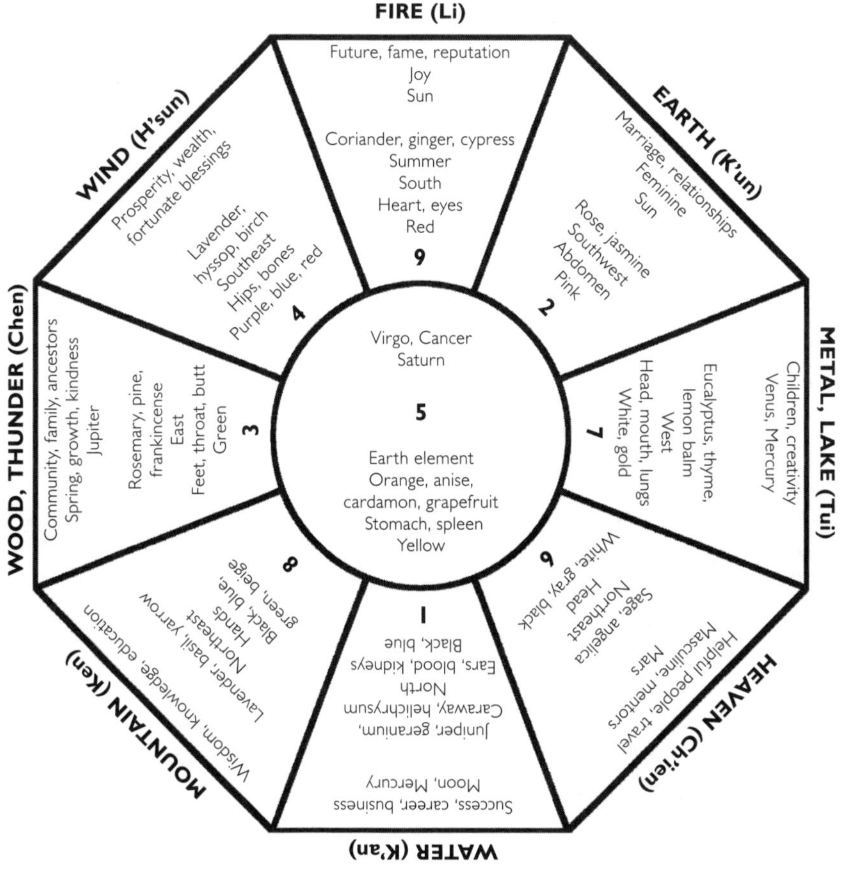

Bagua

in life. The guidelines and tips offered here will carry you a long way toward positive feng shui, but if your interest is not sated, consider having a professional feng shui master come to your home for a consultation.

Activating the Relationship Sector

To attract a new love relationship into your life or improve an existing one, consider energizing the relationship sector, which is the farthest right corner from the entrance to a given room. You can do this in the bedroom and the living room. Paint that sector bright red or hang a red tapestry on the wall, and install red lanterns or red lights. Once a week or during the new moon, light red or pink candles in the relationship sector as a love charm. Outdoors, you can also focus the relationship energy in your yard by placing a bird feeder or a statue of Venus or a loving couple in that sector.

Keeping plants in the relationship sector can attract all kinds of potent sexual energies. Flowers to consider include:

- Hibiscus: to encourage sexual fulfillment
- Gardenias: to attract love and happiness
- Peace lily: for harmony
- Roses: to open the emotional heart
- Orchids: to inspire sexual energy

Flowers should be fresh or made of silk (which should then be dusted regularly); dried flowers are not recommended. When fresh flowers begin to wilt, dispose of them immediately, because decomposing flowers represent dying energy.

Do not keep prickly cacti in the home, as they create "cutting chi," or negative energy. (Kept outdoors, cacti represent protection.) I once noticed that a friend of mine—still single—kept many cactus plants around her bed. I remarked, "Getting naked here looks dangerous. Sharp pointy things do not encourage letting down your pants." Avoid bonsai, as well, because they represent stunted growth. Turning the bedroom into a greenhouse with too many plants creates excess chi and might make it difficult to sleep.

Invite magic and passion into your love life by creating a love altar in the relationship sector. For good love medicine, a shelf or table can include a vase with two fresh or silk flowers and two red or pink candles. Write a love poem, or copy down one of your favorites, and prop it up against a wall or screen behind the altar. Over the altar, scatter pieces of rose quartz (signifying love and equanimity), seashells (representing depth and the feminine aspect), pearls (signifying lasting love), and/or garnets (signifying passion and constancy). You might even consider including two fresh red peppers to signify the spice of life. If you are still in search of a beloved, place an item that symbolizes a loving couple on the altar. If you have already found your beloved, set a photo of the two of you, taken in a time of happiness, in a prominent location on the altar. When you have a gift for your lover, activate it by placing the gift on the love altar for a couple of days before presenting it to your mate.

After you have found your beloved, it's time to change the feng shui energy in the relationship sector from attraction to simple vibrancy. Repaint the area its original color or take down the tapestry. Take down the red lights and install strong, warm indoor lighting. Keep the area clean, uncluttered, and fresh to allow these qualities to imbue the relationship. Do not keep trash or dirty laundry in the relationship sector.

BEDROOM FENG SHUI

Improving the feng shui of the bedroom is a powerful mechanism for improving or attracting a romantic relationship. With proper arrangement and décor, the bedroom becomes a sanctuary of comfort, serenity, and sensuality. We spend one-third of our lives in the bedroom, so make it a wonderful, inspiring place of pleasure. May you wake and sleep in beauty!

The Entryway

Entering the bedroom must be easy; blockages or obstacles at the bedroom door can cause blockages or obstacles in your love life. To minimize disharmony, there should be just one entry to the bedroom, and the door should open inward rather than outward.

Place a plant, wind chimes, or a mobile at the entrance to encourage movement, rather than stagnation, in your love life. A bell will encourage the flow of positive chi. Be sure to ring it once in a while as beautiful sound has a healing energy.

The Bed

A bed that is too large can detract from intimacy. A full size or queen bed might promote more harmony. Your bed should be rectangular and comprised of a standard mattress and box spring or a futon mattress and base. Circular beds lead to disorientation; waterbeds encourage "wishy-washy" support in a relationship. Beds that are made by pushing two smaller mattresses together can cause a subconscious split in the relationship; in this case, place a red sheet that spreads across the breadth of the bed between the mattresses and the box spring(s) to unify the bed and the relationship.

When you're starting a new relationship, a secondhand bed or a bed that has been used for a previous partner can carry negative energy. It is best to purchase a new bed. If you can't do that, sprinkle the bare mattress with 1 cup of baking soda mixed with 30 drops of lavender essential oil and let it sit for a day, with the bedroom windows open. Then vacuum up the baking soda. You can also smudge the bed by burning aromatic herbs such as sage, artemisia, or cedar and waving their smoke over it; use a shell or ashtray to catch the ash. At the very least, get new sheets.

Place the bed so that you can see the room's entrance. Try to avoid having the bed in a corner, as this can make the person who sleeps in the corner feel boxed in or trapped in the relationship. Best not to store items under the bed; they will block the flow of chi. If one side of the bed has a nightstand with a lamp, the other side should also have one, to convey equality.

If the bed shares a wall with a toilet, good fortune will drain from the room. The cure is to hang a tapestry on the shared wall to buffer the effect. The direction in which the foot of the bed points is very important. Traditionally, if the feet are pointing toward the door, the bed is in the "death position," which allows the spirit to leave the body and the home. If the foot of the bed is pointing toward an outside door or the bathroom door, you are more likely to become ill or to have an accident. If one of these inauspicious bed positions is unavoidable, hang a crystal between the door and the bed, and be sure the bed has a solid headboard.

Sleeping under a slanted ceiling or an exposed ceiling beam can cause a split in the relationship or health problems. For example, while lying in bed with your lover and looking up at a ceiling beam that cuts between the two of you, you might both be psychologically programmed to feel that the relationship just won't work out because something will come between you.

Or a beam over your chest may contribute to heart or lung problems. If you cannot avoid placing the bed in such a position, hang a wind chime, a garland of silk flowers, or a crystal over the bed.

Make sure that the edges of bookshelves, bureaus, and other bedroom furniture are rounded, rather than sharp. Sharp edges can create cutting chi and disturb the comfort and security of those who sleep in the bed. Close closet doors and cover open shelves to avoid such disturbances. If a sharp edge cannot be avoided, hang a five-rod wind chime or a crystal between the bed and the sharp object—or soften the sharp edge by draping a pretty cloth over it, or putting a vase of silk flowers above it.

Blankets and Bedsheets

Blankets and bedsheets should be made of natural fibers, not synthetics, so the body can breathe at night. For ultimate comfort, look for cotton sheets with at least a 250-thread count. Organic fabrics are available. Bedspreads should be dark in color and plain in design. Pink in small amounts is good for attracting love. Do not use bedspreads with abstract or geometric patterns, as their pointed symbols give off cutting chi. Spritz the mattress and pillows with an essential oil solution. (See chapter 5 for suggestions.)

BEDROOM DÉCOR

Décor in the bedroom should focus on pairs; solitary items and images promote independence, rather than harmonious relationships. If you keep one teddy bear on the bed, keep two instead. If you have artwork that depicts living beings on the bedroom walls, the beings should be in pairs, including pairs of people. Pairs of birds—especially ducks, geese, peacocks, phoenixes, and swans—carved from precious stones, such as adventurine, jasper, rose quartz, and tourmaline, are especially beneficial feng shui. Two geese flying high is a symbol of togetherness for those already in a relationship; a pair of mandarin ducks attracts new love for those desiring a relationship. If you are looking for a heterosexual relationship, make sure your figurines are of the opposite sex—don't use two male peacocks, for example, unless that's what you're looking for. For good fortune in marriage, keep an image representing the Moon in your bedroom.

If you decorate your home solely as if it were a goddess sanctuary, you shouldn't wonder why it only appeals to women. To attract a relationship with a man, at least one-third of the imagery in your bedroom should represent the masculine. Strong masculine images that I keep in my home include Jesus, Pan, Buddha, Shiva, Merlin, and the Beatles. Likewise, to attract a woman, a small amount of feminine imagery should be featured rather than a plethora of sports posters. For relationship harmony, honor the divine feminine and masculine. *Angels work in pairs.*

If the bedroom is small, hang wind chimes or a multifaceted or heart-shaped crystal in its center to increase the flow of chi. The symbol of water promotes the healthy flow of chi in many areas of the home, but it is not recommended in the bedroom where it might encourage infidelity. Remove fountains, photographs or paintings of water, and all other water symbols, including sheets with water motifs, from the bedroom.

When you open your eyes in the morning, your first sight should be of beauty. Place a beautiful object in the room in the line of vision that you most often wake up to, so that your days begin with truth, beauty, and goodness.

Do not keep photos of relatives overlooking the bed. Great Auntie Em does not need to watch you having oral sex! Also remove mementos of previous relationships, which can create negative energy in the new relationship.

Windows

Weather permitting, open windows during the day to allow the angels of light and air to dance inside and bring fresh chi into the bedroom. Hang crystals in the windows to bring rainbows of delight into the boudoir.

Closets and Storage

Clutter anywhere in the home encourages one to feel confused, uneasy, stressed, and overwhelmed. As you might imagine, these feelings are particularly undesirable in the bedroom. Keep your bedroom space uncluttered. Organize and clean closets. (To attract a new relationship, leave some space in closets and drawers as a symbol that there is room for love in your life.) Keep work-related items, such as computers and phones, out of the boudoir, or at least hide them from view—perhaps with a screen or curtain.

Color Therapy

Color in the bedroom can have a powerful effect on the psyche and the flow of chi. The most arousing colors are reds, ambers, oranges, and purples.

Generally, men find red to be most erotic; women seem to prefer violet. Red, pink, and peach are the best colors for the early years of a relationship. Red symbolizes passion. Pink is a combination of the passion of red muted with the purity of white. Peach blends the passion of red with the wisdom of yellow. However, excess red (such as a room painted red) may be overstimulating and could cause arguments. Blue, yellow, and white are more friendly than sexual.

Different colors can be added to the bedroom in moderation in the form of candles, fresh flowers, pillows, luxurious fabrics, and wall or ceiling hangings.

Lighting

Soft lighting is necessary for romantic occasions. Natural candles work well. Another option is soft pink lightbulbs, which flatter the body and are easy on the eyes. Keep one of these bulbs available for a bedside light. Also consider stringing holiday lights in your bedroom for a joyous illuminating effect.

Mirrors

Mirrors create the impression that there are more than two people in the bedroom, interfering with the harmonious energy between the couple. I know that many of us enjoyed mirrored ceilings in the 1970s, but most of those relationships are over, *n'est-ce pas?* Therefore, there should be no more than one mirror—if any—in the bedroom. If there is a mirror, it should not be visible from the bed.

Televisions should not be kept in the bedroom; they are as reflective as mirrors and can encourage disharmony and infidelity. You will end up falling asleep to late-night talk show hosts and their guests rather than satiated by your lover's embrace. Exercise and electronic equipment are also not conducive to romance. Keep them elsewhere.

According to feng shui tradition, when a mother wants her daughter to find a good husband, she hangs a large picture of peonies in the living room. If you want to attract a man, consider keeping an image of a peony just outside your bedroom door. Once that man is sleeping in your bedroom, however, remove the picture, as the peony energy can encourage a man to have a roving eye.

Create a portable love altar so that you can transport your healthy feng shui energy and a sacred space of passion everywhere you travel. Two friends of mine, after many years of marriage, still travel with their wedding picture, candles, and incense and have been known to place it on the mantels of Holiday Inns!

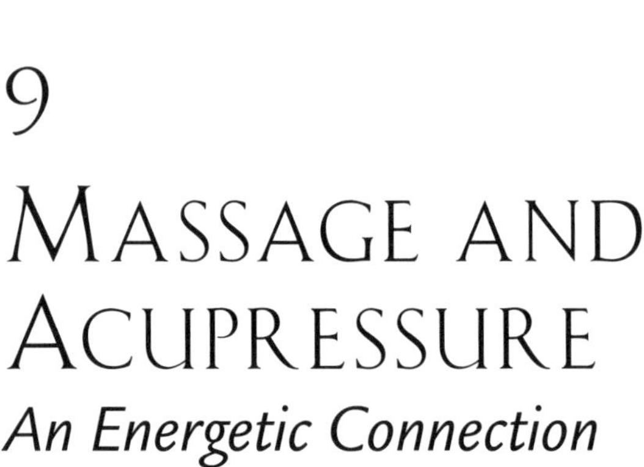

9 Massage and Acupressure
An Energetic Connection

TOUCH IS BELIEVED TO BE the first of the senses to develop in the human embryo, and it defines much of our experience of life. Our skin, the conductor of touch, is the largest organ in our bodies, and it is richly endowed with sensitive nerve endings. In fact, the skin is sometimes described as an external nervous system.

For humans, the awareness of touch is ever-present. Our minds are constantly flooded with sensations like the feel of our clothing against our bodies, the air on our skin, hot and cold, pain and pleasure. Recognizing this, we can understand that the power of massage—the physical healing resulting from hands-on bodywork—is no small wonder. But while we acknowledge that massage is useful for loosening up sore muscles, soothing aching feet, and rubbing out knots in the back, we often forget that the simple power of touch—the caress of body against body—is itself a potent catalyst for energizing, arousing, soothing, and healing the emotions. Most important, touch is an expression of love.

Massage is a wonderful way to build, support, and express the passion you have for another human being. It stimulates secretion of the hormone oxytocin, which promotes emotional bonding. Furthermore, massage boosts circulation of blood and lymph, stretches muscles and connective tissue, releases physical and emotional tension, stimulates the production of endorphins, and builds the immune system. And when your mate is too tired or tense to make love, massage can be an intimate, tender form of connecting with your beloved.

HOW TO GIVE A GREAT MASSAGE

Many people are reluctant to give a massage because they've never done it before and feel that they don't know how to do it properly. Let's set things straight: *Almost* every massage feels good, whether it's the disorganized rubbing of a novice or the probing bodywork of a professional. That's the beauty of massage; even if you don't do it well, your effort will still be well appreciated.

If you and your beloved make massaging one another a habit, your technique will improve rapidly. Even better, you'll soon learn each other's bodies like you've never known them before. You'll know where your lover carries tension, where he or she tends to develop muscle knots, which spots are particularly sensitive, and which spots inspire arousal. When you're making love, such knowledge can carry you and your lover to new heights of desire and release.

You might not always have the time to give or receive a full-body massage. If that's the case, consider a scalp, facial, hand, foot, buttocks, or back massage; all can give exquisite pleasure and relaxation in a relatively short amount of time. Many nights while watching a movie on TV, my husband and I will trade foot massages. You never know what might happen after that!

There are no strict rules for giving a massage; do what seems to feel good to your partner, and try out on your partner those things that feel good to you. Be sensitive to your fingers and to your partner's skin. The following guidelines will help. For more ideas, take a class on massage or watch an instructional video.

Create a Calming Environment

Because the person receiving the massage will likely be naked, make sure the room is warm and free of cold drafts. Use soft lighting; candles are wonderful. Be sure that the surface on which your partner is lying—the floor or the bed—is not covered with a sheet or blanket that you prize. Spilled massage oil usually leaves a stain.

Use Oils to Smooth the Way

A light oil enhances the power of massage, allowing the hands to glide over and feel more deeply into the body. The friction of the massage also causes the oil to warm up; the heat is transmitted to the body, encouraging muscles to relax.

The best oils to use for massage are those that are light, fragrance-free, and moisturizing for the skin rather than clogging. My favorites are almond and coconut. Coconut oil smells great and imparts beauty and radiance when rubbed on the skin. It has a long shelf life and does not form trans-fatty acids, as it is a saturated fat. It can also be used as a sexual lubricant, though not with condoms or other latex forms of birth control.

Do not use heavy, odoriferous oils like peanut or corn oil, mineral oil—which is a petroleum by-product—or oils that have become rancid. Keep your massage oil in a bottle with a flip-top lid; this type of container is easy to close when your hands are full of oil and minimizes the potential for a bottle-tumbling distraction disaster. When you're not using the oils, store them in the refrigerator to keep them fresh.

For an aromatherapy massage, you can add a few drops of essential oil to the base oil. See page 139 for more details.

Warm Your Hands and the Oil

Icy-cold hands on a warm back can produce an unpleasant shock. Before touching your beloved, wash your hands in hot water or rub them together briskly to generate some warmth.

It is also important that the massage oil be warm. Place the container of oil in a bowl of hot water for a few minutes before starting the massage. Alternatively, pour just a drizzle of oil into one hand, then rub the oil briskly between the hands. It's always a good idea to pour massage oil onto your hand first so you can check the temperature.

Let Your Fingers Do the Talking

Before you lay your hands on your lover, draw a deep breath and try to center yourself. Call to mind the love, desire, and tenderness you feel for your beloved. Then allow the love in your heart to be transmitted through your hands to your lover's body.

Use a Variety of Strokes

Incorporate a variety of strokes into the massage, such as circles, short strokes, long strokes, squeezing, and tapping. Just learn a few techniques. Use your fingers to work at small areas and the entire palm of your hand for rolling, broad strokes. Generally speaking, the left side of the body tends to be more sensitive for women, and the right side for men. It's a yin and yang thing. When you find a tension spot—a knot or tight muscle—work at it, starting gently and gradually increasing the pressure. Avoid pressing directly on the spine.

Pay attention to your partner's breathing; deep sighs and soft moans signal that you're on the right track. Encourage your partner to give you feedback.

Encourage Quiet

Receiving a massage can bring you to a blissful place where touch rules the senses. It can be hard to think clearly, and even harder to hold up your end of a conversation. So go deep. As a masseur, you should respect or even encourage that dreamy silence, wherein the only sounds are involuntary sighs and groans drawn forth from a body experiencing true pleasure. If you feel like singing or humming, by all means go ahead, but don't ask for a response from your partner.

Always Stay in Contact

To maintain the bond that has formed between you, don't lose contact with your beloved at any point during the massage. If you have to reach for more oil or shift to a more comfortable position, leave at least one hand on your partner to stay connected.

End Tenderly

A massage leaves a person emotionally open and physically tranquilized, so it is important to end with tenderness. Give your beloved a soft kiss on the forehead or the back of the neck. Whisper sweet nothings in his or her ear. Lie close and be still. Cover him or her. Do whatever feels right in that moment.

Avoid deep massage during infection, after recent surgery, and when skin is infected or inflamed. Use caution during pregnancy, because massage that is overly deep or centered on particular points can induce labor. If your beloved is pregnant, take a class on prenatal massage so that you can proceed with confidence and give your partner some much-deserved comfort. Or give her a gift certificate with someone great.

REFLEXOLOGY

Reflexology affirms that our feet are a map of the body, containing points that connect to each of the body's systems. (See p. 477 for chart ordering information.) A deep foot massage can stimulate the body's internal organs. Reflexology aside, our feet carry us to and fro, support our weight all day long, and too often get stuffed into less-than-comfortable shoes. By caring for our feet, we are caring for ourselves; we can relax and be more open to bliss. There are times when a foot massage might be more desirable than sex!

Foot massages don't require your entire focus, but attention to a few particulars can be helpful. Don't forget to massage the hollows under the anklebones, for instance, since this helps keep the prostate and uterus

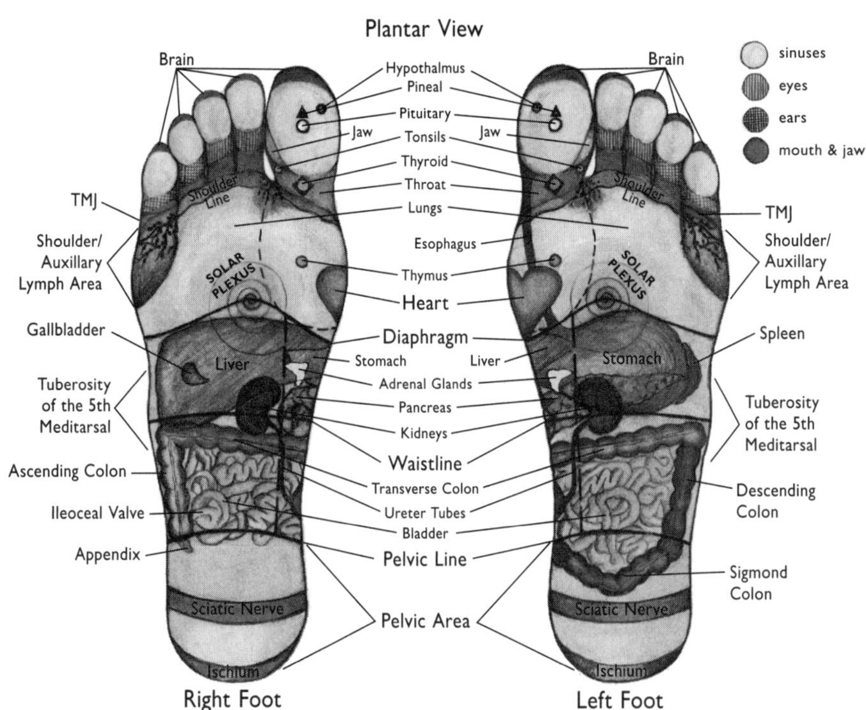

Foot reflexology chart showing correspondences between the soles of the feet and all parts of the body

healthy. Likewise, the heel and the center of the arch on the sole of the foot are linked to sexual vitality; massage in these spots nourishes libido. In general, be sure to massage both feet.

ACUPRESSURE

Acupressure is a noninvasive form of acupuncture. Instead of using needles to tap in to pressure points, the practitioner uses finger pressure. Like acupuncture, acupressure is used to strengthen internal organs and move blockages of energy. In the section below I've described a few acupressure points that can be helpful for sexual and reproductive health. You can massage them on your partner, beginning with a light finger pressure then increasing it gradually. This approach allows the tissues to respond and creates a connection between the giver and the receiver. You and your partner can breathe in unison to help build a stronger connection. Hold each point for one to five minutes.

For more information about acupressure, take a class or read *Acupressure for Lovers* by Michael Reed Gach (Bantam Books, 1997).

Sea of Vitality

Location: On the lower back, two to four inches on either side of the spine at waist level as indicated by the four black dots in the illustration below.

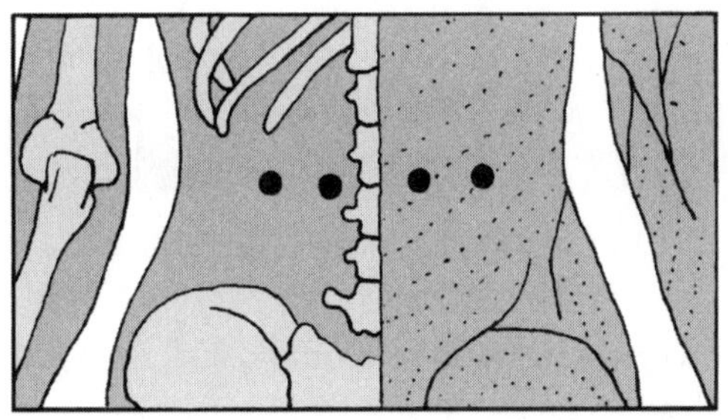

The Sea of Vitality

Stroke: The patient should lie on his or her stomach or stand. Squeeze the Sea of Vitality firmly for one minute.

Therapeutic effect: The Sea of Vitality can help improve many reproductive problems, including erectile dysfunction, premature ejaculation, low libido, infertility, and abnormal vaginal discharge. It also strengthens the immune system and the Kidneys and helps relieve trauma. When you wrap your arms around your lover to give him or her a hug, try pressing your hands on this area.

Three-Yin Meeting Point

Location: Four fingers' width above the inside of the anklebone and one finger's width behind the bone of the leg (the muscle should flex under your finger).

Stroke: Apply deep gentle pressure, gradually increasing in strength.

Therapeutic effect: Pressure on this spot strengthens the reproductive system. If practiced regularly, acupressure here can, over a few months, relieve erectile dysfunction. It also promotes emotional openness and nurturing. This point should not be massaged during pregnancy.

Sea of Intimacy

Location: Two to four fingers' width below the navel as indicated by the three black dots in the illustration below.

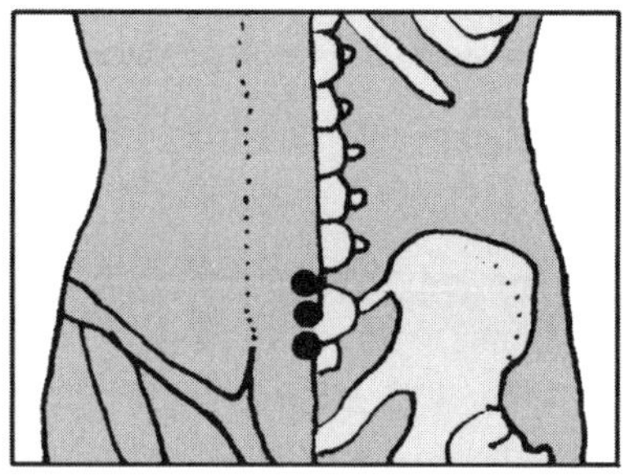

The Sea of Intimacy

Stroke: Have the receiver lie flat on his or her back with knees bent and feet flat on the ground. Press on the Sea of Intimacy so that your fingers sink at least one inch; maintain pressure for one to two minutes. Alternatively, press the edge of your hand crosswise under the navel, and then slide it down toward the genitals. Another effective stroke is to massage this area in a circular motion thirty-six times.

Therapeutic effect: This acupressure point helps relieve erectile dysfunction and premenstrual syndrome.

MASSAGE AS FOREPLAY

When you are giving a massage that you intend as foreplay, use strokes that move toward the genitals, directing blood flow to, and thus increasing sensitivity in, that area. You needn't touch the genitals directly, nor avoid them, but simply include them in your stroking, without obvious sexual intent. Work from the upper body down, relaxing the neck, shoulders, and back before even approaching the pelvic region.

If you think massage may lead to intercourse and you intend to use a condom, be sure to keep massage oil away from the condom and the genitals. Massage oil and essential oils can degrade the structural integrity of condoms, rendering them ineffective as birth control or as protection against the spread of disease.

A lovely game can be made out of blindfolding your partner for a massage session. During the massage, use not only your hands but also a soft paintbrush, silk scarf, or feather to stroke his or her body. Waft under your partner's nose some of the delicate, passion-inspiring essential oils described in chapter 5. Slip a sweet, sensual food—a strawberry, a sliver of kiwi, or a strip of ripe mango, for example—into your partner's mouth. Play soft music, a small chime, or a Tibetan bowl. Turn on all of your beloved's senses to awaken his or her entire being.

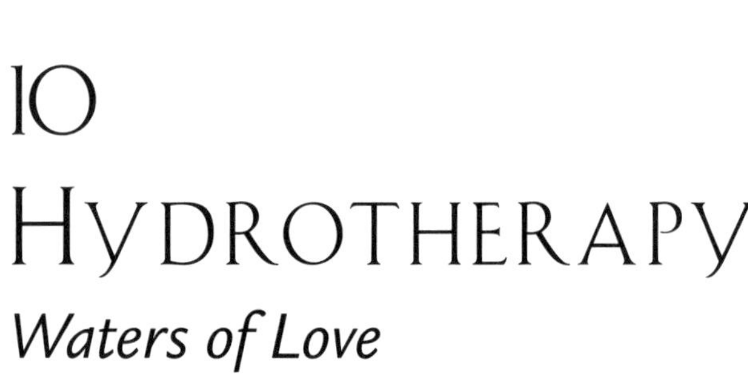

10 HYDROTHERAPY

Waters of Love

WATER, THE MOTHER OF LIFE, is not only a vital ingredient but also a powerful healer and a tremendous aphrodisiac. The sensuous feel of drinking it (water sliding down the throat, penetrating every inch of the body, filling every cell, nurturing the body) or bathing in it (the childlike feeling of weightlessness, the smooth rolling and flowing of it over the skin, the soaking of the skin, water pouring in through the body's outer layer) satisfies the human body in a way that no other element of daily life can.

Except, perhaps, sex. That may help explain why sex, love, health, and water are such perfect complements to one another. My husband and I both watched our first grandchild be born underwater in the Virgin Islands. Water can be infused with affirmation, prayer, and song. May you never thirst!

THE SENSUOUS BATHROOM

If the bedroom is a temple of love, the bathroom is the altar of sensuality. Here we cleanse ourselves physically, emotionally, and mentally so that we enter the sacred bed with washed body, fresh breath, and gentle mind.

The bathroom is so often a neglected space—cramped, cluttered, harshly lit, and often dirty. How much more uplifting and peaceful our homes would feel if the bathroom were, instead, a warm, inviting retreat from the world. Thankfully, it's not difficult to make it so.

First, examine the lighting in your bathroom. The bulbs should emit a warm light, not a harsh glare. If you have a window in the bathroom, leave it open to the air and natural light; if you need to cover the window for privacy's sake, install a light, filmy curtain that allows some natural light to filter through. Install a night-light with a soft red or yellow bulb in a bathroom outlet within easy reach of the door. If you need to use the bathroom in the middle of the night, a night-light will not offend sleepy eyes to the same degree that bright overhead lights do.

The color of the paint or wallpaper in the bathroom should complement your coloring and complexion. For example, if you think you look good in blue, by all means, paint the bathroom blue. We spend a lot of our time in the bathroom looking in the mirror. Let's like what we see!

Not many of us actually enjoy cleaning the bathroom, but it's important to keep it tidy; when the bathroom is clean, we are free to relax, refresh, and purify ourselves in it. Keeping the room clean will be much easier if you first reduce the clutter in it. Get rid of all the potions and lotions that you hardly ever use. Install doors on all cabinets and shelving so that when it's time to clean, you only have to wipe down the doors, not everything on the shelves.

When you clean, use natural cleansers. When you clean with toxic chemicals it can make you feel toxic, because when you smell something, you are inhaling its molecules. Cleaning can become a more pleasant chore when we support our environment, using biodegradable cleansers that smell like uplifting botanical essential oils such as geranium, lavender, mint, orange, or lemon.

Keep a small container of bath salts, a bottle of natural bubble bath, some of your favorite essential oils, and soft sea sponges near the tub. Just sitting there, they'll imbue the bathroom with their delicate aromas, and when it's time for a warm soak in the tub, you can add a scoop of bath salts, a splash of bubble bath, or a few drops of essential oil to the bathwater for pure bathing delight. I love the colorful ritual bath kits by Little Moon Essentials.com.

BATHS FOR TWO

Bathing with a lover indulges the senses, but it's also good love-building therapy for a relationship. Bathing together promotes intimacy, erodes inhibitions, and can help partners develop a sense of tenderness and protectiveness toward each other. For new lovers, bathing together is a gentle way to get to know each other. (It can even be an innocent way to connect with a dear friend of either sex that you may or may not want to be sexual with.)

Time spent together in the bath can encompass much more than washing each other's hair and backs. Try reading to each other, sipping delicious potions, listening to music, practicing deep-breathing exercises, stretching, singing (bathrooms usually have great acoustics), and making love. A joint bath can also be a good time to talk about some of the more difficult issues that you face; it becomes difficult to have an argument with someone when you're lying naked in his or her arms in a warm bath!

Of course, bathing together doesn't have to be limited to the tub. On occasion, think of the 1960s' slogan "Save water—shower with a friend." For a truly sensuous break from the everyday hustle and bustle, stay overnight at a spa or hot springs resort. Indulge with your loved one in soaking, steaming, and other water-based healing therapies; you'll come back feeling refreshed, invigorated, and thoroughly in love.

Footbaths

If you're in the mood to pamper your partner, consider giving him or her the ultimate of honors: a sensual foot washing with scented waters. The feet are among the most sensitive and erogenous areas of the body, and a hands-on footbath is a lovely way to relax the mind and inspire desire.

Have your partner sit in a comfortable chair and place a towel under his or her feet. Fill a basin with warm water and add a few drops of an essential oil of your choice; if you have small fresh flowers, float a few blossoms in the water. Set the basin on the towel and gently place your partner's feet in the water. Use a soft cloth to gently wash each foot in turn; use a small cup to pour water over each foot from time to time. Linger over each toe and every other part of the foot, taking your time and allowing the experience to unfold leisurely. When you're done, pat each foot dry with a soft towel. A foot massage is optional.

Sitz Baths

Sitz baths are often recommended for increasing circulation to the pelvic region. A sitz bath is nothing more than a shallow bath in which one sits upright. The water should cover the pelvic region but not rise above the navel.

Alternating hot and cold sitz baths can work wonders for the circulation. Take three minutes in hot water, then two minutes in cold water. Repeat three times. If you find the baths overheating, try applying a cold compress to your forehead. Afterward, wrap up and keep warm to keep that circulation moving.

A brief soak in a cold sitz bath increases circulation to the genital organs and stimulates the production of sperm and hormones. It is often recommended as a treatment for infertility, fibroids, cysts, hemorrhoids, and other reproductive problems. If cold water on the sensitive skin of your pelvic area makes you squeal, start with tepid water and gradually build up a tolerance.

PART TWO

How to Be a Fantastic Lover

WHEN SEX offers myriad ways to express love and support for a partner, it becomes the building block for a strong relationship, regardless of how strongly or flatly libido is felt at any particular moment. Good sex cannot be reduced to an orgasm rated on a scale of one to ten. Good sex is, rather, healthy sex—a true making of love, with joy and respect. Although you and your partner won't always have equal sexual needs, you can still be compatible as long as you have similarly healthy attitudes and a sincere desire to communicate with each other.

11
Improving Your Techniques

AH, SO YOU'VE DECIDED that you might be interested in improving your techniques. Well, my friend, you've come a long way just to turn to this chapter. Many people are confident that they are already fantastic lovers, and many others are too timid to try experimenting with something new. Now that you're here, I'll let you in on a little secret. The single best way to inject your lovemaking skills with true finesse and masterful expertise is this: Communicate with your lover. That's it. Really. It's not an earth-shattering pronouncement, but it can be a life-changing realization. Your partner isn't psychic, and even if he or she is psychic, he or she might not be adept at reading your mind. He or she will never learn to please you unless you speak up. Most lovers are too shy to speak openly and frankly with each other about what they do and don't like. Many are so taken with the notion of romantic passion that the thought of a "here's what I like" educational lovemaking seminar would horrify them. But I assure you, twenty minutes taken here and there to point out to your lover your likes and dislikes will be time well spent—and your lover will be forever grateful for the insight.

While you're having these honest discussions, practice tact. Rather than criticizing what you don't enjoy, commend what you do enjoy, and suggest new efforts. If you're trying to pull this information out of your lover, ask pointed questions. Queries such as "Does this feel good?" and "Is this better?" are more likely to get you the advice you want than "Tell me what you want me to do."

Above all, pay attention to your lover's body language. Moans, sighs, and smiles are all signs that your lover is enjoying what you are doing. If your lover pulls his or her pelvis slightly away, jerks, or suddenly tenses, you may need to lighten up.

Likewise, making sounds of delight and approval will encourage your lover to pursue techniques that work for you. Sounds of pleasure can become a signal between you and your partner that all is well. In fact, sounds of pleasure are themselves often arousing. They can increase pleasure and function as a form of release as well as a way to go deeper.

SETTING THE STAGE FOR SEX

Love begins anew in every moment. If you wait until you're in bed with your lover to be thinking about sex, you're missing many wonderful opportunities for romance and sexuality. You can create an environment that encourages sexual play just by paying attention to a few essential points.

Timing Is Everything

Men's testosterone levels are highest in the morning, often peaking around 9 a.m. Women's desire levels tend to be highest at night. If couples always waited for sex until they were both in the same states of arousal, it would rarely happen. Be respectful of your partner's level of interest in sex—and your own. It is better to say "no" nicely rather than end up making love with a "no" attitude.

Instead, make time for sex when you can both be present and awake. Quickies are great once in a while and show how physically attracted you are to each other. However, too often love happens after you've already begun to drift off to sleep, or at 7 a.m. when you need to be somewhere by 8. Saving sex for last can indicate it's your last priority. Though these stolen moments can be their own lovely times of connection, leftover time makes for leftover sex.

Make a conscious effort to connect in an intimate way with your mate. Lovely times for such connection are sunset, evenings of the full moon (try

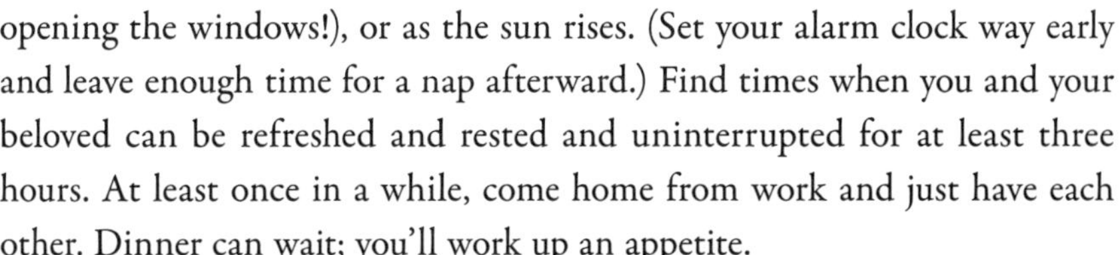

opening the windows!), or as the sun rises. (Set your alarm clock way early and leave enough time for a nap afterward.) Find times when you and your beloved can be refreshed and rested and uninterrupted for at least three hours. At least once in a while, come home from work and just have each other. Dinner can wait; you'll work up an appetite.

Some nights, try setting the alarm clock to go off an hour and a half after you have gone to bed. Then get up, shower, make love, and go back to sleep. Make time for each other. Trade babysitting with other parents or employ a responsible teen.

Holidays can be opportunities to enjoy beautiful, unstructured time with your partner, but you may need to schedule them. Solstices, equinoxes, Sabbath, Sundays, the first snow. Create sacred ways to celebrate the holidays. Rather than starting the New Year with a hangover, have your own intimate celebration. Make a collage together of what you want to manifest in the next year—a vision board, as they say. Rather than toasting, you could be coming at midnight. When you can't be present for a loved one's birthday, celebrate in advance or with a rain check.

It is best to be totally calmed down after an argument before making love. Taoists consider it less than ideal to make love during times of extreme emotional stress, illness, or while intoxicated. These would be less than auspicious times to conceive a child and would deplete the person under duress (as well as a potential child).

When one partner is infirm in some way, plan intimate activities other than intercourse: spend time together by bathing, talking, reading, or napping together. The stronger partner can express his or her love by giving a massage to the one in need. But if it feels right to make love, simply connecting *calmly* can be a way to build chi and strength.

If you are stressed from a difficult day and coming home grumpy; take a relaxing bath, read something upbeat, put on some hot music and enjoy a dance by yourself to unwind before getting together with your beloved.

Try to go to bed together, at the same time, at least a few times a week, to ensure more opportunities for connection. If one needs to stay up, at least tuck in your beloved, share some talk and cuddling before going back to the TV or computer.

Sex is best without a big meal in your stomach. Right after meals it can aggravate hiatal hernias and feel uncomfortable. It is difficult for the body to supply chi (life force) and blood to sex and digestive centers at the same time, so it's better to separate the two activities. However, sharing an invigorating piece of fruit together can really get your chi going. Eating after sex (and sometimes during!) can be delicious. But for the most part it is wisest to avoid lots of food, at least for three hours before bedtime, to avoid interfering with sleep. Instead of eating before bedtime, save some hunger to enjoy your beloved.

Where to Get It On

Beds offer comfort and privacy. Showers and baths can be slippery places for athletic sex, so don't slip! There's always the rug, kitchen countertop, hallway, or couch. Go parking. Make love on a boat or train. Make love in the ocean and defy gravity. (This works best with the man standing and the woman wrapping her legs around him.) Making love in a secluded place in nature can be a cosmic experience. You can touch your lover while seeing the blue sky and the radiance of the clouds, inhaling the scent of wildflowers, and hearing birds sing.

Vacations

Traveling together creates adventure and intimacy. Vacations are a necessary part of life, and though they can be expensive, they are much cheaper than the cost of a divorce. Start a vacation savings account that you both contribute to each month.

Take time for a vacation when the relationship is doing well, rather than waiting until a crisis arises. If you cannot agree on a destination, take turns deciding on the location. Be sure to take romantic vacations in addition to family vacations. Woe to the couple whose only idea of vacation is to visit relatives! Vacations with others can interfere with your own opportunities for intimacy, so try to go away by yourselves once in a while. And try to avoid busy tourist seasons.

Long trips can take a lot of planning, travel, and expense, but they are not the only option; sometimes a more simple adventure can be refreshing. Be a tourist in your own town. Discover wonderful places and their history, making your own daily path more amazing. Try exotic restaurants. Take your beloved back to the town where you grew up—just to look at the old house and school that were a part of your childhood. On any trip, be sure to have plenty of free time for enjoying one another rather than heavy schedules, expectations, and 7 a.m. snorkeling lessons. Freedom from assignment is ideal. And plan ahead: avoid exhausting long drives just for an overnight. With the freedom that a vacation brings, change your routines. Make love at different times of night and day. Create beautiful memories together. Display photos of your happiest times. Make love more and argue less!

HOW TO BE A GOOD KISSER

If sex can be likened to art, then kissing is poetry. A kiss is the sweet, symbolic communication of our passion for another person. You might think that the true measure of intimacy with a lover would be reflected in intercourse, but as it turns out, kissing—more than sex—is our most emotionally intimate expression of desire and love. Studies have shown that couples having relationship problems are more likely to neglect kissing than sex. But kissing is far more than a rich emotional connection. It also has the potential to be incredibly arousing. The tongue, lips, and moist walls of the mouth are richly supplied with nerve endings. In Oriental facial diagnosis, the lower lip corresponds to the genitals and the upper lip to the brain's sex center; when the lips are stimulated, so too is sexual desire. In Oriental tradition, kissing is also a way to exchange and stimulate chi. Using the lips and mouth to kiss encourages sympathy and compassion; stimulation of the tongue inspires joy.

It takes twenty muscles to form a kiss. To strengthen your kissing ability, practice tongue exercises. Stick out your tongue as far and down as possible. Try touching your tongue to your nose, then your chin. Move it from side to side, reaching as far as you can.

Kiss with Love

The Golden Rule of Kissing: Let your kisses communicate love. When you kiss a lover, even casually, make it an expression of how you feel about him or her. You don't have to be physically passionate with every kiss, but endowing each kiss with emotional passion will nurture, sustain, and enrich the love in your relationship. This visualization technique will help: Gather all your love, passion, and desire and visualize it radiating through your lips onto and into your partner. You may actually feel your lips tingle a bit! If you're not feeling particularly passionate, pause, breathe, and call up the memory of passion, even if just for a moment. Let a kiss be a moment unto itself, not necessarily a prelude to sex but a sweet connection nevertheless. In fact, to keep your sex life vibrant, sometimes you have to step back from sex and revert to your "just dating" days. A flurry of soft, small kisses around the eyes, ears, and forehead make a lover feel adored.

Decide with your partner that you will engage in no sexual activity other than kissing for two or three days. Allow yourself time to just make out. And above all, kiss with feeling. As heartfelt kissing fades to quick pecks on the lips so, too, does passion in a relationship fade. One of the easiest ways to keep your love alive is to make every kiss count, as if it were the last one you'd ever give your beloved. A kiss with feeling takes no more time and just a bit more concentration than a quick peck. The payoff—enduring passion and a strong relationship—is enormous.

Kissing to Arouse

Kissing can be a potent and fun foreplay technique. The trick is knowing where your lover's most sensitive spots are and making good use of them, caressing the body with your lips in a way that promises more to come. Generally speaking, the human body is most sensitive to stimulation in the following areas:

- Lips
- Chest
- Ears
- Navel
- Cheeks
- Along the spine
- Eyelids
- Lower back and over the kidneys
- Neck
- Buttocks
- Palm of the hand
- Genitals

Of course, different people have different sensitivities, and over time those sensitivities can change. Explore your lover's body as if you were on a treasure hunt, mining those areas that elicit soft sighs, goose bumps, and the arching of the back that indicates high arousal.

How you kiss can be just as important as where you kiss. Shallow kissing gives the mind space to wander, to fantasize about the lovemaking to come and to feel the warmth and movement of the beloved's body. Deep kissing, also known as French kissing (although, interestingly, the French call it "English kissing"), initiates an escalation of passion. It is a rehearsal for sexual congress and provides an opportunity for a woman to penetrate a man. Deep kissing can be terrifically arousing, but the effect usually wears off quickly, and the longer you keep it up, the more it tends to seem just sloppy, rather than exciting. So use your tongue with delicacy. Don't force yourself into someone's mouth until you know that he or she enjoys—and is ready for—deep kissing.

When you're kissing to arouse, alternate between shallow and deep kisses. Brush your tongue against your beloved's lips. Kiss the upper and lower lips in turn. On occasion, suck gently on your beloved's upper lip, running your tongue over the frenulum, the small membrane that stretches from the inside of the upper lip to the gums just above the front teeth.

Some people enjoy having their lips bitten when they are aroused; ask your beloved whether he or she enjoys being bitten and, if so, whether you should use gentle or firm pressure.

If you're feeling daring, shuffle across a carpet and slowly lean in to your lover, allowing your lips to be the first point of contact. This "electric" kiss will cause sparks to fly, both figuratively and literally. Give hot and cold kisses, taking a sip of a cold or hot drink before pressing your lips to your lover's. In the heat of summer, pass an ice cube from mouth to mouth as you kiss. The cool, slippery surface can incite passion at a time when you might otherwise think it was just too hot to roll around in bed with someone.

Don't focus exclusively on your lover's lips; kisses all over can be beautiful and arousing. When you kiss your lover's body, alternate between soft and vigorous kisses. Barely graze the skin with your lips, then practice deep kissing on the surface of the skin. Gently touch your lips to the skin and hum a little tune; the vibration can be stimulating. Lift your partner's hair and kiss him or her on the nape of the neck. Give a little lick, then pull back and blow warm breath upon it. Warm breath meeting cooling moisture at one of the body's most sensitive spots will have your lover melting in your arms.

A butterfly kiss is where you gently flutter your eyelashes by blinking a few times on a sensitive part of your beloved's skin like the cheek or thigh. Enjoy kissing in the beginning, middle, and end of lovemaking. Drive each other pleasurably wild with kisses!

Sweet Breath Is Essential

Your kissing quota is guaranteed to double if you have the sweetest breath your lover has ever tasted. (The opposite is also true.) Be sure to floss, and brush your teeth (includng the tongue) twice a day. Keep a small tin of anise seed, cardamom seeds, cloves, and fennel seeds by your bed; suck on a pinch of this spicy-sweet mixture to freshly flavor your mouth.

If you suffer from chronic bad breath, take three chlorophyll capsules daily, eat a small handful of fresh parsley, or drink a glass of wheatgrass juice every day. Have your teeth examined by a dentist. Monitor your diet; if you have difficulty digesting certain foods (dairy foods are a common culprit), you could develop bad breath after you eat them. And if you can't banish bad breath on your own, enlist the help of your health care provider.

MASTURBATION

Masturbation, or self-pleasuring, is an ideal way to find out what you find pleasing so that, in turn, you can help a lover please you. Masturbation can help you overcome inhibitions, discover which parts of your body are most sensitive, learn to achieve orgasm, and, perhaps, become multiorgasmic. Masturbation is especially important when you are not in a relationship; not having a partner is no reason not to feel sexually alive and active. It can also be helpful in cases where your partner is absent, feels fatigued, has a lower libido than you, or is ill. For men that ejaculate more quickly than they'd like, masturbating can be an opportunity to practice delaying orgasm, so they can last longer with a partner.

The goal of masturbation is usually orgasm, but there's no need to rush headlong toward it. Masturbation is as much about making yourself feel like a sexually desirable and desiring being as it is about orgasm. Make a ceremony of it, no matter how small. Light a candle. Bathe luxuriously. Create a sacred space that is warm, private, and comfortable. Undress and look at yourself in the mirror. When we look in the mirror, we usually focus on those things that we don't like about our bodies. This one time, at least, focus on those things that you do like about your body. See and feel yourself as a desirable being. If you've never examined your genitals closely, do so at least a few times. Women should use a mirror and part the labia to reveal the clitoris, vaginal entrance, and urethra. Touch yourself. Run your hands over your chest, navel, and hips. Pleasure yourself. Breathe deeply. Take your time. Experiment. Practice. Learn. Enjoy.

Over time, vary the methods of self-stimulation, learning to experience pleasure in a multitude of ways. Masturbate slowly, taking fifteen to twenty minutes to reach orgasm. When you are close to orgasm, stop, rest, and practice Kegels (see page 118). Try using lubricant. Most of all, enjoy this time of being available to yourself. Remember that you are truly making love to yourself.

Masturbation during Sex

Though it may take some bravery, masturbating in front of your partner, and having your partner do the same in front of you, can be a tremendous turn-on. Watching your partner touch his or her own body is the best opportunity you will have to find out what really pleases him or her. If your lover feels shy, hold him or her close to you, and help out by kissing and caressing your lover's face, neck, and upper body.

Masturbating while a lover holds and kisses you can be an extremely beautiful and tender form of sex. It is also a wonderful way for a couple to keep their sex life vibrant in times when one person is unable to participate or has a lower libido than the other.

Too Much of a Good Thing

There are a thousand and one myths about the dangers of masturbating: "If you masturbate too much, your penis will fall off." "Nice girls don't masturbate." "You only have so much semen. You'll use it all up if you have too many orgasms." "You'll go blind." (Can I just do it until I need glasses?) If you haven't heard these lines, I'm sure you've heard others. Most people see them for what they are, silly fabrications cobbled together to inculcate the human psyche with the idea that sex for pleasure is wanton or immoral.

But as with most things, too much masturbation can be harmful. A preoccupation with masturbation doesn't give you much incentive to go out and interact with people. If you feel isolated or shut out from the social world, you may turn to masturbation for relief. This can develop into a progressive inward cycle. Excessive masturbation may also prevent you from devoting energy to creative activities that stimulate the mind and please the spirit. It may also satiate—and thus dampen—your sexual desire, which can undermine the sex life you have with your lover.

According to Taoist tradition, *jing* is life essence in our bodies. It is present in blood, ova, sex hormones, and sexual fluids. Menstrual fluid is a physical manifestation of jing in women. Sperm is a physical manifestation of jing in men. For men, excessive ejaculation can cause a loss of jing and weaken the life-force and sexual energy, as well as deplete the Kidneys, bones, teeth, hair, and sense of hearing.

What's excessive? It depends. Some people have an abundance of sexual energy and may, in fact, need to masturbate every day in order to satisfy it. Others may find that if they masturbate more than once or twice a week, they lose interest in having sex with their lover. Take some time to find and maintain your own balance. Enjoy the pleasure of masturbation without guilt, but avoid excessive indulgence so that your sexual, social, and creative energies remain vibrant.

FOREPLAY

Foreplay is composed of anything that happens before intercourse that gets you "ready." It is truly one of the secrets to great sex. By activating the body's meridians, foreplay in effect activates the entire being, both internally and externally, and leads to fuller presence in the moment. Foreplay generates chi, invigorates yin, and calms yang. It also relaxes the body. (You can have much better sex when your body is relaxed than when it holds tension.) It decreases performance pressure, helps men develop stronger erections, and enables women to have better vaginal lubrication.

A Taoist truism says that foreplay "helps bring the waters to a boil while keeping the fire burning slowly." Man is compared to fire, quick to ignite and quickly extinguished. Woman is like water, slow to come to a boil and slow to cool down.

The most common complaint from women is that their partners do not engage in enough foreplay. The key to pleasing a woman is bringing pleasure to her slowly. There is a time and a place for wild, fast, hard sex, but if you're worried about your ability to please a woman, take your time. That includes a long, slow, unhurried session of foreplay.

Foreplay All Day Long

Foreplay can encompass much more than five minutes of heavy petting before intercourse. Indeed, you might say that foreplay is a way of life. Great foreplay constitutes a state of mind that ignores human fault, practices loving-kindness, helps with chores, and acknowledges great joy in the everyday presence of a lover.

Foreplay can happen with words, looks, acts of helpfulness, shared activities, and physical affection. It starts when you open your eyes in the morning and look upon your beloved with love in your heart. It continues throughout the day, manifesting as dishes washed because your beloved didn't have time to do them, a smile shared as you head to the bathroom with toddler in tow and your beloved heads to the laundry with a heaping basket, a tire changed, or a hand held on the porch as you watch the evening pass. It does not end when you climb back into bed together, happy to be with this person for whom you care so dearly, but continues through the night, in stray caresses, shared breathing, and the warmth of the bed.

It's true that foreplay is important to sex. But it's also true that foreplay is important to a good relationship. Foreplay is an expression of love and affection that tells your beloved that he or she is an essential part of the joy you find in life.

The "Other" Erogenous Zones

Foreplay is exactly that: For play. Instead of having specific goals, play for play's sake. Don't just jump for the genitals! Neglecting foreplay is said to be akin to walking right past the host at a dinner party and helping yourself to the food before it has been served.

The entire body can be a playground for touch and sensuality. Every zone can be an erogenous one. We'll focus here on those that are the most energetically potent.

THE KIDNEYS

In the tradition of Oriental medicine, the Kidneys govern sexual vitality. Strong Kidneys contribute to strong libido and sexual ability. To activate the energy of the Kidneys, have your partner lie on his or her stomach. Place your hands in the small of his or her back and rock them back and forth.

This energetic massage can be particularly helpful in encouraging a sexually uptight person to relax.

THE EARS

Massaging the ears can greatly increase sexual vitality. The ears are not only delightfully sensitive, they also correspond to the Kidneys and therefore to sexual energy. An Oriental proverb says, "In order to be a good listener, one must have strong Kidneys." And as anyone who's experienced it will know, having your ears orally massaged—by a partner using his or her lips and tongue to nibble and delicately lick—can be an incredibly arousing experience. Nibble on earlobes sweetly. Most people do not enjoy wet or sucking kisses over the ear itself as it can impair your hearing for a few minutes.

THE PALMS AND THE SOLES

The palms of the hands and the soles of the feet are extremely sensitive; the hands alone contain forty thousand nerve endings. The hands and the arms are extensions of the Heart meridian. Stimulating them opens both the physical heart and the emotional heart to love.

According to reflexology, the entire foot is like a map of the body, each part of the foot corresponding to a portion of the anatomy. The uterus and the prostate correspond to the inside of the heel, while the ovaries and testicles correspond to the outside of the heel. The Achilles tendon correlates to the reproductive organs. Massaging the feet feels wonderful and can increase circulation to these and other parts of the body.

THE BREASTS

Women's breasts and men's breasts both contain several acupuncture meridians, including the Pericardium (the tissue surrounding the heart), the Liver, and the Stomach meridians. The breasts should be touched gently at first; as passion increases, the stimulation can become more vigorous. Many women find having their breasts squeezed, sucked, pinched, or otherwise overstimulated before they are sufficiently aroused to be very agitating. Find out what your woman really enjoys. Waiting until she is ready to climax to stimulate the nipples can greatly intensify her pleasure. Of course, a woman can also stimulate her own nipples.

Be aware that a woman's breasts may be especially tender before her menses; approach them more gently at that time.

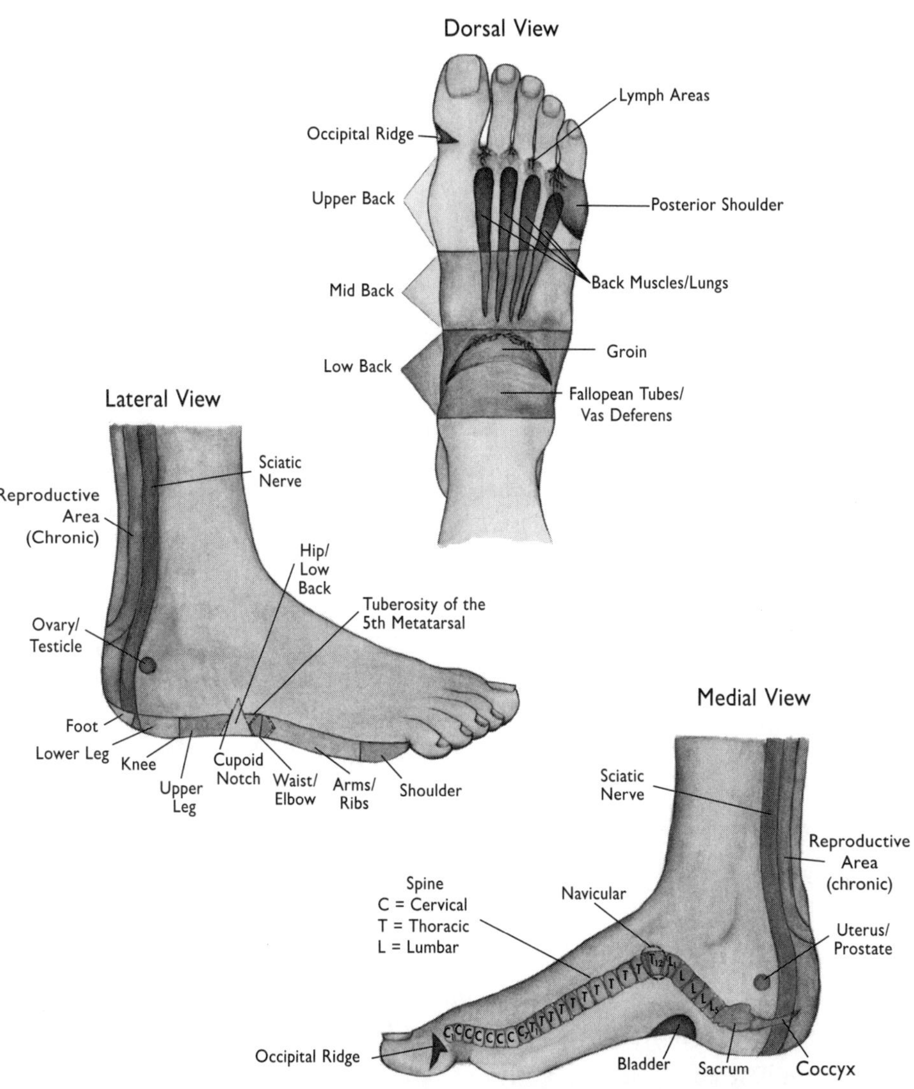

Side and top views of the feet showing the reflex points for the reproductive organs

The Pleasures at Hand: Genital Massage

Foreplay doesn't always have to end with intercourse. A couple can regularly engage in foreplay just for the joy of building sexual energy, feeling pleasurable sensations, and connecting. Genital massage can be an erotic alternative to sexual intercourse. Use whichever of the techniques below that suit your desire, then just relax, enjoy the experience, and be willing to return the favor!

FOR HER

A woman is like a flower with her genitals hidden. If you show a woman patience and tenderness, the flower will open lovingly. You can even start through her underwear. Caress her abdomen, hips, and thighs before arriving at the genital area. Touch the inner thighs, mons pubis, and vaginal lips. Stroke the pubic hair. Warm and calm the area by placing your entire hand over the closed lips and rubbing in a circular motion; this also gently stimulates the clitoris without being too intense.

The labia majora (the fleshy outer lips) are less sensitive than the clitoris but very responsive to touch. Gentle tugging on them can be very pleasing and opening. The hidden inner sides of the labia minor (the inner lips) are richly supplied with nerve endings. Part the labia and tap along the insides of each. Gently pull down on both sets of labia, gradually increasing pressure. As your partner becomes aroused, tenderly part the labia and slide your fingertips up and down over the inner labia, using long, slow movements that just barely touch the clitoris at the top of the stroke. Wait for the woman to part her legs to invite you to touch her before going any further.

Place the three middle fingers over the vagina and gently press and rub in a circular motion. This can be internal acupressure! Your partner will let you know when her clitoris is ready to be touched by opening her legs more, raising her pelvis, or pushing against your hand. Wait to be encouraged, as the clitoris is highly sensitive and touching it too soon can cause your partner to pull back from you. The clitoris spends most of its life tucked away behind a hood and protected by the labia, making it supersensitive when it comes out to play. Many women want their clitoris stimulated directly only when they are about to have an orgasm. And others don't. Ask what does it for her.

Make gradual teasing circles around the clitoris. Draw the circles smaller and smaller until they are about the circumference of a quarter, and occasionally brush against the clitoris. Touch the hood, base, and sides of the clitoris. Because the clitoris is not self-lubricating, overstimulation can cause dryness and pain, so proceed cautiously and use a lubricant if needed. If a circular rubbing motion seems to make your partner uncomfortable, try a gentle pulsing movement. Some women may prefer to have pressure on the inner labia rather than directly on the clitoris.

After your partner is very aroused, roll the clitoris between the fingers, at a pace of about one cycle per second. If she is well lubricated, slide a finger or two inside the yoni while keeping up the clitoral stimulation. If she wants you to lie close to her while you're doing this, you'll have to use just one hand—fingers inside the yoni, thumb stimulating the clitoris. If you find this difficult, ask her to touch herself, while you lie close and continue to stroke inside the yoni.

Use your fingers to create sensuous circles inside the vagina. Massage around, as if the vagina were the face of a clock, stroking at one-hour intervals until you have circled the clock. Try this at different depths. For many women, twelve o'clock is the most sensitive and six o'clock the least. Begin gently, then stroke more vigorously as orgasm approaches.

FOR HIM

As with genital massage for women, begin a man's massage with foreplay. Touching through clothes, then underwear, can be quite erotic. Touch the man's inner thighs and stomach, building his desire. (Some men and women find a tongue in the navel very teasing.) The pelvic region abounds with sensitivity. The crease between the thigh and groin is especially sweet. Tease him. Run your breasts or hair over his man root. See if you can get him erect and wanting more without making genital contact. Honor the man in him.

The secret to great manual sex for men is warmth, lubrication, and a snug fit. Use a nice natural lubrication on both hands. (On occasion, you can use bubbly mineral water to give a fizzy genital massage.)

The most sensitive parts of the penis are the glans (the skin at the tip of the penis) and the rim of the glans, also known as the coronal ridge. The seam of blood vessels on the underside of the penis that runs from the shaft to the scrotum can also be supersensitive. The tiny slit at the tip of the penis, called the urethral meatus, is worthy of attention, as is the sensitive frenulum, also referred to as the F spot, at the underside of the penis where the shaft and the glans meet. Here are some ideas for love play.

Tap gently over the lingam (the penis) like gentle rain, and tap the head of the lingam against your palm or against your partner's tummy. Use one hand to hold down the skin at the base of the penis, thus exposing more nerve endings higher up. Work upward with a massaging stroke, making a twisting motion when you reach the head of the penis and continuing to "sculpt" the shaft in an uninterrupted flow. When massaging in a downward stroke, use a more open grip so that the penis isn't shoved into the torso.

The penis is actually rooted two to four inches inside the body. Massage deep and gently into your partner's root. Try rubbing, tapping, and pressing the area. Make a "fire" by gently rolling and rubbing the lingam between your hands, starting at the base and working upward. Throughout, avoid choppy, jerky movements. Vary the pressure and speed of hand motion. Stay in contact, leaving at least one hand on the penis if you need to replenish your lubricant.

Try fifteen strokes on the shaft, including the head, then fifteen strokes on the shaft only. As your partner's arousal builds, do thirty strokes on the shaft and five on the head. Start slowly and gently; increase speed and pressure as he becomes more excited.

Most men love having their testicles handled—carefully, of course. Cupping the scrotum while giving a genital massage may add to your partner's pleasure. Try holding the testicles together in the palm of your hand and using the fingers of your other hand to make gentle figure-eight movements over the scrotum. Roll the testicles gently and slowly between the thumb and forefinger of your hand, with a light touch of the fingertip pads.

Another method of testicle massage begins with making a ring with your fingers around the scrotum where it attaches to the groin. Gently squeeze the thumb and forefinger together and pull the scrotal skin taut, though not tight. With the fingertips of your other hand, make small and big circles, using a gentle, tickling touch. Some couples find it erotic to insert the lingam just inside the woman's underwear, and just tease each other.

INTERCOURSE

Like other aspects of sex, good intercourse requires good communication between lovers. Instead of performing, be present with yourself and your beloved. Focus on what is happening rather than what isn't. If you're thinking, "I wish he/she would . . . ," you're missing out on the passion of the moment, the potential for a true connection of souls. If you've communicated well in earlier lovemaking sessions, your lover will know what does and doesn't please you. Be willing to try new things all your life.

Most important, have realistic expectations. Lovemaking isn't designed to give you an orgasm worthy of a fireworks display every single time you have sex. It's a means of connection, of communicating your love to a person,

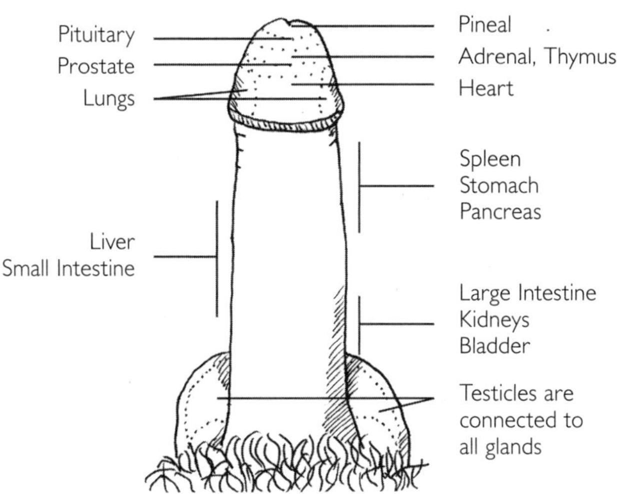

The penis and the acupressure points it contains

of opening to him or her. In its highest sense, sex provides an opportunity for at-oneness with the Divine. Great sex is that which opens the doors to your emotional and spiritual consciousness, draws you deep inside yourself, and lays you bare before your lover, all at the same time. But stronger still is the deep connection of love, manifested in the physical joining of two lovers.

Intercourse as Therapeutic Massage

Intercourse is an opportunity to give each other a mutual acupressure treatment. As the yoni and lingam connect, each stimulates the other's internal organs to bring about health benefits. For women, shallow thrusts into the yoni massage a point that corresponds to the Kidneys, building sexual vitality. For men, the penis contains more than one acupressure point, each corresponding to a particular body system.

Sexual Positions

Sexual positions, also known as sexual asanas, can enhance genital connection, leading to a deeper union, enhanced pleasure, and more soulful bonding. The descriptions that follow address the classic sexual asanas. The point is not to instruct in their usage—I'd guess that most people have tried almost all of them—but, rather, to offer you some ideas for improving your

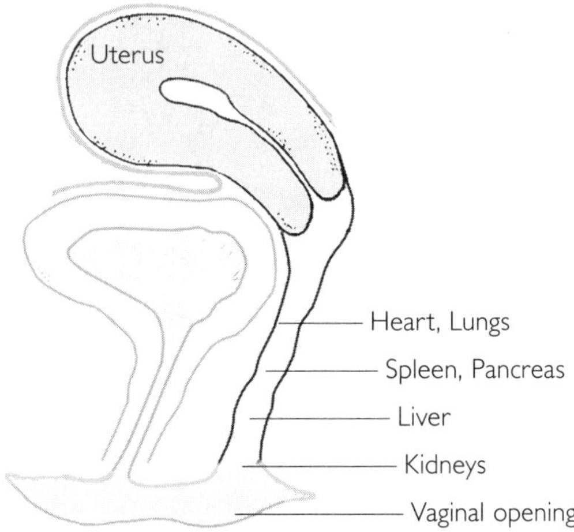

The vagina and the acupressure points it contains

connection in these positions and to encourage you to expand your palette of lovemaking techniques. Being comfortable with four or five different styles allows you to make love in a way that suits your mood and energy at a particular moment. For example, you and your lover may rely on one method of lovemaking when you are tired and another when you want to strengthen your emotional connection.

But more important than any position is the energy that flows between the people engaged in lovemaking. Without that heart-to-heart connection, it's less possible for any physical configuration, no matter how simple or contorted, to bring true satisfaction.

MISSIONARY

This is an excellent position for strengthening an emotional connection, because it allows for verbal communication, eye contact, kissing, deep penetration, and a heart-to-heart connection. Simultaneous orgasm is most likely to happen with this position.

The woman lies on her back and the man lies over her, facing her, with his pelvis between her thighs. Placing a pillow under the woman's hips raises the vagina and allows deeper penetration. To trigger the G-spot while making love in the missionary position, press down on the woman's belly just above the pubic mound.

The missionary position impedes manual stimulation of the clitoris. One solution is to have the woman lie with her pelvis at the edge of the bed. The man lies over her but keeps his feet on the floor. This position allows greater freedom of movement between the lovers in the pelvic area. Also experiment with the woman raising her legs to the ceiling, then closing them together around her beloved for a close connection. Opening the yoni lips manually can open a woman to bliss states.

WOMAN ON TOP

The man lies on his back, and the woman straddles him, facing forward. Many women find that this is an excellent method for achieving orgasm; they can control the depth of penetration and stimulate their clitoris against the man's pubis or manually. For good G-spot stimulation, the woman should try sitting on top of the man facing his feet.

Men with large stomachs, men who have trouble maintaining erection, elderly men with heart trouble, and pregnant women will find that the woman-on-top method of lovemaking is easier than most others.

Some men claim that they have more control over ejaculation when their lover is on top of them. Women may tire easily in this position, but men won't. Just breathe in chi. You can share deep inhalations of essential oils with your lover. Much safer than amyl nitrate. Women must be careful to avoid bending and hurting the erect lingam. To avoid putting too much pressure on the man, the woman may want to support some of her weight with her arms or knees.

COITAL ALIGNMENT TECHNIQUE

Coital alignment can be accomplished in the missionary position. To achieve alignment the man lifts himself farther up the length of his lover's body so that his thrusts make contact with her clitoris, creating a greater likelihood of female orgasm. At the same time the base of the man's penis is also being stimulated. Sex occurs from a higher angle than usual; with thrusting pressure on the woman's clitoris the couple rocks back and forth together, maintaining constant contact between the man's pubic bone and the clitoris.

SIDE BY SIDE

The couple lies side by side facing each other. She has one leg between his and one leg bent over his hips. By turning her hips, she can increase or decrease the depth of penetration. This position requires minimal effort and allows for kissing, facial contact, and heart-to-heart connection.

SPOONS

The couple lies side by side with the man spooning the woman's backside and penetrating her from behind. This position allows for a snug fit, and the man can massage the woman's breasts and clitoris to bring her to orgasm. This can be a relaxed way to make love; it's not uncommon to fall asleep this way, still connected. Keep in mind that spooning, with one partner's groin area snuggled up to the partner's rear, is a tender way to hug, connect, and heal. The partner who needs the most nurturing at the moment should take the inside position.

WORKER'S POSITION

The woman lies on her back, and the man lies on his side, facing her. She then lifts the leg closest to her partner and places it over his pelvis, giving the man's penis access to her vagina. This position allows the man to suck on the breast closest to him. It's a low-effort lovemaking position that's useful when couples are exhausted but still want to connect.

X POSITION

The man and the woman sit facing each other, with legs extended, and hook up. They clasp hands and help each other lie down on their backs with their genitals connected, making a sort of X formation, with the heavier partner having his or her legs on the bottom. With a bit of movement you can sustain delightful pleasures. This is an excellent position for outdoor sex; you both can lie facing the sky, where clouds sing.

WHEELBARROW (BUTTERFLY)

This lovemaking method enables deep genital contact. The woman lies on her back. She lifts her buttocks off the bed as far as possible and the man stands as he enters her. Place pillows under the woman's lower back to help support her. She can also wrap her legs around her lover's waist.

REAR ENTRY

The woman supports herself on her hands and knees. The man kneels behind her and enters from behind, pulling her buttocks toward his pelvis.

For deeper penetration, the woman should lift her bottom or lower herself onto her elbows and lower her head.

Another possibility is for the man to sit in a chair with the woman on his lap, facing the same direction, so that his chest is pressed against her back. This position allows for G-spot stimulation and deep penetration. It also enables the man to manually stimulate the woman's breasts and clitoris during penetration, which can help her achieve orgasm. The rear-entry position is ideal for men who have difficulty inserting their lingam because of weak erection. However, it can make ejaculatory control more difficult.

WOMAN LYING ON STOMACH

The woman lies on her stomach with her buttocks raised by pillows, while the man lies over her, laying his chest on her back. This is considered a very easy method of lovemaking. Although penetration is not deep, the couple is connected along the entire length of their bodies.

SITTING IN A CHAIR

An upholstered chair without arms is ideal for this asana. The man sits in the chair, and the woman straddles him, facing him. She sets the pace by lowering and raising herself with her feet.

This position is not strenuous for the male and can help him control ejaculation. It can also be used in cases of male paraplegia.

STANDING

Though standing during intercourse can be fatiguing, it increases muscle use and can quickly build excitement. The couple stands facing each other. The woman lifts one leg, turning it slightly outward, to provide the penis access to the vagina. Once the man has entered her, he can lift the woman by putting his hands under her thighs as she holds on to his neck. She can cross her legs behind his back to contribute to her support. If the woman is pressed against a wall for support, thrusting can be more vigorous.

YAB YUM

Yab yum is Sanskrit for "father mother" and refers to this position's union of the father and mother aspects of God. The couple sits facing each other, with the woman sitting on top of the man's thighs. The legs can be bent or straight. For comfort, try placing a pillow under the woman's buttocks to help support her.

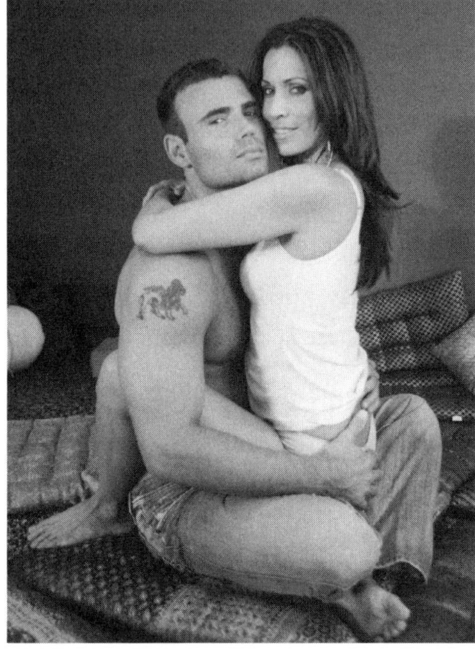

Yab yum

This position is excellent for building a heart-to-heart connection and practicing synchronized breathing (see page 125). Some people consider it an excellent technique for mystical sexual experiences, because the spines of the lovers are aligned with heaven and earth.

Kneeling yab yum is an alternative. The man kneels down and pulls his beloved onto his thighs, facing him. She wraps her legs around him.

CHANGING POSITIONS

It can be rewarding to try several different positions during a single love-making session. The trick to staying connected while changing positions is as follows: While in the missionary position, the woman wraps her left leg around the man's waist, and hooks her left arm under his shoulder. She pushes off with her right arm, keeping gripped to her guy, and rolls him onto his back toward the bed's right side in one sweeping motion. If you disconnect, just reconnect.

OTHER TECHNIQUES

Certain lovemaking techniques are known to build sexual energy, increase arousal while delaying orgasm, strengthen orgasms, and nurture the cosmic union between two lovers. Feeling skeptical? Try one. You just might be surprised.

Eye Contact

Staying connected by looking into each other's eyes during intercourse allows for a deep union of souls.

Sets of Nine

Sets of Nine is a delightful technique for providing a restorative massage to the vagina and penis. The man makes nine shallow thrusts into the vagina, using just the head of the penis, then one deep thrust. Next are eight shallow thrusts and one deep thrust. Then seven shallow and two deep, six shallow and three deep, and so on, until he makes nine deep thrusts. Then he reverses the process—one shallow and eight deep, two shallow and seven deep, and so on, making his way back to nine shallow thrusts. At no point should he withdraw the penis completely.

Try doing at least three complete sets of nine before allowing either partner to orgasm. The woman can also deliver Sets of Nine from a position on top of the man.

Kegel Congress

Kegels can add great pleasure to intercourse and possibly strengthen orgasms. To start, both man and woman should perform one Kegel per thrust. (For Kegel instructions, see page 118.) With the inward thrust, both should relax the pubococcygeus muscles. With the withdrawal, both should tighten the pubococcygeus muscles. This is a wonderful way to practice Kegels together!

Kegels can also constitute an alternative to thrusting. The man should thrust forward and then relax as the woman squeezes him with her love muscles. This Kegel exercise helps bring a woman closer to orgasm while giving a man endurance.

Karezza

Karezza (pronounced ka-ret-za) is derived from the Italian word for caress. This technique is said to have originated in Persia (now Iran). Also known as coitus reservatus, it involves making love without orgasm, thus conserving the male seed. Ahead of time, the couple agrees to avoid orgasm. Intercourse consists of long periods in which the couple is united but passive, mostly lying still. They connect in a relaxed fashion, experiencing calmness and bliss; it is a magnetic connection with love, rather than lust, as its focus, allowing the couple to enjoy the union of their souls.

ORAL PLEASURES

Oral love play can provide special pleasures and deepen intimacy. It can be a prelude or an alternative to intercourse. It can even be a form of birth control, allowing two people to enjoy each other without risking pregnancy. And performing fellatio on a man gives him a unique opportunity to let go of performance anxiety.

As is often the case with other forms of sex, it is best to refrain from jumping right in. Instead, use foreplay to excite your beloved. It is delicious to kiss, lick, and nibble the abdomen, navel, and insides of the thighs, working slowly toward the genitals. Making eye contact as you tease and then begin to give oral pleasure can help build an especially profound sense of connection between you and your lover.

It's best to start out slow and increase the speed of stimulation gradually. Avoid biting or rough play—you're working in a sensitive area! Keep up the same technique for a while, allowing sensations to build, instead of changing your stroke every few seconds.

Receivers of oral pleasure should let their partner know when he or she is on the right path by moving their hips, caressing their partner's hair, and making appreciative sighs and sounds. It's important for givers of oral pleasure to let their lover know they are enjoying what they are doing. Be demonstrative, showing a desire for and relish in what you are doing.

Many couples enjoy orally pleasuring each other simultaneously. (It's called "69" because of the way the two digits fit together, head curled into the other's tail—like a yin/yang symbol.) Others enjoy just taking time out to savor the feeling on an individual level. Whatever your preference, be willing to give as well as receive. If you want to get more, give more!

If you and your partner are not in a monogamous relationship or have not both tested negative for STDs, use dental dams or nonlubricated condoms when performing oral sex.

Playful Dimensions

Hot and cold can add pleasurable dimensions to oral sex. Fill your mouth with ice water or warm it with hot tea before going down on your partner. Or slip a spicy mentholated herbal lozenge into your mouth. Let it dissolve partially so that your mouth is well coated before taking in your beloved. Chewing a pinch of cardamom seeds will yield a similar sensation.

Fellatio

EUPHEMISMS FOR FELLATIO: PLAYING THE FLUTE • SUCKING A MANGO • MOUTH CONGRESS

If the man is standing or sitting in a chair, sit, kneel (on a pillow or mat), or crouch in front of him. If he is lying down, stretch yourself out next to or on top of him. Begin with light foreplay, stroking and kissing his belly, thighs, and chest. Give the lingam gentle butterfly kisses with your eyelashes. Roll it against your cheek, your hair, and your breasts.

Make him hunger for you to take his sex into your mouth. Sucking on the lingam when it is soft gives you the opportunity to feel it grow in your mouth. Use your lips to cover your teeth so you don't scratch or bite the penis.

When you're ready to begin, flick the head of the lingam lightly with your tongue. Gradually progress to longer strokes of the tongue, as if you were licking an ice cream cone. Use both the top and underside of the tongue. Swirl your tongue around the head, first clockwise, then counterclockwise.

Try giving gentle "lip pinches." Use your teeth to gently comb over the glans. Lick. Nibble. Suck, moving the lingam in and out of your mouth. In general, short intense sucks are better than long ones. When taking the lingam in your mouth, try twisting your head in a gentle corkscrew motion to give even more stimulation. Try humming with the lingam in the mouth to create stimulating sound vibrations. Run the tip of your tongue over the little hole at the top of the penis. If your man has been circumcised, pay special attention to the scar that marks where the foreskin used to be. If your mouth becomes tired, use your hands for a while.

The thick cord running the length of the penis's underside is an important erogenous zone. Try lightly flicking your tongue over this ridge; this is called the "butterfly flick."

To perform the vacuum technique, which most men find extremely pleasurable, take in as much of the lingam as is comfortable. You can hold the base of the lingam with one hand to keep yourself from taking it too deep in your mouth and setting off the gag reflex. Make a seal around the shaft with your lips and then pull your head back, creating a vacuum like effect. If you can, hold the lingam so that your knuckles point downward; this brings extra stimulation to the sensitive underside. Use your free hand to caress the root of the lingam, the scrotum, the perineum, the buttocks, and the area from the navel to the pubic bone.

It's been scientifically proved that men are especially turned on by visual stimulation. Of course, the long and successful history of "men's" magazines could have told us that. In any case, when performing fellatio on a man, keep in mind that visual stimulation can be as important as physical stimulation. Don't hide what you're doing. Consider performing in front of a mirror. And try giving oral pleasure in various states of undress. You might be surprised by what really turns on your man!

OVERCOMING THE GAG REFLEX

Many people have a difficult time taking a penis into their mouth without gagging. If this is your situation, try breathing through your nose and keeping the penis to the side of your mouth, rather than the center, where it is more likely to stimulate the gag reflex. Make a fist around the base of the lingam, with your little finger resting on the pubic bone, to give yourself a buffer zone against gagging.

Another quick trick is to gargle beforehand with 1 cup of warm water to which 1 teaspoon of salt has been added. The salty mixture has an astringent effect, temporarily tightening the loose tissue at the back of the throat that initiates the gag reflex. Always remember to breathe.

IT'S NOT A MARATHON

When a couple is having intercourse, a man often tries to pace himself, wanting to last long enough to please his partner. However, during oral sex, the giver can tire easily, so this is not the ideal time for a man to show off his endurance.

If you're the giver and your jaw becomes fatigued, rest your head on your lover's thigh or encourage him to lie on his side so that you can curl in a semifetal position near his hips, where the penis is at mouth level. Take brief breaks and kiss his thighs and abdominal area. Prolonged sucking and caressing can be fatiguing for muscles unused to such work. When you need a rest, use gentle tongue and lip stimulation on the ridge along the underside of the shaft, where the penis is particularly sensitive.

EJACULATION

When a couple is familiar with each other, a man's partner may be able to tell when he is about to ejaculate by his body language. One giveaway, for example, is that testicles ascend when orgasm is imminent. A man can also let his partner know when he is close to orgasm through some prearranged signal.

A man should not take it for granted that his partner wants ejaculate in the mouth. Some people simply don't enjoy it, and a man should restrain himself and ejaculate outside the mouth until the invitation is extended. In addition, unprotected oral sex puts the giver at high risk of STDs; it should not be undertaken until both partners are sure that they are free of disease. Very arousing oral sex can be had while using a nonlubricated condom.

If the relationship is monogamous and the partners have taken reasonable measures to determine that they will not transmit STDs to each other (see chapter 19 for more information), then barrier-free fellatio becomes a possibility. If you don't want to swallow your man's ejaculate, keep a towel close by, so that you can spit the ejaculate into it. If you do want to swallow the ejaculate, your man may feel thrilled that you would lovingly accept his fluids. For a woman, swallowing ejaculate is a wonderful opportunity to receive yang fluids as a chi tonic. As your man is erupting, place your lips as far down the shaft as possible, and stay there calmly until orgasm is complete.

The average ejaculate contains between five and thirty-six calories. It is composed mainly of protein and fructose, but it also contains vitamins C and B_{12}, potassium, sulfur, and zinc. Sperm makes up only 2 to 5 percent of semen.

The flavor of a man's ejaculate can be a reflection of his health. Normal semen tastes sweet. If a man's ejaculate tastes excessively sweet, he may be eating too much sugar. A bitter flavor may indicate the presence of toxins, drugs (including tobacco), or other chemicals in the body.

If the ejaculate tastes truly unpleasant, the man should eliminate coffee and alcohol from his diet for several weeks and stop or reduce smoking as well. He should add to his diet plenty of celery, green leafy vegetables, pineapple, strawberry, mango, and citrus fruits. If the semen continues to taste unpleasant, the man should consult with a health care provider, because he may have an undiagnosed infection.

Cunnilingus

EUPHEMISMS FOR CUNNILINGUS: SIPPING AT THE VAST SPRING • DRINKING FROM THE JADE FOUNTAIN

For women who have difficulty achieving orgasm, oral sex may be the answer. However, the technique of performing pleasurable oral sex on a woman is often considered one of the Great Mysteries. It's actually not that difficult, provided you know where to look and have the patience to be persistent.

You may find that cunnilingus is most pleasurable when the woman lies on her back, while you lie with your head between her thighs. Your woman may also enjoy kneeling over you, again with your head between her thighs.

PATIENCE, PATIENCE, PATIENCE

The vagina is primarily an internal organ. All that's left outside the body are the lips, or labia. Even the clitoris, the most sensitive part of the vagina, is hidden under a hood. All this tucking away is done for a reason: a woman is best approached slowly and gently. In most cases, she needs to be warmed and teased and aroused before she can even come close to orgasm. So reread the section on foreplay, beginning on page 182 and put some of those tips into practice.

Gently separate the outer and inner labia with your tongue. Use your tongue to massage the sensitive inner sides of these lips, moving up and down as well as in and out. In general, the woman will derive more pleasure when you use your entire tongue than when you use just the tip, although you may want to switch back and forth occasionally.

Once a woman is aroused and has become "wet" (her vagina has started to secrete sexual fluids), the clitoris should become the focus of your attention. The clitoris is the primary vehicle of pleasurable sensation, but you must be careful not to overstimulate it, because it can be very sensitive. The tip and underside of the clitoris tend to be the most sensitive areas; some women find oral stimulation in that area orgasmically divine, while others cannot tolerate it. If your partner suddenly jolts, it may be that you have stimulated her too intensely. If this happens, retreat for a bit, using your lips rather than tongue until your woman warms up again. Using one type of pressure for a minute or so, rather than switching from spot to spot and stroke to stroke every five seconds, often yields better results. Some women prefer hard pressure, others soft pressure, and still others variations of the two. There's no way to tell for sure unless you just flat-out ask. Your beloved will most likely be glad to tell you.

ORGASM SECRETS

If you're having trouble bringing a woman to orgasm while giving oral pleasure, try the following:

- Push up on the mons veneris, the mound atop the pubic bone. This can expose the underside of the clitoris at a new angle.
- Insert one or two fingers into her vagina; simultaneous stimulation from outside and inside the vagina can often bring a woman to orgasm. I do believe this ranks as a favorite.
- Use a free hand to stimulate your lover's nipples. There is a direct nerve connection between the nipples and the clitoris, and taking advantage of it can bring a woman great pleasure.

ELIMINATING VAGINAL ODOR

The vagina normally smells slightly musky and tastes somewhat salty. If a woman's vagina has an unpleasant odor or taste, she should eliminate coffee, alcohol, and dairy products from her diet for several weeks and stop or reduce smoking as well.

The woman should consider adding chlorophyll, which is a natural deodorizer, to her diet. Wheatgrass juice is loaded with chlorophyll; taking a shot of it daily may help eliminate odor. She should also eat plenty of dark green, leafy vegetables. Acidophilus capsules can be taken orally and used as a vaginal suppository to help. (See page 250 for more details.)

As further treatment, the woman should bathe regularly in a tub; add 7 drops of lavender essential oil to the bathwater. Lavender essential oil is not only pleasantly fragrant but also mildly antiseptic and antifungal. In addition, it's very mild, which makes it safe to use in close proximity to the delicate mucous membranes of the yoni. If the unpleasant odor or flavor persists, the woman should consult with her gynecologist to rule out a possible infection.

ANAL SEX

There's a certain "taboo" surrounding anal sexual pleasures. For some, anal stimulation is highly erotic; for others, it's uncomfortable and deflates arousal. Whatever your preference, it's important to recognize that no person should be coerced into anal sexual pleasures if he or she isn't comfortable with them. If you haven't experienced anal sex but would like to try it, talk to your lover about it. If he or she seems open to the idea, read through this section so that you're both comfortable with the precautions anal sex requires.

Anal pleasuring can make lovers more open, trusting, and receptive to each other. It also can be very opening emotionally, if it is done slowly and respectfully. For some people it is just as likely to bring up fears or tears as it is to bring arousal. In this case, use the intimacy created by anal pleasuring to support your lover. Hold your beloved close, remind him or her that you are there, and allow him or her to undergo the cleansing of stored negative emotions in the safety of your arms.

Anal sex carries a much higher risk of disease and infection than vaginal and oral sex does. It may expose you to fecal matter, which can be a risky business. In addition, the walls of the rectum are made of very thin tissue that tears easily, exposing you to blood. Therefore, safety precautions are a top priority for anal sex. Any item—penis, finger, sex toy, and so on—inserted into the anus must be washed before it is introduced to the mouth, the vagina, or any other part of the body. For anal stimulation and intercourse, latex gloves and condoms are imperative.

Anal Stimulation

The body becomes aroused from front to back, so wait until your lover is very aroused before attempting to stimulate the anal area. Unless you and your partner engage regularly in anal pleasuring, it's usually a good idea to ask him or her for permission before approaching the anal area. Always allow your lover to feel in control of what you're doing.

Cupping the testicles gently and pressing them into his torso is a sweet way to start. Moisten a finger with lubricant. Press or massage around the perineum (the area between the anus and the genitals) and over the outside of the anal opening. Imagining the anus as the face of a clock, press gently yet firmly at all the hourly positions. Ask if any of these areas feel sensitive.

Most people find that the regions around ten o'clock and two o'clock are the most sensitive.

Stimulation of the outer rim may satisfy your lover, so that you will not proceed any farther. But many people find anal penetration to be highly erotic. Ask permission to enter your beloved's vulnerable place. If he or she assents, replenish the lubrication on your finger. Insert it just slightly into the anus. Hold it still until the area becomes relaxed before proceeding.

For most people penetration itself is not a means of stimulation. Some movement is required. Initially, practice only circular and front-to-back, "come hither" motions inside the anus, avoiding in-and-out and side-to-side motions until your lover is quite comfortable with anal stimulation. If your initial stimulation is well tolerated, try using the fingertip to gently stretch the anal entrance. Keep the heel of the hand gently pressed against the perineum.

To put your lover at ease, try simultaneously touching a familiar place of pleasure, such as the penis, vagina, or clitoris.

When you are ready to exit the anus, your lover may find it more comfortable to ease away from your finger slowly, rather than having you pull it out.

The Male G-Spot

The male version of the G-spot is sometimes identified as the prostate gland stimulated from the back of the upper wall of the anus. It feels like a firm mass about the size of a walnut. Stimulation of the prostate gland in this manner, with a lubricated thumb or knuckle, can trigger a rapid and intense orgasm, particularly if the stimulation takes place during intercourse or oral sex. See the section on the female G-spot on page 215 for ideas on tenderly tending to this power spot.

Anal Intercourse

Before attempting anal intercourse, practice finger penetration until the receiver is quite comfortable with it. Thrusting of the penis in the anus should not be as deep or as rapid as it is in the vagina; remember, anal tissue is quite thin and fragile, and with rough play it can tear. Be sure to use plenty of lubricant on the penis to avoiding damaging the anal tissue.

To protect against the spread of disease, a condom must be used for anal intercourse. Use an extra-strength condom, which is better suited to the rigors of anal sex, and spread lubricant over the outside of it.

AFTER PLAY

In the blissful state after your last orgasmic gasp, you may still be in a highly receptive mode. Using the senses of sight, smell, sound, taste, and touch at this time can extend the lovemaking experience. However, men and women may have a refractory period after lovemaking, during which additional stimulation can be uncomfortable. This period can last from thirty seconds to several minutes or an hour or more, so be sensitive to your own and your lover's needs. (Then again, there are those memorable times when you're ready again right away.)

After orgasm, the body is suffused with sexual energy. Blood is flowing freely through the circulatory system, endorphins are sweeping through the body, and the mind is released of tension. To fully absorb the influx of energy, the body must rest.

Indulge in this time of sweetness after love. Allow your mind and body to relax and soak up the sexual energy of your beloved. Enjoy the feeling of peace. Orgasm triggers production of the hormone prolactin, which can cause you to feel satisfied and sleepy—this is one reason that men often doze off after sex. Sleep if you both can, for lovemaking often calls forth a deep and blissful slumber.

If you don't want to sleep, the urge to do so may pass in a few minutes. Some people feel energized after orgasm and may need to expend some creative energy before they can rest. Share some gourmet chocolate, fresh fruit, or juice.

Others cry after experiencing a powerful release, and they may be frightened by a perceived loss of control. Be there for your lover, supporting the emotions and energies that arise. If lovemaking has taken your beloved to a distant emotional place, speak tenderly, using his or her name to call him or her back to you. Stay with your beloved, maintaining physical contact, which increases oxytocin.

If you must get up, sustain the mood and the flow of energy by sharing an activity. Eat together. Go for a walk. Enjoy some music. Garden. Rejoice in a blessed soul connection with your partner. Allow your lovemaking to be an opportunity to create more love and bliss. Bask in the afterglow!

12 Controlling and Intensifying Orgasms

THE WORD *ORGASM* IS derived from the Greek *orgasmos,* meaning "to grow ripe, swell, or boil over." The French refer to orgasm as *le petit mort,* or "the little death." In Sanskrit, orgasm is referred to as *urja,* meaning "power" or "nourishment." It has been described as an altered state of consciousness, resplendent with waves, colors, light, warmth, and energy. It is said that the first mystics had glimpses of enlightenment at the moment of orgasm. Of course it doesn't need to happen this way, but simultaneous orgasms are believed by some to be one of many secrets to long-lasting love.

Sounds like pretty powerful stuff, right? Not sure whether you've ever experienced an orgasm quite that cosmically altering? With a little help, you could. Read on.

ORGASM FOR WOMEN

As a woman becomes aroused, blood begins to circulate more quickly through her body. Her face and chest may flush. Her muscles may tense; her breasts swell, and her nipples become erect. Blood engorges the labia, which become red, enlarged, and sensitive. The labia secrete mucus and become moist and slippery. The clitoris becomes hot and swollen.

At the point of orgasm, muscles in the lower third of the vagina, which is suffused with blood, contract involuntarily in intense, rhythmic, pleasurable waves of spasm. For most women, the contractions take place at a rate of about one every 0.8 seconds. Muscles in the rectum may contract in sync with the vaginal muscles. Veins and arteries in the pelvic area constrict. A woman's entire body may become rigid as the spasms continue, then totally relax as they subside and pulse, circulation, and breathing slow down.

ORGASM FOR MEN

As in a woman, arousal in a man causes blood circulation to speed up. Increased blood flow to the penis combined with the constriction of arteries and veins that allow outflow of blood from the area cause the penis to become engorged with blood. Muscles in the penis contract, and it grows erect. A man may become flushed on his lower abdomen, face, neck, chest, forearms, and thighs. He may sweat. His testicles will draw closer to the torso as orgasm approaches. The glans may darken.

The prostate and Cowper's glands may secrete a few drops of pre-ejaculate—a clear alkaline fluid that lubricates the urethra, easing the passage for sperm and neutralizing any acid that may remain from the passage of urine. When ejaculation is inevitable, the prostate contracts rhythmically, squeezing out the alkaline fluid that forms the base of semen. The seminal vesicle empties its contents into the urethra, also contributing to the seminal fluid. Sperm travels from the epididymis through the prostate and into the urethra. A series of powerful muscular contractions causes the forcible ejection of 2 to 5 ml of semen, which spurts from the tip of the penis.

After ejaculation, the muscles at the base of the penis relax. Blood flow from the penis is restored, and penile tissue becomes flaccid once again. Ejaculate that dribbles rather than shoots out may indicate a weak prostate, while a very small amount of semen may indicate digestive or muscle weakness. Semen that is clear may indicate a digestive disorder.

INTENSIFYING ORGASMS: THE SIX-STEP PROGRAM

Achieving great orgasms involves a commitment to good health, a few simple techniques, and an awareness of how to use sexual energy. Many of the sexual techniques outlined in chapter 11 and the love therapies presented in part 1 will carry you a long way on the path to intensifying orgasms. The six steps outlined here, if undertaken with goodwill and patience, can help speed your progress.

1. **Support sexual energy.** Read through chapters 1, 2 and 3, which deal with nutrition, herbs, and supplements that can be used to build and support radiant sexual health. Work with your lover to make some of the practices suggested in these chapters a part of your daily life. Try the recipes. Live healthfully. Great sex will soon be yours—naturally.
2. **Exercise the love muscles.** Practice Kegels to strengthen the muscles that control orgasm. See page 118 for more information.
3. **Be patient.** Allow yourself (or your lover) to achieve a high level of arousal before permitting orgasm. Approach and pull back from orgasm at least three times.
4. **Relax.** Let the orgasm come to you; don't force it by tightening up your muscles, though if it helps, tighten for now, until you can learn to relax more.
5. **Stimulate the nipples.** In women, the nipples share a nerve response with the clitoris; stimulating the nipples just before orgasm brings an almost leaping response of arousal from the clitoris. Men's nipples are also very sensitive to arousal just before orgasm. For either gender, try rolling the nipples between your fingers or taking them into your mouth.
6. **Visualize.** Just before orgasm, visualize sexual energy building in the genitals, radiating up the spine, and streaming into all the cells of your body. You may see that energy as a current of light or a stream of color. Breathe deeply, and direct the energy in and around your connected bodies. See yourselves enveloped in dazzling rainbow light!

Beyond these simple tricks, recognize that having great sex involves an opening of the mind. In order to be more orgasmic in love, we should be more orgasmic in life—laugh more, love more, and experience the rush of life!

Controlling Orgasm

In order to approach and then pull back from orgasm (step 3 above), we must learn to control our body's responses. One of the best ways to establish control over orgasm is to breathe more deeply and fully. Slowing down the breath promotes calmness and increases sexual stamina.

A normal heart rate is approximately 70 beats per minute; during orgasm, the heart rate can reach 140 to 180 beats per minute. Breathing rates also increase, from an average of twelve breaths per minute to thirty or forty. When you get to the brink of orgasm and want to pull back, you need to disperse the highly charged energy that suffuses your body. Try doing Kegels while pressing your tongue to the roof of your mouth. (In the tradition of Oriental medicine, touching the tongue to the soft spot of the palate helps delay ejaculation by causing energy to flow down the front of the body to the navel.) Look up or roll your eyes several times in each direction.

To delay a man's ejaculation, reach between his legs and grasp his testicles. Circle the top of the sac with your thumb and forefinger while gently tugging the testicles down, away from the torso. Men should relax enough to allow an erection to deflate somewhat at least once every twenty minutes. This allows healthy circulation of blood to move into the genitals.

Premature Ejaculation

Premature ejaculation, also referred to as rapid ejaculation or involuntary ejaculation, is sometimes defined as the inability to delay ejaculation long enough to satisfy one's partner 50 percent of the time. Other sexologists define it as ejaculating within thirty seconds, not being able to maintain vaginal contact for at least two minutes, or not being able to endure fifty strokes. Many definitions!

In fact, research has shown that the biological response of most men is to ejaculate within two minutes of vaginal penetration. Because few women can reach orgasm within that time, most men could be qualified as having premature ejaculation and could please their partner by learning to delay ejaculation. As an alternative solution, if a man learns to please a woman by oral or manual stimulation (see chapter 11) before initiating intercourse, she may not care how long he lasts, which can relieve the pressure on him. Positioning the woman on top during intercourse will cause less genital friction for the man, enabling him to hang in there longer. The woman can take frequent pauses.

Causal Factors

Stress can often be a factor in premature ejaculation. Do your best to slow down in other aspects of your life, and you may find that you'll slow down in the bedroom as well.

Premature ejaculation can also be related to diet. Excess consumption of salt and animal products (meat, dairy, and eggs) can be excessively stimulating, contributing to overexcitement. Try cutting down on salt and switching to a more vegan diet. Prostate malfunction may also be a contributing factor. See "Improving the Health of the Prostate" on page 328 for tips on supporting healthy prostate function.

In traditional Oriental medicine, premature ejaculation is considered a deficiency of the Kidneys, which can be aggravated by chronic fatigue (yin deficiency), stress, and digestive problems. If yin is deficient, the body cannot retain yang and sex will be completed quickly. Herbs that can help nourish the Kidneys include damiana, hops, ho shou wu, nutmeg, oatstraw, and saw palmetto; look up these herbs in the herbal compendium in chapter 2 to find out how to use them.

Delaying Ejaculation

A good exercise to practice delaying ejaculation is to masturbate with a dry hand. Concentrate on the sensations. Stop before you lose control and ejaculate. Breathe. Do Kegels. Continue, starting and stopping as needed, for fifteen minutes. Get a sense of what strokes and rhythms affect you. Have a goal of being able to arrive at the brink of orgasm without going "over the edge" three times within one fifteen- to twenty-minute session. When you can masturbate in this fashion reasonably well, try it with lubrication.

Because a second erection generally lasts longer than the first, some men masturbate two to four hours before intercourse. Other pre-intercourse tricks include urinating (a full bladder will increase the desire to ejaculate) and practicing the Taoist exercise called the Deer (see page 119) just before making love.

During intercourse, try to keep your buttock and pelvic muscles relaxed. When you feel the urge to ejaculate, breathe deeply and contract the abdominal muscles. Exhale deeply after the urge passes. A female partner can help you survive the moment by minimizing or stopping movement and relaxing the vaginal muscles. Also useful in preventing premature ejaculation is for the man to practice Kegels, both during intercourse when the urge to ejaculate occurs, and as a general endurance-building exercise. Kegels have an effect similar to that of the squeeze technique (see below) and are totally safe.

Another simple technique is to dip the lingam in a bowl of cold water until the erection decreases by about half. Some use a technique of rubbing an ice cube over the shaft to cool things down. As you do this, continue to caress your partner to keep the momentum of sexual energy flowing.

Some men find wearing one or two condoms decreases sensation enough to delay ejaculation. You can also try applying Clove Anesthetic Balm (see below).

CLOVE ANESTHETIC BALM

Combine 1 or 2 drops of clove essential oil with 1 or 2 ounces of coconut oil. When massaged onto the genitals, this aromatic oil brings a warm glow and has a pleasant numbing effect, which can allow for prolonged lovemaking. (Not latex friendly, though, so don't use this with a condom.)

Also highly regarded is the "squeeze technique," which helps retrain the brain to control ejaculation. Before the man reaches ejaculation, either thumb is placed firmly on the frenulum (the area underneath the head of the lingam). The first and second fingers are placed on the ridge of the glans, on the lingam's upper side, or pressing back to front at the base of the lingam. This must be done firmly enough and with constant pressing, until the urge to ejaculate has passed. Repeat for up to twenty minutes. The man must have an empty bladder before engaging in the squeeze technique. Though this is a well-known practice, it is not a first choice because it is potentially dangerous.

Orgasm without Ejaculation

Orgasm is defined by its contractions, rather than by fluid release. For men, orgasm can be achieved without erection or ejaculation. In some cases, those who have experienced nerve injuries and lost genital sensation may still experience orgasm in other parts of their bodies, including the face, lips, necks, chest, arms, and back. A whole-body orgasmic experience might include the back, legs, toes, neck, face, and brain.

Although ejaculation is often referred to as *coming, going* might be a more appropriate term for it. Ejaculation moves energy outward and can leave a man fatigued, both physically and emotionally. In the Taoist tradition, one drop of semen is considered to have the life force of one hundred drops of blood. By not ejaculating, a man can conserve the powerful energy that orgasm produces and turn it toward the development of creativity and spiritual growth. This is also an important tenet of Tantrism, a religious practice that, simplistically put, combines meditation and sex.

Some Oriental traditions encourage avoiding ejaculation one time to strengthen essence, two times to improve vision and hearing, three times to cure diseases, and more than that to have a religious experience. A plant that does not go to seed outlives the other plants in its surroundings. Likewise, a man who conserves his seed may stay healthier than he otherwise might. This is particularly true for older men or men with a weak constitution; for them, having orgasm without ejaculation can provide a reservoir of energy and vitality to draw from. In general, strong, young men can ejaculate freely without risk of harm to their health. Even these strapping men, however, would benefit from occasionally drawing in the strength of orgasm, rather than sending it out with ejaculation.

It's important to ejaculate after vigorous sex to avoid undue stress to the prostate gland. However, when lovemaking is relaxed, avoiding ejaculation should not be stressful.

If a man does not ejaculate, semen is broken down and reabsorbed by the body. It is not a waste product that needs to be eliminated. In fact, semen contains many hormones and proteins that can stimulate the pituitary gland and other creative brain centers. When analyzed, semen and brain matter have many similarities, including a rich supply of magnesium, phosphorus, sodium, and chlorine. If not ejaculated, the nutrients from semen are carried to every part of the body, including the brain.

Preventing ejaculation during orgasm requires practice. One key is breathing more slowly, through the nose and into the belly, which will slow down the heart rate. You can feel the sexual energy released by orgasm being drawn up the spine, into the brain, and throughout the entire body.

To learn more about ejaculatory control, take a tantra workshop. See the resources section on page 480.

Inability to Orgasm

Inability to orgasm during sex is a common female complaint; it is rarely experienced by men except when they have a physical dysfunction. Between 10 and 15 percent of women claim that they have never reached orgasm, and a great majority of women have had difficulty with it at one time or another. If you have never had an orgasm, don't give up hope! Consider yourself preorgasmic rather than nonorgasmic.

Most women experience their first orgasm through self-stimulation. Learning to orgasm by masturbation can teach a woman what brings her pleasure so that she can better inform and help her partner please her. If you've never had an orgasm, make a commitment to practice self-stimulation every day for two to three weeks. (See page 180 for advice.) If after this time you still haven't experienced orgasm, try using a vibrator. If that, too, doesn't help, consider consulting with a sex therapist. The American Association of Sex Educators, Counselors, and Therapists (see the resources) can help you find one in your area.

If you can experience orgasm through masturbation but have trouble achieving it consistently or during sex, read on.

Identifying Anti-Orgasm Factors

There are a variety of physical and emotional factors that can impede orgasm. Most can be resolved through lifestyle changes or natural therapies or with the help of a sex therapist.

HISTAMINE DEFICIENCY

People who have a hard time achieving orgasm may suffer from inadequate histamine release. Most of us recognize histamine release as the result of an allergic reaction. However, histamines are also contributors to the intensity and frequency of orgasms. They cause dilation of capillaries and contraction of smooth muscles. Supplementation with niacin may contribute to histamine production. See page 108 for more details.

DIETARY IMBALANCES

A diet that is overly rich in saturated fats may make a person less sensitive physically, which can have a detrimental effect on orgasmic ability. Fats have a tendency to insulate the body and decrease nerve sensitivity. They also impair circulation, which is vital to arousal and orgasm. Try eating more fruits, vegetables, nuts and seeds, and whole grains; avoid fatty meats, fried foods, and heated oils.

Supplementation with niacin has the opposite effect of a high-fat diet. It increases circulation and sensitivity to touch and can, in some cases, intensify orgasms. See page 108 for more information.

EMOTIONAL ARMORING

Be sure you are not withholding enjoyment in bed as a way of having power over your lover, or because you feel resentment toward your lover or fear losing control of yourself. Make sure you feel entitled to pleasure and are comfortable with your body. Communicate openly with your partner about your feelings and physical needs.

If you have doubts about your emotional openness and suspect it might be having a negative effect on your orgasmic ability, consider consulting with a sex therapist or other counselor.

INTELLECTUAL DISTANCING

You may have difficulty reaching orgasm if you pay too much attention to the process instead of becoming lost in the connection. That's a tough challenge for women who have difficulty achieving orgasm; of course you're going to be concerned about the process if you're concerned about your potential for orgasm. Try to relax into the lovemaking. Follow the advice given in the next section, but when it comes to the time of stimulation, do your best to enjoy the pleasure of connection rather than worrying about the outcome.

Flower essences may be helpful for those who experience emotional armoring and intellectual distancing. With the strength of their dual connection to body and mind, flower essences can be a powerful tool in the quest for orgasm. See chapter 7 for more information.

Achieving Orgasm during Sex

If you know that you're able to achieve orgasm but your lover is unable to bring you there, it's time to step up to the plate. Be responsible for your own orgasm. Stimulate yourself, or show or tell your partner how to do it. You can have wonderfully intimate lovemaking with orgasm if you will take the initiative to touch yourself during intercourse.

In fact, most women need clitoral stimulation to achieve orgasm, and it may be difficult for a lover to provide that during lovemaking, depending on the position. Only about 30 percent of women are able to achieve orgasm from penetration alone, and many of those find that the orgasm is intensified if the vaginal pressure is accompanied by clitoral stimulation.

It may be that only certain positions can bring orgasmic release for you. During intercourse, consider woman-on-top (see page 191) or rear-entry (see page 192) positions, which offer G-spot stimulation. If you're most comfortable in the missionary position, try the coital alignment technique (see page 191), which can bring the man's pubic bone in contact with your clitoris. Many women find that the only method by which their lovers can bring them to orgasm is oral sex. If you are lying on your back, try placing pillows under your pelvis to arch the clitoris toward better stimulus. Find out what works and communicate with each other about it.

Try massaging your breasts or nipples, or having your lover do so, when you have reached a just-preorgasmic state of arousal. Bear down with the vaginal muscles upon your man's penis or fingers. Make sounds of pleasure as you approach orgasm; sometimes sound can help you let go into bliss.

Women are often more orgasmic around ovulation. If you're tired of trying and failing to reach orgasm, you may want to designate the week or so after menstruation ends, when ovulation usually happens and sex hormones are highest, for the lovemaking sessions in which you make a real effort to achieve orgasm. And remember: It's not necessary to experience orgasm every time you have sex. Expecting to do so is unrealistic and sets you up for disappointment. Whether or not orgasm occurs, we can still experience extreme levels of pleasure and a deep connection with a lover.

Female Ejaculation

When deeply stimulated, some women emit a fluid that is called, technically, female ejaculate but that is more poetically named in various traditions amrita (Sanskrit for "immortal"), moon flower medicine, or female nectar. In the Hindu tradition, female ejaculation stimulates a tremendous release of kundalini, or life force, which travels up the woman's spine and down to her yoni, blessing the woman, her lover, and the planet.

About one in ten women are able to achieve female ejaculation. And more are learning to do it every day! The ejaculate is a spurt of fluid released through the urethra. It is believed to originate from the ductus paraurethrales, also known as the Skene's glands, which are vestigial organs located behind the vaginal wall. (Not all women have them.) The liquid is similar to prostate fluid, containing high levels of glucose and acid phosphatase.

Female ejaculation seems to occur more frequently with the second or third orgasm. It is most likely to be achieved when a woman's G-spot is stimulated.

The G-Spot

The G-spot is named after Ernest Grafenberg (1881–1957), a German gynecologist practicing in the United States who published a paper about it in 1950. Yet long before Dr. Grafenberg's time, this sacred spot was known to Indian, Chinese, Roman, and Japanese cultures, as well as many others, I'm sure. This is an area that can give intense pleasure when stimulated but can release strong emotions that have been stored within it, creating an ultimate, sometimes life-changing, experience.

The G-spot can be felt from inside the vagina, on the front of the vaginal wall, 1½ to 2 inches up from the entrance. The tissue there is spongy and has many tiny folds that cause the skin to feel bumpy. A woman can reach inside herself to feel it, but it's usually a stretch, so it can be difficult to stimulate the G-spot during masturbation.

This G-spot area is richly endowed with nerve endings, ducts, and glands, and when a woman is aroused, it swells to about the size of a dime. The swelling appears to help protect the bladder and urethra from injury and stress during intercourse.

To find a woman's G-spot, have her lie on her back, knees apart and slightly elevated. Start by massaging her belly, and then the areas around her genitals to help her relax. Ask permission to enter, then insert a finger into her yoni with the pad of your finger facing up. Feel for the pubic bone at the front of the vaginal wall; there's a small "ledge" of sorts there, and the G-spot is just above it. Fold your finger forward in a "come hither" motion and you'll find it. You'll know you have it when the pressure of your finger causes the woman to feel an urge to urinate, even if she has just done so. If you keep up the pressure and the woman relaxes into it, the urge to urinate will pass, transformed into sexual pleasure. She can stimulate her clitoris at the same time.

The most effective way to stimulate the G-spot is to apply prolonged steady pressure and stroke it gently from left to right, pulse against it, or massage the spot in a circular motion. Gently pushing down on the mound of Venus (mons veneris) with your other hand can enhance your lover's pleasure. If she experiences pain, move to another area, then come back to the painful area briefly.

For a woman experiencing G-spot stimulation, it is important to breathe. Let go of having to control. Surrender to a supreme pleasure that can enable you to have more creativity, trust, and bliss. It is not unusual for G-spot stimulation to trigger a release of emotions or memories. Be there to comfort and support your partner if this occurs. Thank your lover for trusting. Allow the surfacing of old emotions to be healing and cleansing.

To stimulate the G-spot through intercourse, the best positions are rear entry, man on top (with the woman's feet on his shoulders), yab yum, woman on top, or woman lying on her stomach. (See "Sexual Positions" beginning on page 189 for explanations.)

A corollary to the G-spot in men is the prostate gland, located about three inches inside the anal canal. It swells when aroused and can increase a man's sexual pleasure.

The A-Spot

Stimulation of the A-spot, more formally known as the anterior fornix or *fornix vaginae,* can trigger women to have copious vaginal lubrication and also, as has been reported, multiple orgasms. The A-spot is located above the G-spot on the front wall of the vagina, between it and the cervix. To locate the A-spot, moisten two fingers, insert them into the vagina, and find the G-spot (see previous section). Continue upward until you find the cervix, which feels like the end of a nose sniffing down into the vagina. Bring your fingers back down to a spot about one-third of the way down from the cervix to the G-spot. If you can find a smooth area of the wall here that your lover says feels sensitive, you've found the A-spot. Try stimulating this spot in a circular or up-and-down motion.

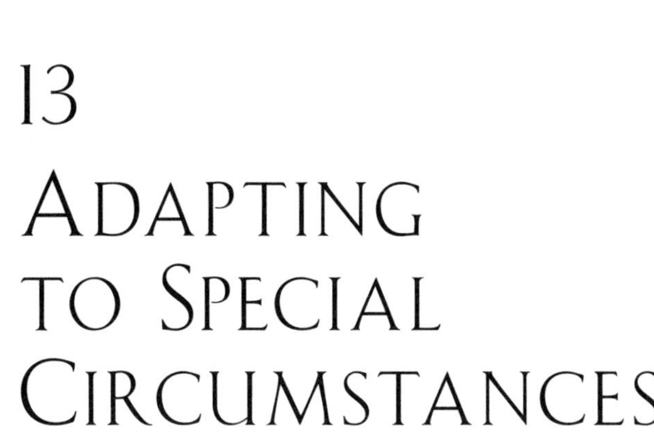

13 Adapting to Special Circumstances

DURING A LIFETIME, MANY special circumstances arise that can affect sexuality. Menstruation, pregnancy, illness, and disabilities can all challenge the sexual habits you and your lover are accustomed to. You may find yourself with a lover whose large or small build must be accommodated. And as you grow older, you'll find that your sexual needs and abilities also grow and change, requiring new ways of thinking about sexuality.

Humans are sexual beings. Thankfully, we are also amazingly adaptable. When we find ourselves faced with circumstances that challenge our sexual comfort zone, we figure out a way—usually with great speed—to handle them. This chapter offers ideas for handling some of the more common "special" circumstances.

LOSING VIRGINITY

You will always remember your first time, so do your best to create a moment worth remembering, with someone worthy. If you and your lover are both virgins, learning together and teaching each other can be one of the sweetest pleasures on earth. An intact hymen is an indicator of virginity for a woman, but a woman who is a virgin may not necessarily have an intact hymen. Athletic pursuits and even tampon use can stretch and even break the hymen. If the hymen has not been broken, the woman may experience some pain and bleeding the first time she has intercourse. If you're concerned about the potential for bleeding and staining the sheets, place a thick towel underneath you.

Allow for plenty of time, privacy, and freedom from interruptions. The missionary position is a good choice for your first time, because it allows good eye contact and verbal communication. Make sure that the woman is sufficiently aroused and has good vaginal lubrication before penetration. Penetration itself should be slow and gentle, and thrusting should also be gentle. Prolonged pressing and pushing can be painful for a woman during her first experience with intercourse.

Women may not experience orgasm during their first time, though most men will. Men tend to orgasm very quickly their first time.

Do all you can to make the experience of losing your virginity safe and pleasant. It can color how you feel about sex for years to come. Remember that sex can definitely get you pregnant—even your first time—so be sure to use adequate birth control. See the section on contraception on page 227.

SEX DURING MENSTRUATION

Many people enjoy making love during a woman's menstrual time. However, sex during menstruation is considered taboo by Native American, Jewish, and Arab cultures, among others. And traditional Oriental medicine cautions that having intercourse during the menses "brings illness to both men and women."

These warnings come for a reason. Having sex during menstruation does carry risks, although they are relatively low. The vagina is normally acidic, which helps destroy invading bacteria. During the menses, it becomes more alkaline, which can leave a woman susceptible to infection. In addition, menstrual blood washes away some of the naturally occurring mucus that covers the cervix, making it easier for infection to penetrate her reproductive system.

Intercourse during menstruation can push menstrual flow back into the uterus and fallopian tubes, which can be a contributing factor to endometriosis. For this reason, those who are prone to reproductive disorders or who have been diagnosed with endometriosis should avoid intercourse during menstruation. If you do engage in intercourse, the woman-on-top position has a lesser likelihood of pushing blood back inside the woman's uterus.

But you'll notice that these warnings apply only to intercourse, in which the penis penetrates the vagina. Manual stimulation does not offer any risks to the woman, nor does oral sex. (If you practice oral sex, use a dental dam or other barrier device to prevent oral-blood contact.) But as my beloved Floridian husand once said, "Honey, if mah thang was dripping blood, wouldn't you want to wait a few days?"

Beyond sex, it's a loving gesture to be especially considerate of a woman just before and during her menstrual time. For many women, menstruation causes cramps, bloating, fatigue, and mood swings. So treat your beloved with extra kindness, speak softly, do your best to minimize stress, and try to avoid being demanding yourself.

SEX DURING PREGNANCY

Kidney chi works to support pregnancy and can give women a healthy, beautiful glow. Some women also experience an increase in libido due to increased blood flow to the pelvic region. Others experience a decrease in libido due to hormonal changes, fatigue, morning sickness, and the body's desire to conserve Kidney chi.

Sex during pregnancy is a given for most couples. It's nine months, after all! However, there are some precautions. Women who have a history of miscarriage may be cautioned to refrain from intercourse in the early months, until the pregnancy is well established. Some physicians may suggest that lovers use a condom during pregnancy, because hormone-like substances in ejaculate may trigger contractions and pose a risk of infection for the woman. And when a woman is late in her pregnancy, intercourse should be approached gently; recent research indicates that rough, vigorous intercourse late in a pregnancy may be linked to premature labor and respiratory disease in newborns.

Approached gently, sex generally will not induce labor unless it is already about to begin. However, avoid intercourse if you experience uterine bleeding or vaginal pain, or if your water has broken—that is, if the membrane enclosing the amniotic fluid has ruptured.

Massage, oral sex, and manual sex can all become a greater part of lovemaking during pregnancy. Anal intercourse is not recommended during pregnancy because it causes the rectum to be pushed against the vagina, which could initiate labor.

Sexual positions that can accommodate a woman's belly during the later stages of pregnancy include woman on top, rear entry, and spooning. Of course, no position is prohibited; you just have to get creative.

Most women can resume intercourse six weeks after giving birth vaginally; healing after a cesarean section may take longer. When you do resume lovemaking, go very slowly and gently, and use lubrication.

Breast-feeding does inhibit fertility, but it doesn't prevent it. If you have sex while you're breast-feeding, use contraception. When my husband was only six weeks old, his mother became pregnant with his brother! Are you ready for two babies in diapers?

New parents must work hard to find alone time and ways to keep the love that brought them together in the first place flourishing. Make an effort to show and share love for each other. See the techniques for keeping your love alive in chapter 21.

SEX FOR SENIORS

As long as you're in good health, sexual activity need never end. Despite the physical changes that accompany aging, sex and orgasm can feel as pleasurable as ever for older folks. Some couples say that the older they get, the better sex gets. Indeed, sex itself can ease the aging process. Research has shown that humans are likely to die at younger ages if they are deprived of touch. And practicing nonejaculatory sex (see page 210) can help a man build sexual chi and improve his energy level.

Testosterone levels—a factor in sexual desire in both sexes—decrease with age. On the other hand, as men age, they often are able to extend the duration of erection, experience longer periods of high sexual excitement, and become more emotionally open with others. They will also experience viropause (also known as andropause), the male version of menopause; sperm production normally ends while men are in their seventies.

The healthier life you lead, the better things will go. Older men may need longer and more direct stimulation to achieve erection, and their erections may be less firm and less upright. The scrotal sac may not bunch up during arousal as much as it used to, and testicle size may diminish. There may be less ejaculate and less ejaculatory force. Frequency and desire for masturbation may also decrease. A man's refractory period (the time needed between ejaculations) may also become longer. As throughout their lives, however, men's sex drive will be highest in the morning; that's often a good time for older couples to make love.

For women, fear of pregnancy ceases to be an issue after menopause. However, women can become pregnant during menopause, so be sure to use contraception for twelve months following a woman's last period. After the menopausal drop in estrogen levels, blood flow to the vagina may diminish; vaginal walls may become thinner and less elastic and may take longer to produce lubrication. The vagina may shorten in width and length. However, these changes do not equate to changes in sensitivity or orgasmic ability. In fact, women often become more orgasmic as they age. You go, girl!

Staying physically fit can help older men and women stay sexually active. At this stage of life, exercise and a healthy diet are more important than ever. Avoid habits such as smoking and heavy drinking. Be aware of the side effects of any medication you are taking. Many prescription drugs decrease libido and sexual ability; if your health care provider prescribes one of these medications for you, ask him or her if there are alternative treatments that do not diminish libido as a side effect.

When you do make love, spend some extra time on foreplay, allowing the woman adequate time to accumulate sufficient vaginal lubrication. Use a lubricant if necessary. Mutual masturbation and oral sex may become increasingly easier than intercourse. Laugh and play together to keep your love alive.

SEX DURING ILLNESS OR DISABLEMENT

Like everybody else, people with a disability have a fundamental need for intimacy. Whether a disability is temporary or permanent, it does not preclude the possibility of being sexual with a lover. If you have any particular concerns, discuss them with your health care provider. Otherwise, get creative and experiment!

It's important to let go of the belief that sex must be spontaneous. A love exchange with a person who is ill or disabled often requires some planning. At the very least, you'll need to discuss what hurts and what can and cannot give pleasure. You may also need to gather props to help minimize discomfort and maximize the connection and pleasure that you feel. The stronger partner should take the more dominant role, although the disabled partner may need to take the responsibility of communicating his or her needs.

If your lover is in pain, allow him or her to lie, sit, or stand in a position that is most comfortable, and find a lovemaking position that accommodates it. (See "Sexual Positions" on page 189 for suggestions.) Use chairs, pillows, or whatever else is needed to cushion vulnerable areas such as the knees, neck, or back. Make love slowly, while the stronger partner visualizes sending healing energy into his or her beloved. A person with heart disease should avoid lying facedown or on his or her left side, as these positions increase pressure on the heart.

If a disability is new, begin slowly with manual pleasuring and work up to intercourse only when you feel ready. If illness or an accident has caused loss of sensation in the genitals, it is very possible that other areas of the body will increase in sensitivity and enjoy stimulation. If intercourse isn't the ticket, there are plenty of other possibilities. Pleasure can be experienced by all parts of the body! Keep communication open, and share with each other your thoughts on what hurts and what feels good. The counsel of a marriage or sex therapist may be helpful.

A loving, open-minded partner is a true blessing for anyone, but especially for a person with a disability. Let your partner know that you appreciate his or her help and patience. Allow your inner radiance to shine.

SIZING DIFFERENCES

Men and women come in all different shapes and sizes. Many men take great pride in the size of their penis, but the size of one penis compared to others matters little. All that matters is the fit of penis and vagina together. Vaginal tissues are elastic and can accommodate almost any size. In certain situations, however, couples have to make some adjustments to ensure a pleasurable fit. Finding ways to fit together is part of the challenge—and delight—of a loving relationship!

Large Penis/Small Vagina

When the lingam is much larger than the yoni, engage in plenty of foreplay and use plenty of lubricant. If possible, bring the woman to orgasm with manual or oral stimulation before penetration, so that the vaginal passage is naturally lubricated.

The man should insert the lingam in stages and proceed slowly until the woman is receptive. She should breathe slowly and relax. If the penetration becomes uncomfortable, the man and woman should lie motionless for a few seconds, until the vagina has adjusted to the penis. The woman may enjoy the woman-on-top position, because it gives her greater control of the penetration.

If the lingam is too long rather than too wide, try having intercourse with the woman lying on her back, with her legs straight and close together, and the man on top, with his legs placed outside hers. This position prevents overly deep penetration. The side-by-side position may also be comfortable.

Small Penis/Large Vagina

In this situation, both partners should practice Kegels (see page 118). For a woman, the Kegels will strengthen the muscles in her vagina that contract around the penis, holding it to her. For a man, the Kegels will increase endurance, allowing him to last longer and maximize his ability to please a woman through intercourse.

As always, penetration is not the best method for bringing a woman to orgasm, and in this situation it is especially true. The man may wish to pleasure the woman with manual or oral stimulation before intercourse.

To encourage a tight fit during intercourse, employ sexual positions in which the woman's legs are kept close together. For the missionary position, place pillows under the woman's back to allow the man deep access in the pelvis. The woman might try wrapping both legs over the man's shoulders, which will constrict the yoni and allow for deeper access. Other beneficial positions include rear entry and woman on top, leaning slightly backward.

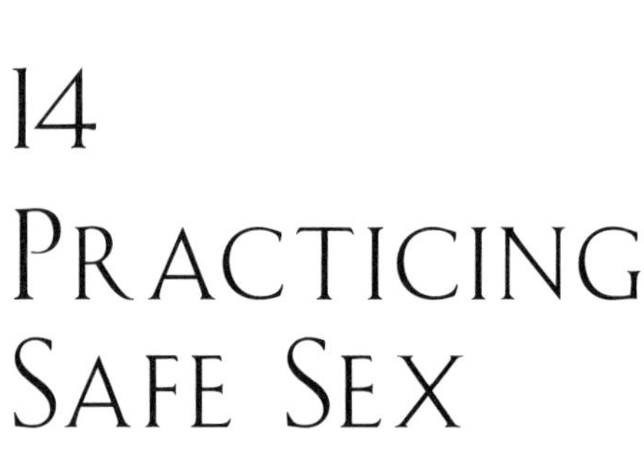

14 Practicing Safe Sex

BIRTH CONTROL HAS BECOME a ubiquitous fact of Western civilization. Condoms are available at every corner store; the Pill, as it's called, is covered under some health care plans. Even the Roman Catholic Church, known for its firm stand against birth control, advocates and teaches "fertility awareness," a natural method of avoiding pregnancy. The pregnancy rate in the United States is dropping, and it's not because we're having less sex. Contraception enables family planning, and more and more people are choosing to have fewer children, and to have them later in life.

But pregnancy isn't the only risk of sex. Sexually transmitted diseases (STDs) are among the most contagious diseases known to afflict humankind. They are widespread and often asymptomatic (meaning that they don't produce symptoms), and their effects range from irritating to debilitating to deadly.

Certain types of contraception are supposed to safeguard users against these infectious diseases. But if contraception is so widely available, why, then, do STDs continue to spread so quickly? Hepatitis C and HIV—each a very scary disease—have infected vast populations of people. Genital herpes affects one-sixth of all sexually active people. The numbers are staggering.

The reasons for this are twofold.

1. Most sexually active people don't know enough about STDs. They don't know how they're spread, what their symptoms are, or which activities can and cannot put them at risk of contracting an STD.
2. Most sexually active people resist using contraception to its full potential. They focus on preventing pregnancy rather than STDs, even if they are having sex with multiple partners. Many pursue this reckless path because they believe that "safe" equates to "boring." Not so, my friends. Proper use of contraception can be as much a part of foreplay and arousal as kissing. You just have to open your mind to it.

PROTECTING YOURSELF AGAINST STDS

There are two categories of contraception: contraception that protects you against pregnancy alone and contraception that protects you against STDs and pregnancy. If you are not having monogamous sex, you must employ the latter.

Both men and women need to be responsible for taking measures to ensure safe sex. In most heterosexual relationships, the responsibility for contraception falls to the woman. That's unfortunate, because the best prevention against STDs is a condom. Men may complain that the condom barrier reduces the pleasurable sensations of intercourse, but honestly, that's a lousy excuse for exposing a partner to possible STD infection. If lovers want to engage in barrier-free sex, they should get tested and begin a monogamous relationship.

If you and a partner want to have a monogamous relationship, get tested together. Practice safe sex for six months, using STD-prevention contraception, and remain monogamous. Get tested again. If the results are negative, then enjoy each other freely and delightfully, using a nonbarrier method of contraception if you wish to avoid pregnancy.

No method of contraception is absolutely foolproof against pregnancy or STDs, but they sure do cut down your risk. Remember: It takes only one unsafe sexual encounter to expose yourself to a disease that could stay with you for life.

Minimizing Risk

Risk-free activities include:

- abstinence;
- hugging;
- massage (see page 159);
- kissing, so long as neither person has gum disease or open sores in the mouth;
- genital massage (see page 185), so long as your partner does not have any genital sores; and
- masturbation.

Low-risk activities include:

- monogamous sex with a partner who is free of disease.

High-risk activities include:

- vaginal intercourse without use of a condom;
- anal intercourse without use of a condom;
- sexual activity in which semen, vaginal secretions, or blood are exchanged;
- oral-anal contact;
- moving an item (including a finger) directly from anal to genital contact, without washing it first;
- oral sex without use of a barrier, such as a condom or dental dam;
- sharing sex toys or douching supplies; and
- sexual activity with an infected partner without use of proper safeguards to prevent transmission of disease.

Safeguards against STDs

The only sure way to eliminate your risk of contracting an STD is abstinence, plain and simple. For most of us, that's not an option. The following methods, however, can substantially reduce the STD risk.

STD TESTING

Before engaging in unprotected sex, you and your partner should undergo a thorough physical, including examination and testing for STDs. Practice safe, STD-prevention sex for six months and go through another round of testing before abandoning your concerns about potential STD infection.

CONDOMS

Condoms, including female condoms, are key to STD prevention. They should be used for vaginal, anal, and even oral sex. (Condoms designed for oral sex come in many flavors.) They should be used once and then discarded.

DENTAL DAMS

Dental dams are small squares of latex used by dentists that have been appropriated as an effective barrier for vaginal-oral and anal-oral contact. In a pinch, household plastic wrap can also be used. They should be used once and then discarded.

SPERMICIDES

Spermicidal creams, foams, and jellies were designed to reduce the risk of pregnancy, but they have also been shown to kill herpes, syphilis, gonorrhea, and Trichomoniasis organisms. The active ingredient in most spermicides sold in the United States is nonoxynol-9. In laboratory studies, nonoxynol-9 has been shown to kill HIV; however, whether it can offer increased protection against HIV in the vagina has yet to be proved. The compound does sometimes irritate vaginal tissue, which can make a woman susceptible to HIV infection.

DIAPHRAGMS

Diaphragms are rubber vaginal inserts that cover the cervix, denying sperm access to a woman's ova. They can offer some protection against diseases that tend to affect the cervix, such as chlamydia and gonorrhea. They are best used in combination with a spermicide. They can be reused, provided that they are removed and washed after each use.

CONTRACEPTION

Once barrier-free sex is possible, heterosexual lovers have two choices: try for pregnancy or use birth control. The latter is described here.

Much of the traditional wisdom about herbal contraceptives has disappeared, though it surely must have existed in the past: although having kids is natural, individual people have always had to find ways to keep it from getting out of hand. I hope the future introduces healthy, sex friendly, and effective methods of birth control as all of the current choices have concerns. New methods become available every few years, though they all vary in effectiveness. Each method's rate of success as a means of birth control is given in the descriptions that follow.

Condoms

EFFECTIVENESS AS A METHOD OF BIRTH CONTROL: 85–98 PERCENT

Condoms are designed to sheath an erect penis. To be effective, they must be put on before the penis comes in contact with the vagina, because even preseminal fluid can contain sperm. For maximum effectiveness, they should be used in combination with a spermicide; the spermicide should be placed in the vagina before intercourse.

Condoms are available just about everywhere—pharmacies, grocery stores, convenience stores, and so on. They're even available in some public bathrooms, although I wouldn't recommend taking advantage of this convenience unless the condom dispenser offers high-quality, name-brand condoms. Condoms of unknown origin are of unknown quality and, therefore, unknown effectiveness.

If you keep condoms in stock, store them away from extremes of heat and cold, and honor the expiration date posted on the packaging.

Lubrication on the outside of the condom can help prevent it from breaking. An additional drop of lubricant placed on the head of the penis before the condom is rolled on can create a soft, moist, pleasant sensory experience. Some condoms are prelubricated; with others, you have to add the lubricant yourself. Use only water-based lubricants, since oil-based products, including lotions, mineral oil, and petroleum jelly, can quickly degrade the latex barrier. You can purchase water-based lubricants at most pharmacies and at any store that sells "sensuality" supplies.

Putting on a condom can be worked into foreplay. A man's partner can help him slip one on, giving him a genital massage at the same time. If the man is uncircumcised, gently push the foreskin back first. Then expel the air from the tip of the condom and place it over the head of the penis. Slowly unroll the condom down over the shaft of the penis, leaving just a pinch of space at the tip of the penis, so that when the man ejaculates, there is room for the ejaculate in the condom. (Otherwise, the condom may burst.)

When unrolled completely, the condom should fit smoothly over the penis and extend almost to the base of the shaft.

After ejaculation, the condom must be removed carefully—before the man's erection has completely subsided—to prevent semen from leaking into the vagina. The man should withdraw from the vagina while holding the condom securely at the base. Take care that any semen that may end up on the fingers or hands is not transferred into the vagina. Do not flush the used condom down the toilet; it is not biodegradable and can cause the plumbing to back up.

Don't suggest that you and your partner use a condom; assume that you will. Both men and women should carry condoms. Just imagine—if someone tries to convince you to have unprotected sex, he or she will likely have convinced others. And that means that he or she has been at risk of contracting an STD.

A common male rationale for not using a condom is that it isn't big enough to fit him. There's a quick fix for that situation. Open the condom and unroll it over your hand, wrist, and arm, being careful of your fingernails. Most condoms are quite stretchy and can reach your elbow. Ask your "big" man how much bigger than that he is.

ALTERNATIVES TO LATEX

Many people have a sensitivity to latex. In that case, lambskin and polyurethane condoms are options. Many people feel that lambskin condoms offer a man greater penile sensitivity than either latex or polyurethane ones. However, lambskin is more porous than latex and may not prevent transmission of HIV. If a man is sensitive to latex, he can apply a lambskin condom first, then a latex one over it. If a woman is sensitive to latex, her partner can apply a latex condom first, then a lambskin one over it.

Polyurethane condoms have a porosity similar to that of latex. They are also safe to use with any kind of lubricant, including those that are oil based.

IF A CONDOM BREAKS

If a man senses that a condom has broken or is coming loose, he should pull out immediately. If the condom has broken or come loose before the man has ejaculated, simply remove it and apply another one. If the malfunction occurs during or after ejaculation, the woman should urinate immediately. Do not douche or insert spermicidal creams into the vagina, as they may actually push sperm along in their journey. Wash with soap and water, apply some spermicide to your outer genitals, and consider taking emergency contraception ("the morning-after pill"), especially if you are near ovulation.

Female Condoms

EFFECTIVENESS AS A METHOD OF BIRTH CONTROL: 76 PERCENT

A female condom looks like an enlarged, unrolled male condom. It has a ring at either end; one end is open, and one end is closed. The ring at the closed end is inserted into the vagina and helps hold the sheath in place during intercourse. The ring at the open end provides passage for the penis. Female condoms are made of polyurethane, are usually prelubricated, and do not need to be used in combination with a spermicide. Although they are somewhat less effective than the male condom at preventing pregnancy, they are good protection against both pregnancy and STDs, and they're available just about everywhere male condoms are sold.

The female condom can be inserted up to eight hours in advance of intercourse. You may wish to apply a drop or two of a lubricant (oil- or water-based) to the closed end to ease the insertion. Squeeze the ring at the closed end and insert it into the vagina, pushing it up just about as far as it will go. When the ring is let loose, it springs back into shape and covers the cervix. The other end of the sheath remains outside the vagina, partially covering the labia.

To remove the condom after intercourse, twist the outer ring to trap semen inside the sheath and gently pull it out. Female condoms are designed for one-time use, so dispose of the used condom. Do not flush it down the toilet, because it can clog the plumbing.

Diaphragms and Cervical Caps

EFFECTIVENESS AS A METHOD OF BIRTH CONTROL: DIAPHRAGM, 80–94 PERCENT; CERVICAL CAP, 74–91 PERCENT

Diaphragms and cervical caps are soft, rubber cups that fit over the cervix and prevent sperm from passing through the cervical opening. A diaphragm looks like a small saucer; a cervical cap is the size of a large thimble. Each comes in different sizes and must be fitted to the user; your gynecologist or a practitioner at a family-planning clinic will assist you in choosing one and learning to insert it. Diaphragms and cervical caps must be used with a spermicide. They offer some protection against STDs that affect the cervix, such as chlamydia and gonorrhea.

A diaphragm or cervical cap can be inserted up to eight hours before sex. Spread a layer of spermicide over the inside of the cup. Squeeze the sides of the cup together and, while squatting or standing with one leg raised, insert the cup into the vagina, pushing it up and back toward the cervix. You should feel it lock into place. Confirm that the diaphragm or cervical cap is in the correct position by reaching in and making sure you can feel the cervix behind the rubber cup. A properly fitted cup should not cause any discomfort.

The diaphragm or cervical cap should be left in place for at least eight hours after intercourse to give the spermicide time to do its work. If intercourse is repeated, use of a diaphragm will require that you first insert more spermicide into the vagina, without removing the cup. With a cervical cap, additional spermicide is not necessary for repeated intercourse.

A diaphragm should be removed within twenty-four hours; if it's left in for longer than forty-eight hours, toxic shock syndrome becomes a risk. A cervical cap can be left in for up to forty-eight hours.

To remove a diaphragm or cervical cap, simply reach inside the vagina and gently pull it out. Wash the device carefully in warm, soapy water. Check for tears or holes. If you don't find any, let it dry, and store in a cool place. If you do find perforations in the cup, discard it and see your gynecologist for a replacement.

The fit of a diaphragm or cervical cap should be reexamined by your gynecologist in the event that you gain or lose twenty pounds or more, or after miscarriage, childbirth, or pelvic surgery.

Diaphragms and cervical caps have very few negative side effects. Some women report an increased rate of bladder infection. Others report a sensitivity to the rubber material. And, of course, the cups are not foolproof. They may shift around during intercourse and are not a guaranteed method of birth control. They are best used in combination with a condom. They should not be used during the menses, as they can contribute to toxic shock syndrome. Note that the cervical cap has a high failure rate in women who have given birth but a very low failure rate in women who have not.

Vaginal Contraceptive Film (VCF)

EFFECTIVENESS AS A METHOD OF BIRTH CONTROL: **90** PERCENT

VCF is a fairly recent arrival in the U.S. marketplace, although it has been around for years in Europe. It's a thin film that contains spermicides. Simply fold the film in fourths and insert it into the vagina, pushing it up as close to the cervix as possible. The film must be applied at least ten minutes before intercourse, and a new film should be applied if intercourse is repeated. The film dissolves; it does not need to be removed. This method of birth control is less messy than some other spermicide methods, but frequent use may cause vaginal irritation.

Contraceptive Sponge

EFFECTIVENESS AS A METHOD OF BIRTH CONTROL: **84–91** PERCENT

This is a method that combines a barrier with a spermicide. It is effective for twenty-four hours and can be used multiple times without removing. However, it does not protect against STDs.

Emergency Contraception

EFFECTIVENESS AS A METHOD OF BIRTH CONTROL: **76–99** PERCENT

Emergency contraception is often referred to as the "morning-after pill," but in fact it can be an effective method of birth control up to seventy-two hours (three days) after unprotected sex. It should be reserved for emergency situations in which a woman has forgotten to use birth control, the chosen method of birth control did not work properly, or a woman was raped.

Emergency contraception consists of a concentrated dose of hormones that stops the ovary from releasing an egg, and changes the lining of the uterus so that the egg cannot implant there. Two doses are taken, the second dose coming twelve hours after the first. Do not use emergency contraception if you are pregnant and think you might continue the pregnancy. Possible side effects include nausea, vomiting, dizziness, headache, and spotting. Taking the pill with food will minimize the side effects. If you suffer from nausea, drink ginger tea to settle your stomach. If you throw up within thirty minutes of a dose or become too sick to complete the second dose, seek the guidance of the clinic from which you obtained the contraception.

OBTAINING EMERGENCY CONTRACEPTION

For information on health care practitioners in your area who can provide emergency contraception, contact the Emergency Contraception Hotline: 1-800-584-9911.

Fertility Awareness

EFFECTIVENESS AS A METHOD OF BIRTH CONTROL: 80–95 PERCENT

Fertility awareness is a method of natural birth control effective only for the disciplined, organized woman. It involves tracking the fertility cycle and practicing abstinence or using contraception during the times when a woman is able to conceive. To avoid pregnancy, a woman should not have unprotected sex from seven days before ovulation to three days after.

With this method, there are three signs to keep track of: basal body temperature, cervical mucus, and the menstrual "rhythm." Monitoring all three signs can offer a very effective means of birth control. As a side benefit, a woman practicing fertility awareness will become more familiar with her body's rhythms.

New fertility awareness tools are becoming available that help you view your saliva through a handheld microscope. During fertile times, saliva forms an easy to discern fernlike pattern. One brand available is called Ovu-Tech. This method should be used in conjunction with charting one's temperature and cervical mucus.

BASAL BODY TEMPERATURE

Basal body temperature is the temperature of the body at the beginning of the day. (*Basal* means "of the base" or "of the foundation.") To monitor your basal body temperature, you can use a basal body thermometer, which can measure temperature in tenths of a degree. A regular thermometer is fine, however (and less expensive), as long as it distinguishes temperatures by tenths of a degree. Take your temperature every morning, before you even get out of bed. Keep track of your body's temperature over the course of a few cycles. Most women's basal body temperature rises slightly, just less than one degree Fahrenheit, just after ovulation. It remains elevated until menstruation begins, and then it slowly drops back down to the pre-ovulation temperature.

CERVICAL MUCUS

Women normally experience a vaginal discharge—mucus produced by the cervix—at different times in their fertility cycle. The fluid varies in texture and quantity depending on the stage of the fertility cycle. Monitoring cervical mucus, then, is an excellent way to monitor a woman's fertility. This method is sometimes called the Billings or ovulation method.

Cervical mucus is thought to be an expediter of sorts for semen; it smoothes the passage of sperm from the top of the vagina to the traveling ovum. Below is a list of the various types of mucus as they appear during a woman's cycle.

1. Menstruation begins. Menstruation generally signals the end of a fertile cycle. The endometrium is being shed, and new eggs are developing in several follicles. For many women, particularly those who often or occasionally experience short cycles, menstruation is not a safe time for intercourse. Sperm can survive for several days inside the vagina, and sperm ejaculated during the time of menstruation can fertilize the egg of a woman who ovulates quickly after menstruation. If a woman begins to discharge cervical mucus toward the end of menstruation, the mucus may not be noticed until menstruation stops.
2. Menstruation ends. Most women experience several "dry" days after menstruation, when no cervical fluid is present. A woman is not fertile during a dry period.
3. Mucus appears. The first sign of cervical fluid is a sign of approaching ovulation. The mucus will grow in volume and become more slippery over the course of the next few days. A woman is fertile during this time and should refrain from intercourse if she does not wish to become pregnant.
4. Mucus disappears. When slippery cervical fluid becomes dry or tacky and opaque and gradually disappears, a woman's time of fertility has ended. From this point until the time of her next menses, she cannot conceive.

THE RHYTHM METHOD

The Rhythm method (sometimes called the Calendar method) involves keeping close track of menstruation. Generally speaking, the period of fertility is assumed to fall halfway between the first bleeding day of one menses and the first bleeding day of the next menses. The woman assumes she is fertile from four days before to four days after the halfway point. For this method to work, of course, you must be reasonably certain of when your next menses will occur, and so your menses must be regular. Chart your cycles for six to twelve months to establish the pattern before relying on this method.

If these natural methods of birth control appeal to you, find a competent fertility awareness counselor who can offer instruction and guidance. The techniques I've described here are only a brief sketch; successful fertility awareness requires further training in the methodology.

INJECTABLE CONTRACEPTIVES

EFFECTIVENESS AS A METHOD OF BIRTH CONTROL: 99 PERCENT

There are two types of injectable contraceptives currently available in the United States. One, currently marketed under the trade name Depo-Provera, is a progestin (a progesterone-like hormone). The other, marketed under the trade name Lunelle, contains both progestin and estrogen. They are very effective methods of birth control. However, they do not offer any protection against STDs.

There are several other injectable contraceptives that are not currently approved for use in the United States. They can be classified in either the progestin or the progestin-and-estrogen category.

If, after reading the descriptions that follow, you think you'd like to use injectable contraceptives, consult with your gynecologist.

DEPO-PROVERA (PROGESTIN)

Depo-Provera contains depot-medroxyprogesterone acetate, a man-made hormone that greatly resembles progesterone. This progestin prevents ovulation and also thickens cervical mucus so that sperm can't penetrate it. It gives no protection against STDs. The injection is given once every three months; you'll need to schedule an appointment with your gynecologist for each injection.

More than 80 percent of women who use Depo-Provera stop menstruating after three to four injections. When you stop using Depo-Provera, it can take nine to eighteen months for menstruation and fertility to return.

Depo-Provera should not be used if you are pregnant, have unexplained vaginal bleeding, have or have had breast cancer, are taking certain medications, or have diabetes, liver dysfunction, high blood pressure, heart disease, or serious depression.

Side effects can include depression, weight gain, irregular menses, absence of menses, headache, breast tenderness, nausea, appetite change, skin rash, hair loss or growth (on the face or the body), dizziness, abdominal distress, nervousness, and change in libido.

LUNELLE (PROGESTIN AND ESTROGEN)

Lunelle contains both progestin and estrogen. The progestin, like that found in Depo-Provera, prevents ovulation and thickens the cervical mucus. The estrogen promotes a monthly menstrual cycle. The Lunelle injection must be received every month. Lunelle holds an advantage over progestin-only methods of contraception in that fertility is recovered quickly after the contraception is discontinued. Ovulation and predictable menstrual cycles begin one to two months afterward.

Lunelle should not be used if you are pregnant, have abnormal vaginal bleeding, are taking certain medications, have a history of breast or uterine cancer, or have high blood pressure, elevated cholesterol levels, heart disease, liver dysfunction, or diabetes. Women over the age of thirty-five who smoke heavily are also discouraged from using Lunelle.

Side effects include nausea, breast tenderness, skin changes, and fluid retention. Women who use a contraceptive method containing estrogen, such as Lunelle or the Pill, are at risk of developing blood clots. The risk is low, but it must be recognized. Symptoms of a blood clot include: sudden, severe chest pain; unexplained shortness of breath; sudden vision problems; numbness or weakness in the extremities; and severe pain in the calf or thigh. If you experience any of these symptoms, get to a health center immediately.

Intrauterine Devices (IUDs)

EFFECTIVENESS AS A METHOD OF BIRTH CONTROL: 97–99 PERCENT

An IUD is a small plastic or metal device inserted into the uterus via the cervical opening. One or more strings hang down from the IUD and can be felt in the upper vagina. IUDs are usually available from and inserted by a family planning practitioner.

Some IUDs contain copper, which is thought to cause inflammation in the uterus. As a result, the immune system kicks into gear, and the resulting overflow of white blood cells, enzymes, and prostaglandins interferes with a sperm's ability to fertilize an egg. IUDs with copper can be left in place for years at a time.

Other IUDs contain progestins, which cause the cervical mucus to thicken so that sperm cannot pass through it. These IUDs must be replaced yearly. Mirena is a newer progestin IUD that lasts five years.

Neither type of IUD offers protection against STDs.

The most common problem with IUDs is expulsion—that is, sometimes they fall out. The danger here is that a woman may not know that she expelled an IUD, which can lead to an unplanned pregnancy. IUD expulsion is most likely to take place in the first three months after insertion and most common in women who have not given birth. Check weekly to make sure that your IUD is still in place by reaching up into the vagina. You should be able to feel the IUD's strings. If you cannot, schedule a visit with the practitioner who made the insertion.

IUDs should not be used if you have abnormal vaginal bleeding, a recent genitourinary infection, a recent abnormal Pap smear, any immune-compromising disease (such as AIDS), or an artificial heart valve.

Possible side effects include pain, discomfort, bleeding, fever, and discharge. There have been cases of pelvic inflammatory disease resulting in sterility. If a woman does contract an STD, the danger of the infection traveling deeper into her reproductive organs is greater if she has an IUD. There have also been cases in which IUDs have perforated the uterine wall, requiring a surgical repair. Seek medical attention if you have severe abdominal pain, fever, and chills of unknown origin, pain or bleeding during intercourse, or a foul-smelling vaginal discharge.

The long list of side effects may cause concern about the safety of this method of birth control, but it is important to note that most of these side effects are rare. The World Health Organization considers the IUD a safe, effective means of birth control.

If an IUD fails and you become pregnant, seek medical attention immediately. Having an IUD in place during pregnancy puts you at risk of serious infection or tubal pregnancy.

Contraceptive Implants

EFFECTIVENESS AS A METHOD OF BIRTH CONTROL: 99 PERCENT

Contraceptive implants are hormone-containing capsules that are inserted under the skin; the hormone is slowly released from the capsules and affects the user's reproductive system. Norplant is the most common contraceptive implant. It is implanted in the fleshy skin on the underside of the upper arm. Its active ingredient is the progestin levonorgestrel, which causes the cervix to thicken, prevents the ovaries from releasing eggs, and thins the endometrial lining so that it cannot support egg implantation.

If the implants are removed and not replaced (which can take place at any time), ovulation and menstruation generally begins anew within the next month. Implants do not offer any protection against STDs.

Side effects of contraceptive implants vary depending on the mechanism that they employ to prevent pregnancy. Consult with the practitioner who provides you with the implant for information about side effects. In general, you should not use implants if you are pregnant, are taking certain medications, or have a history of unexplained vaginal bleeding, blood-clotting problems, breast cancer, stroke, heart disease, or liver disease. Seek medical attention if you experience extreme vaginal bleeding, absence of menses (if you are accustomed to having them regularly), or severe abdominal pain; if you spot pus or infection at the site of the implant; or if an implant comes out.

Oral Contraceptives

EFFECTIVENESS AS A METHOD OF BIRTH CONTROL: 95–99 PERCENT

The oral contraceptive known as "the Pill," introduced in 1959, contains both progestin and estrogen. The progestin thickens cervical mucus so that sperm cannot penetrate it and also prevents proper development of the endometrium so that if, by chance, an egg is fertilized, it will not be able to implant in the endometrium. The estrogen is at a high enough level that it stops the pituitary gland from producing follicle-stimulating hormone (FSH). FSH triggers the follicles in the ovaries to begin developing. If there's no FSH, there's no follicle development and, thus, no egg.

There are many different kinds of combination pills that contain both estrogen and progestin in varying proportions; your health care provider can help you select the type that is best suited for you. Monophasic pills contain the same amounts of estrogen and progestin in each pill. Triphasic pills are designed to mimic one's natural cycle and vary the proportions of estrogen to progesterone throughout each month. Another type of oral contraceptive is the mini-pill, which contains only progestin. As a means of birth control, it is generally not quite as effective as combination pills, but it can be useful for women who are sensitive to estrogen therapy.

The Pill must be taken faithfully every day, preferably at a set time. If you miss one pill, take it as soon as you remember. If you miss two pills, take two a day until you are caught up, and use a backup method of contraception. If you miss three or more pills, call your health care provider. He or she will probably suggest that you use another form of birth control until after your next period, at which time you can begin the Pill cycle anew.

The Pill may increase, but often decreases, a woman's sex drive (by suppressing testosterone) and can cause vaginal dryness. Other side effects may include headache, nausea, breast tenderness, weight gain, bleeding between cycles, and depression. Positive side effects include menses that are lighter, less painful, and more regular. Some oral contraceptives also help to clear acne.

There may be more risk in taking the Pill if you are obese, if you are a smoker (particularly if you are over thirty-five), or if you have a history of diabetes, liver disease, cancer, heart disease, or blood-clotting disorders. If you are taking antibiotics or medications for treating epilepsy or tuberculosis, consult with your health care provider to make sure that they won't interfere with the Pill's effectiveness. Seek medical help immediately if you experience sudden chest, arm, or abdominal pain; severe headache; shortness of breath; blurred vision; severe depression; or swelling or pain in the legs.

Birth control patches worn on the skin have become available. Patches deliver a combination of progestin and estrogen from a two-inch piece of adhesive that releases hormones into the skin. The patch is applied to the arm, torso, stomach, or buttocks. A new patch is reapplied every three weeks. Also new are intravaginal rings that contain hormones. They are available by prescription and release estrogen and progesterone directly into the vaginal walls. A flexible ring (about two inches in diameter) is inserted and removed after three weeks. Guess we'll see how their health history unfolds.

Spermicides

EFFECTIVENESS AS A METHOD OF BIRTH CONTROL WHEN USED ON ITS OWN: 74 PERCENT

Spermicidal creams, jellies, foams, and suppositories contain sperm-killing chemicals, most notably nonoxynol-9. They are inserted directly into the vagina before intercourse. Spermicides should not be used on their own as a means of birth control, since they are not reliably effective, but they make a powerful partner for other methods of birth control, such as diaphragms, cervical caps, and condoms. They also offer some protection against syphilis, gonorrhea, and trichomoniasis.

Each spermicidal product has unique properties and applications. Read the product label for instructions. About 5 percent of women who use spermicides experience a localized allergic reaction that manifests as vaginal irritation, soreness, or discharge.

Tubal Ligation

EFFECTIVENESS AS A METHOD OF BIRTH CONTROL: 99 PERCENT

Tubal ligation is a surgical procedure for sterilizing a woman. It is an option only for women who are positive that they do not want to conceive children in the future. It does not offer any protection against STDs.

There are five different surgical procedures for tubal ligation. All, in one way or another, seal off the fallopian tubes (from which comes the colloquialism "getting your tubes tied").

In rare cases, a woman becomes pregnant after tubal ligation. In these cases it is thought that the fallopian tubes may have reconnected. Pregnancy in this situation is likely to be tubal, and dangerous. If you have had tubal ligation and experience severe abdominal pain, or miss a period and test positive for pregnancy, contact your health care provider immediately.

Vasectomy

EFFECTIVENESS AS A METHOD OF BIRTH CONTROL: 99 PERCENT

Vasectomy is a surgical procedure for sterilizing a man. It involves sealing off the vas deferens, which carries mature sperm from the epididymis to the seminal vesicle ducts. It does not offer any protection against STDs.

A vasectomy can be a simple outpatient surgery that takes about twenty minutes. It does not alter a man's sex drive or the appearance of his semen.

There may be short-term bruising or swelling near the testicles, and small lumps may form near the testicles, occasionally requiring medical treatment. In rare cases, the vas deferens may recover, making a man fertile again.

After a vasectomy, some sperm may remain in the man's testes, and he must be considered fertile for at least the next fifteen to twenty ejaculations. He should be tested before engaging in unprotected sex to determine for certain that he is not ejaculating sperm. A man can freeze his sperm at a sperm bank in case he wins the lottery and decides he wants more children.

Abstinence cannot make you pregnant. Neither can same-sex sex. Otherwise, you are just going to have to figure something out.

PART THREE

Achieving and Maintaining Sexual Health

EACH OF US is our own best primary health care provider. After all, who else can better monitor our physical and emotional health, feel our feelings, and gauge the effectiveness of healing therapies? The body is not a simple machine but a loving home for our soul—and we are the most appropriate ones to learn how best to care for our temple.

Making a commitment to self-care is one of the important steps to take to reclaim harmony among ourselves and with the planet. Therefore, the healing techniques and remedies in this chapter focus on self-care as a first solution for sexual health problems. You'll find that the at-home techniques are simple in design and, over time, potent in effect. You may wish to find a holistic health care provider with whom you can consult when more serious illnesses manifest in you or a member of your family.

A healthy lifestyle is the most important precept of good self-care; it prevents disease, which relieves you of the responsibility to treat it. So live life fully but wisely. Develop harmonious relationships and seek fulfilling livelihood. Eat healthfully, exercise regularly, and get plenty of fresh air, and use herbs and natural therapies on a daily basis to build the health of your body and mind.

HERBAL DOSAGES

You'll find many recommendations for herbal therapy in this part of the book. Unless stated otherwise, the therapeutic adult dosage for a recommended herb is:

- *1 cup of tea three times daily;*
- *1 or 2 capsules three times daily; or*
- *1 dropperful of tincture three times daily.*

To figure out an appropriate dosage for a child, take the child's weight and divide by 150. For example, for a 50-pound child divide by 150, which reduces to one-third of the adult dosage.

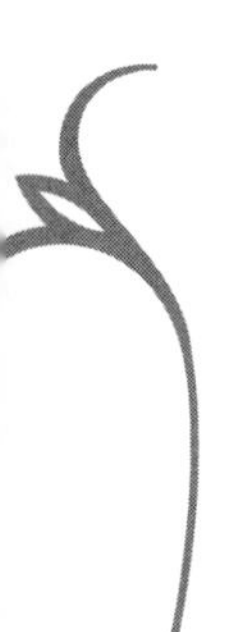

15 Women's Health

IN ADDITION TO MAKING diet and lifestyle choices that support your general health, women must also be aware of the specific conditions that can affect sexual and reproductive organs and tissues. The vagina being a moist and sensitive area, it is particularly vulnerable to irritation and infection; therefore, it's a good idea to have a general understanding of common symptoms and natural treatments for them.

Some regular habits are particularly important in maintaining health in the female genitals. These include:

- Wear loose-fitting, natural-fiber clothing and undergarments. Tight-fitting and synthetic-fiber clothing prevent the skin from breathing, contributing to the buildup of yeast and other bacteria.
- Minimize sitting around in wet underclothing; change into dry clothing as soon as possible.
- Wipe from front to back after using the toilet. This helps keep the organisms that live in your rectum from moving into your vagina.
- Minimize douching, and never douche with chemically scented or flavored douches. These douches introduce toxins to the vagina, leaving you more susceptible to infection.

- Avoid chemically scented bubble baths, feminine deodorant sprays, or deodorant tampons.
- Use only undyed, unscented toilet paper.
- A five-minute air and sunbath on the genitals (where it is safe and won't get you in trouble) can have a powerful healing effect in clearing up infections and healing gynecological concerns.
- When you must take antibiotics, add to your diet fermented foods such as plain yogurt and unpasteurized sauerkraut, apple cider vinegar, miso, and tamari. These foods support and replenish the friendly bacteria in the body. Follow antibiotic therapy with a two- to three-month course of probiotics (see page 249).

From time to time, many women will experience adverse health conditions that affect their sexual energy and enjoyment. What follows is a list of some of the most common ailments, along with suggestions for natural treatment using a wide variety of methods.

BARTHOLIN'S GLAND CYSTS

Bartholin's glands, a pair of small glands located between the labia minor and the vaginal wall; produce mucus when a woman is sexually aroused. If the glands become blocked, cysts may develop. The cysts do not usually lead to more serious infection or permanent injury, but they may cause discomfort.

Symptoms

Cysts are indicated by heat and swelling. When you run a finger against the labia minor, you may feel a hard lump in the area where the Bartholin's glands are located. Gonorrhea can trigger the development of cysts in the Bartholin's glands, so check with your gynecologist to find out whether you have contracted the disease.

Treatment

Support your body's battle against the infection by eating plenty of fruits and vegetables and avoiding white flour and saturated fats, which contribute to congestion. The following natural therapies will also be of assistance. These healing treatments may temporarily increase the discomfort caused by the cyst, but the discomfort will soon pass.

SITZ BATHS

Take alternating hot and cold sitz baths. (For information on sitz baths, turn to page 169.) The resulting increase in circulation to the pelvic area can help clear the blockage in the Bartholin's glands.

CALENDULA-GOLDENSEAL SALVE

Apply a salve containing calendula and goldenseal to the area to reduce swelling and speed up healing. Calendula-goldenseal salves are available in most natural food stores and herb shops. You can also make your own, following Cascade Anderson Geller's instructions on page 99.

CLAY POULTICE

At night, mix cosmetic-quality green clay with enough water to make a paste and apply to the skin over the cysts. This healing poultice draws toxins from the skin as it dries.

OIL MASSAGE

Massage the area with 1 ounce of almond oil to which 10 drops each of chamomile, lavender, and peppermint essential oils have been added. This oil blend helps fight infection and reduce inflammation.

CLEAVERS TEA

Prepare an infusion of cleavers herb (*Galium aparine*) following the instructions on page 50, and drink 4 cups daily. Cleavers cleanses the lymphatic system, clears heat, and relieves inflammation, all of which make the herb very effective for resolving glandular cysts.

HOMEOPATHIC REMEDIES

When Bartholin's gland cysts are accompanied by any of the conditions described below, try the suggested homeopathic remedy. The usual dosage is 4 pellets, or as many liquid drops as the package label recommends, taken under the tongue four times daily. Rather than swallowing the pellets whole, allow them to dissolve slowly.

BARYTA CARBONICA. The glands are swollen but not infected.

BELLADONNA. The cysts are accompanied by vaginal dryness and early, heavy periods.

MERCURIUS SOLUBILIS. The patient has a strong constitution but feels mentally exhausted from overwork. The patient feels rawness or stinging in the genital area, perhaps accompanied by yellow or greenish vaginal discharge.

CANDIDIASIS

Candida albicans is a one of many yeast fungi that grows on the mucous membranes of most living organisms, including people. Candida is usually present on the surface of the skin and in the intestinal tract, vagina, and rectum, living in harmony with many other microbial species. The presence of other flora and the highly acidic vaginal environment—which ranges in pH from 3.5 to 4.5—normally keep Candida growth in the vagina under control. When vaginal pH becomes more alkaline, when excess sugar is available to feed the yeast, when the immune system is weakened, or when the species of bacteria that keep Candida growth in check are removed, Candida proliferates wildly, and vaginal candidiasis—otherwise known as a yeast infection—results. Seventy-five percent of all women have a yeast infection at some time in their lives; about half of these women have the infection more than once.

There are many known factors that cause these changes to the vaginal environment, and probably many more that have yet to be discovered. What we do know is this: Menstruation, pregnancy, birth control pills, some antibiotics, hormone supplements, and diabetes all lead to an increase in vaginal alkalinity. Excess sugar and simple carbohydrates in the diet offer yeast a veritable feast. By stressing the body's cleansing and immune systems, common toxins such as environmental pollutants, fluoride, chlorine, and mercury dental fillings can all encourage the growth of yeast. And antibiotics—particularly broad-spectrum antibiotics—destroy the "friendly" bacteria in the vagina, allowing Candida to spread unchecked.

Symptoms

Symptoms of vaginal candidiasis include vaginal discharge, vaginal itching, vaginal odor, rectal itching, a craving for sweets, depression, mood swings, endometriosis, frequent urination, lack of sexual desire, lethargy, and even premenstrual syndrome.

Treatment

Natural therapy is just as effective, if not more so, than standard medical care for vaginal candidiasis. It's based on three precepts.

1. Restore the balance of vaginal flora.
2. Normalize vaginal pH.
3. Support the immune system.

When you begin a yeast-control program, it's not unusual to feel worse at first. The proteins made available by dead yeast can stimulate a histamine reaction, resulting in further irritation of the vaginal tissues and feelings of anxiety and malaise. This is a temporary side effect; taking powdered vitamin C in 1,000 mg doses two or three times daily will help clear the symptoms.

It is vital that you stick with the treatment program. Candida is resilient. If you stop the treatment too soon, you sabotage the cure, and the infection will soon return.

REFRAIN FROM SEXUAL CONTACT

Yeast infections can be spread by oral, vaginal, and anal sex, so refrain from sexual contact until the infection has cleared. Men carry genital Candida underneath the foreskin and in the prostate; if you pass Candida to a male partner, he may later pass it back to you, allowing the yeast to circumvent and thus survive the treatment protocol you've undertaken. Researchers do not really agree on Candida transmission, but it is more likely to occur if either partner is immune-compromised.

PROBIOTICS

Yeast, bacteria, and other microbial organisms maintain a finely poised balance in the body. Antibiotics destroy "friendly" bacteria, allowing opportunistic Candida to expand. Probiotics replenish and support bacteria, bringing balance back to the flora of the body.

The bacterium *Lactobacillus acidophilus,* more commonly known as acidophilus, is among the most effective probiotics for treating yeast infections. Acidophilus and Candida have similar binding sites in the intestinal tract. The more acidophilus present, the less room there is for Candida. Acidophilus also produces lactic acid, which helps normalize the acidity of the vaginal environment, and competes with Candida for food sources.

Another useful bacterium is *Bacillus laterosporus,* which seems to destroy yeasts and support friendly bacteria. Both *Lactobacillus acidophilus* and *Bacillus laterosporus* can be taken as supplements, in either powdered or pill form. Most natural food stores carry these probiotics.

While you are taking antibiotics, incorporate fermented foods, such as plain yogurt and unpasteurized sauerkraut, apple cider vinegar, miso, and tamari, into your diet. Fermented foods are a good source of probiotics. Eat at least one serving a day. After a course of antibiotic therapy, begin a course of probiotic therapy. Take one or two capsules of *Lactobacillus acidophilus* or *Bacillus laterosporus* three times daily (not with meals) for three to four months.

SUPPOSITORIES

Vaginal suppositories are very effective for treating yeast infections; they introduce the cure directly to the infected area. A garlic clove makes a potent suppository for treating yeast infection. At bedtime, peel the skin from a single clove of garlic and insert it into your vagina. Do not cut the clove, as the potent juices can be irritating to the delicate tissues. In the morning, remove the clove. You shouldn't have any trouble removing it, but if you're overly concerned, place the clove in a square of cheesecloth, gather the corners of the cloth, and tie it off with dental floss, leaving a string of floss hanging out far enough to aid retrieval.

Boric acid is another effective anti-yeast suppository. Insert a "0" capsule filled with boric acid high into the vagina five to seven nights in a row. (Do not ingest boric acid, as it is mildly toxic.)

Probiotic suppositories help resupply the vagina with friendly bacteria. Try using two "00" capsules of acidophilus or, preferably, a broad-spectrum probiotic formula containing acidophilus and *Bifidobacterium bifidum* (sometimes called "bifidus") or *Lactobacillus bulgaricus.* Insert the capsules high into the vagina five to seven nights in a row.

Plain yogurt can also be used as a vaginal suppository to introduce acidophilus directly to the vagina. At bedtime, insert a small amount into the vagina; the applicator that comes with spermicidal cream or jelly makes this an easy task. Wear a cotton menstrual pad to prevent the yogurt from dripping over the bed sheets. Repeat for five to seven nights.

CAUTION

If you are pregnant, do not insert anything into your vagina, including suppositories and douches, without consulting your health care provider.

DOUCHES

Douches, like suppositories, introduce the cure directly to the point of infection. For an effective anti-yeast douche, mix 1 quart of water with *one* of the following:

- ¼ tablespoon of apple cider vinegar
- 1 teaspoon acidophilus powder
- 1 teaspoon salt and 1 teaspoon 3 percent hydrogen peroxide

Douche just twice daily; getting overzealous with this treatment can wash away friendly vaginal flora. Follow up with a plain yogurt suppository.

ANTIFUNGAL TEAS

After bowel movements or urination, wipe the perineal area and then squirt onto it some antifungal herbal teas, such as calendula, echinacea, garlic, myrrh, rosemary, thyme, or yarrow tea.

These teas should be stored in the refrigerator, where they'll keep for up to a week. However, you certainly don't want to squirt cold tea on your sensitive parts. Instead, every morning pour a day's supply of tea into a container. Cover it, and keep it in the bathroom. What isn't used by the end of the day should be discarded.

DIET

For every book that discusses how to treat Candida, there's a different dietary theory. There's no need to dip in to the sophisticated underpinnings of nutritional science to understand what sort of diet supports or counteracts a yeast infection. Instead, follow these six simple, commonsense guidelines.

1. **Avoid simple sugars.** For yeast, sugar is food, and simple sugars make that food readily available. So don't eat sweets; if you must use a sweetener, try using stevia, an herb that has twenty times the sweetening power of sugar without the simple sugars. Avoid fruit juices, sodas, or alcohol; they're packed with sugar. Simple carbohydrates are another source of simple sugars. Avoid anything made with white flour or gluten-rich grains such as wheat, rye, and barley. Also avoid high-carbohydrate vegetables such as peas, potatoes, winter squashes, and lima beans.
2. **Avoid common allergens.** Whether or not you have a bona fide allergy, common allergens stress the immune system and prevent it from focusing its attention on the Candida infection. This is another reason to avoid foods that are rich in wheat and gluten, both common allergens. Also avoid peanuts, pistachios, and cashews. (Substitute almonds, hazelnuts, pine nuts, and sunflower and pumpkin seeds, which are not common allergens.)
3. **Alkalize your system.** A good method for this is to start each day by drinking a pint of warm water to which the juice of a fresh lemon has been added.
4. **Eat high-fiber foods.** Fiber encourages healthy bowel movements. High-fiber foods include vegetables, fruits, nuts, and seeds. Most whole grains are rich in fiber, but because they are also rich in carbohydrates, they should be avoided.
5. **Eat foods that warm the system.** In Oriental medicine, a yeast overgrowth is considered a damp heat condition that obstructs the flow of chi. The remedy is to increase warmth and the circulation of chi. Warming culinary herbs fit the bill. Try seasoning your food with black pepper, cayenne, cinnamon, cloves, curry powder, garlic, ginger, oregano, and turmeric, all of which help dry damp conditions and inhibit yeasts.
6. **Support friendly flora.** Rather than killing Candida, simply help the "opposition" outnumber it! Fermented foods, such as plain yogurt, unpasteurized sauerkraut, unpasteurized apple cider vinegar, and miso, help defeat Candida by supporting and replenishing friendly bacteria

in the body. Chlorophyll-rich foods such as barley grass and wheatgrass juices also support healthy intestinal flora and help cool the heat of this damp condition. Also consider seaweeds, which contain beneficial yeasts that compete with Candida.

BIOTIN

Biotin, a member of the vitamin B complex, helps prevent Candida from developing. Take 300 mcg daily. Avoid vitamin formulas that use yeast as a base.

HERBAL THERAPY

Several herbs can be used to inhibit Candida growth.

Aloe vera (*Aloe vera, A. barbadensis*). Squeeze the juice from the leaves and apply to the irritated tissue. Aloe is antifungal, anti-inflammatory, antiseptic, demulcent, and rejuvenative. Avoid internal use during pregnancy and in cases of intestinal inflammation.

Asafoetida (*Ferula foetida, F. assa-foetida, F. rubricaulis*). This resin is warming to the digestive tract and counteracts Candida overgrowth. It is an antiseptic, a carminative, and a digestive tonic. In rare cases, it may cause diarrhea. Avoid therapeutic doses during pregnancy and in cases of ulcers.

Black walnut (*Juglans nigra*). The hull contains juglone, an antifungal compound. It is alterative, antifungal, anti-inflammatory, antiseptic, antiparasitic, and astringent.

Calendula (*Calendula officinalis*). The flower is a time-tested remedy against chronic infection. It is alterative, anti-inflammatory, antifungal, astringent, and vulnerary.

Cayenne (*Capsicum annuum*). The fruit dries cold, damp conditions. It is antifungal, alterative, anti-inflammatory, antioxidant, antiseptic, circulatory stimulant, and tonic. Avoid contact with eyes and mucous membranes. Avoid therapeutic doses during pregnancy and while nursing.

Chaparral (*Larrea tridentata*). The leaf inhibits the growth of molds, bacteria, and pathogens. It also dries dampness in the body. It is alterative, antifungal, antioxidant, antiseptic, and immunostimulant. Avoid in cases of liver or kidney disease, including cirrhosis or hepatitis, and during pregnancy. Discontinue use if nausea, fatigue, fever, or jaundice occur. Do not use for more than a month at a time. Consult with your health care provider before use.

Cubeb (*Piper cubeba*). The berry helps eliminate bladder mucus and clears cold and dampness. It is antiseptic, carminative, a stomach tonic, and a yang tonic. Avoid in cases of acute digestive or kidney irritation.

Echinacea (*Echinacea purpurea, E. angustifolia*). The root stimulates the immune system and inhibits fungal growth. It also dries dampness. It is an alterative, antifungal, anti-inflammatory, antiseptic, carminative, digestive tonic, and vulnerary.

Evening primrose (*Oenothera biennis*). The oil of the seeds stimulates the T cells of the immune system.

Garlic (*Allium sativum*). The clove cleanses mucous membranes and helps clear yeast infections. It can be used as a suppository and incorporated in liberal amounts into the diet. It is alterative, antifungal, antioxidant, antiseptic, carminative, immunostimulant, and a yang tonic. Some people are allergic to garlic. Excessive use can cause emotional irritability and irritation of the stomach and kidneys. Avoid therapeutic doses during pregnancy, and avoid during the first three months of nursing, as it can cause breast milk to become unpalatable for infants. Avoid use for one week before any surgery.

Goldenseal (*Hydrastis canadensis*). The root clears infection and increases blood supply to the spleen. It is an alterative, antifungal, anti-inflammatory, antiseptic, bitter tonic, and cholagogue. Goldenseal is very bitter, and most people find it easiest to ingest in capsule form. The tea can be used as a douche. Goldenseal salves and powders can be applied topically. This herb is endangered in the wild, so do not use wildcrafted supplies. Avoid during pregnancy.

Marsh mallow (*Althaea officinalis*). The root soothes and moistens irritated mucous membranes and stimulates white blood cell production. Use as a tea or a douche. It is alterative, demulcent, immunostimulant, nutritive, rejuvenative, and vulnerary.

Nettle (*Urtica dioica, U. urens*). The herb increases the oxygen available to mucous membranes, which helps make them stronger and less susceptible to infection. It also dries dampness and helps lessen the effect of food sensitivities. It is an adrenal tonic, alterative, astringent, cholagogue, circulatory stimulant, Kidney tonic, mucolytic, and nutritive. Contact with the fresh plant will irritate the skin. Use only dried herb. Wear gloves when collecting.

Oregano (*Origanum vulgare*). The herb inhibits the growth of Candida. It is antifungal, anti-inflammatory, antiseptic, carminative, cholagogic, and a digestive tonic. Oregano-infused oil is often available in natural food stores and herb shops and can be applied topically. Avoid therapeutic doses of this herb during pregnancy.

Oregon grape (*Mahonia aquifolium*). The root contains antiseptic properties that are especially beneficial to the skin and intestinal tract. It is an alterative, anti-inflammatory, antiseptic, astringent, bitter tonic, cholagogue, digestive tonic, immunostimulant, and Liver tonic. Avoid during pregnancy, and do not exceed the recommended dosage.

Pau d'arco (*Tabebuia impetiginosa*). The bark contains antifungal compounds, strengthens a weakened immune system, and dries dampness. It is alterative, antifungal, anti-inflammatory, antioxidant, antiseptic, and immunostimulant.

Prickly ash (*Zanthoxylum americanum, Z. clava-herculis*). The bark improves circulation to mucous membranes and inhibits yeast overgrowth. It is an alterative, antiseptic, astringent, carminative, circulatory stimulant, and digestive tonic. Avoid during pregnancy and in cases of stomach inflammation.

Spilanthes (*Spilanthes acmella*). This herb counteracts yeast infections and thrush. It is antifungal and antiseptic. Avoid during pregnancy.

Turmeric (*Curcuma longa, C. aromatica*). The rhizome helps heal ulcerated intestinal mucous membranes and stabilizes microflora, thus inhibiting yeast overgrowth. It is an alterative, antifungal, anti-inflammatory, antioxidant, antiseptic, astringent, cholagogue, circulatory stimulant, digestive tonic, and vulnerary.

Usnea (*Usnea barbata*). This lichen is often recommended in treatments for deep-seated infections of the body. It is antifungal, antiseptic, and immunostimulant.

Yarrow (*Achillea millefolium*). The herb opens pores and aids in the elimination of wastes, helping flush toxins from the body. It is an anti-inflammatory, antifungal, antiseptic, astringent, bitter tonic, carminative, cholagogue, circulatory stimulant, digestive tonic, and urinary antiseptic. Avoid during pregnancy.

HOMEOPATHIC REMEDIES

When a yeast infection is accompanied by any of the conditions that are described below, try the suggested homeopathic remedy. The usual dosage is 4 pellets, or as many liquid drops as the package label recommends, taken under the tongue four times daily. Rather than swallowing the pellets whole, allow them to dissolve slowly.

BORAX. The infection is diagnosed as thrush.

CALCAREA CARBONICA. Vaginal itching occurs just before menses. The infection is accompanied by a milky discharge. The patient experiences headache, anxiety, and depression. The symptoms improve in the morning and worsen before and after menses, after exertion, between 2 and 3 a.m., and whenever the weather is cold, damp, and windy.

CANDIDA. Using homeopathic Candida can stimulate an immune response to fight Candida yeast. It is especially effective against intestinal and vaginal yeast overgrowth.

IPECACUANHA. The infection is accompanied by diarrhea and profuse mucous secretions. The patient experiences nausea. The symptoms worsen in heat and humidity.

SEPIA. The infection is accompanied by a foul-smelling, whitish discharge and vaginal itching, soreness, and burning. The patient is irritable and tearful. Symptoms improve after sleep, eating, exercising, and application of heat to the vulva region. Symptoms worsen in the cold, when the patient is fatigued, during exposure to smoke, during intercourse, and in the early morning and the evening.

SULFUR. The infection is accompanied by a yellow or whitish discharge and vaginal itching, soreness, and burning. The patient experiences pain in the vagina during intercourse, constipation or diarrhea, and anal itching. Symptoms improve with fresh air and dry warmth. Symptoms worsen after spending excessive time standing, in cold and damp conditions, with consumption of alcohol, and in the morning and the night.

THERAPEUTIC BATHS

Therapeutic baths are beneficial for both men and women. They are especially well suited for pregnant women, who should not use douches or suppositories.

Fill the tub with warm water, then add the following ingredients:

- 1 cup of unpasteurized apple cider vinegar (to support and replenish friendly bacteria)
- 1 pound of salt (to inhibit yeast)
- 7 drops of allspice, chamomile, cinnamon, cloves, eucalyptus, geranium, lavender, patchouli, rosemary, or tea tree essential oil (to inhibit yeast)

When bathing, use coconut-based soaps. Coconut contains caprylic acid, which has anti-Candida properties. Avoid soaps and lubricants that contain glycerin, which is sweet and can feed yeasts.

CERVICAL DYSPLASIA

Cervical dysplasia is an abnormal precancerous cellular growth on the cervix. Though its causes are unknown, cervical dysplasia has been linked to having intercourse at an early age, having had numerous sexual partners, birth control pills, hormonal therapy, smoking, and sexually transmitted diseases, including venereal warts. If caught in its early stages, cervical dysplasia is benign.

Practices that may lessen your risk for developing cervical dysplasia include using barrier methods of contraception (such as condoms and diaphragms), washing before and after intercourse, and maintaining a strong immune system.

Having cervical dysplasia is not the same thing as having cancer. In fact, most cases of cervical dysplasia resolve themselves, returning to normal without treatment. However, once a Pap smear has shown that you have cervical dysplasia, you will require regular Pap smear testing for the next year to monitor the condition. You should have regular follow-ups with a health care provider.

Symptoms

Cervical dysplasia most often yields no outward symptoms, although in some cases it may cause bloodstained discharge or bleeding between periods, with defecation, or after intercourse. In late stages, the condition may cause a foul-smelling discharge. A Pap smear usually detects the problem.

Treatment

Natural therapies for treating cervical dysplasia focus on supporting the liver and immune system, preventing cancerous growths, relieving irritation of mucous membranes, and reducing inflammation. Overall, they encourage the dissolution of cervical growths.

The most important treatment for cervical dysplasia is getting healthy. If you're on hormone replacement therapy, talk to your doctor about stopping. Give up addictions. Enforce a healthy diet. Eliminate sources of stress. And consult with a holistic health care provider to create a personalized health care program that supports vibrant health.

NUTRITIONAL THERAPY

The following nutrients can have a positive effect on cervical dysplasia. Try to incorporate natural sources of these nutrients into your diet; you may also wish to use supplements. Good sources of each are listed in chapter 3.

Antioxidants. Antioxidants prevent free-radical damage in the body, which is believed to contribute to cancerous growths. They also strengthen mucous membranes and help the body resist infections. Antioxidants are best absorbed through natural sources such as colorful fresh fruits and vegetables that provide the nutrients beta-carotene, vitamin C, vitamin E, selenium, and superoxide dismutase.

Folic acid. In some cases, an irregular Pap smear results from a folic acid deficiency. This is most often the case for women on the Pill, because the synthetic estrogens tend to have a combative effect on folic acid levels. Take 400 mcg daily. Also add plenty of leafy greens, a great source of folic acid, to your diet.

Vitamin A. Vitamin A can prevent cells from becoming malignant. The best source of vitamin A is beta-carotene, which is a precursor to vitamin A. Take 25,000 to 50,000 IU of beta-carotene daily. Better yet, incorporate natural sources of beta-carotene into your diet.

Vitamin B_6. Vitamin B_6, also known as pyridoxine, supports healthy cellular growth and may encourage normal cells to replace dysplastic cells on the cervix. Take 50 mg daily.

HERBAL THERAPY

Herbs that can be used to treat cervical dysplasia include the following:

Burdock (*Arctium lappa*). Burdock root supports proper functioning in the organs of elimination and relieves lymphatic congestion. It is alterative, antifungal, antiseptic, anti-inflammatory, antitumor, choleretic, demulcent, diuretic, laxative, nutritive, and rejuvenative.

Celandine (*Chelidonium majus*). The root and leaves contain berberine, an alkaloid that fights infection. They have alterative, anodyne, anti-inflammatory, and cholagogic properties. Use only in small doses; 2 or 3 drops of tincture three times daily is adequate. Consult with your health care provider before use, and avoid during pregnancy.

Chaparral (*Larrea tridentata*). The leaf inhibits the growth of some cancer cells. It is alterative, antifungal, antioxidant, antiseptic, antitumor, and immunostimulant. Avoid in cases of liver or kidney disease and during pregnancy. Discontinue use if nausea, fatigue, fever, or jaundice occur. Do not use for more than a month at a time. Consult with your health care provider before use.

Dandelion (*Taraxacum officinale*). The root improves liver function, which relieves stagnation in the reproductive organs. It is antifungal, antitumor, cholagogic, and a Liver tonic.

Echinacea (*Echinacea purpurea, E. angustifolia*). Echinacea root stimulates T-cell production and macrophage activity in the immune system. It also dilates peripheral blood vessels, thus increasing circulation to the genitourinary area and helping to flush toxins from the pelvic region. It is alterative, antifungal, anti-inflammatory, antiseptic, antitumor, and depurative.

Goldenseal (*Hydrastis canadensis*). The root inhibits a wide range of pathogens. It is alterative, anti-inflammatory, antiseptic, cholagogic, a deobstruent, and a hemostatic. Goldenseal is very bitter, and most people find it easiest to ingest in capsule form. The tea can be used as a douche. This herb is endangered in the wild, so do not use wildcrafted supplies. Avoid during pregnancy.

Licorice (*Glycyrrhiza glabra, G. uralensis*). The root helps the body produce interferon, its own anticancer treatment. It also inhibits the production of prostaglandin E2, which contributes to inflammation, and soothes irritated mucous membranes. It is an anti-inflammatory, antiseptic, antitumor, chi tonic, demulcent, nutritive, and rejuvenative. Avoid during pregnancy and in cases of edema, high blood pressure, or diabetes. Do not use in combination with digoxin drugs. Excessive use can cause sodium retention and potassium depletion.

Lomatium (***Lomatium dissectum***). The root is an anti-inflammatory, antiseptic, and immunostimulant. In rare cases, lomatium root may cause skin irritation. This herb is endangered in the wild; do not use wildcrafted supplies.

Pau d'arco (***Tabebuia impetiginosa***). The bark inhibits cancerous growths and improves liver function. It is alterative, antifungal, anti-inflammatory, antioxidant, antiseptic, antitumor, and immunostimulant.

Red clover (***Trifolium pratense***). Clover blossom is an excellent lymphatic cleanser. It is alterative, anti-inflammatory, and antitumor.

Red raspberry (***Rubus idaeus***). Raspberry leaf tonifies the uterus and the cervix. It is an alterative, antiseptic, hemostatic, hormonal regulator, and yin tonic.

SUPPOSITORIES

Purchase capsules that contain vitamin A in liquid form. Every night for one week, saturate a pure cotton tampon with 25,000 IU of vitamin A and insert it as high as possible into the vagina. Remove the tampon in the morning.

After one week, make an herbal vaginal bolus from the Radical Resistance Yoni Suppository formula described below. Every night for one week, insert it as high as possible into the vagina. Wear a cotton menstrual pad to avoid any leakage on your bed sheets.

When the week is up, begin with the vitamin A treatment again. Alternate weekly between the vitamin and herbal applications for at least three cycles. Take a break during menses.

RADICAL RESISTANCE YONI SUPPOSITORY

This vaginal suppository helps deter infection and yeasts.

1 part yellow dock root
1 part chaparral leaf
1 part echinacea root
1 part calendula blossoms
1 part pau d'arco bark
½ part witch hazel bark
½ part black walnut hull
1 drop cedar leaf essential oil or infused oil (usually sold as thuja oil)

1 drop cypress essential oil

Coconut oil

Combine the herbs with enough coconut oil to make a thick paste. Roll into a suppository shape the size of your pinkie, and store in a glass jar in the refrigerator. Insert before bedtime.

OVARIAN CYSTS

There are two types of functional (as opposed to neoplastic) ovarian cysts. A follicular ovarian cyst may develop when a follicle has grown—as one or more does every month as part of the menstrual cycle—but does not rupture and release its egg. A luteal ovarian cyst may develop from the corpus luteum if it does not deteriorate as it should after ovulation.

Cysts are by definition filled with fluid. They're quite common, and most are benign and resolve on their own. In some cases, however, ovarian cysts produce large amounts of sex hormones, are painful, or cause irregular menses. Sometimes they rupture, which can be very painful and cause bleeding. In the rare cases where ovarian cysts become extremely painful or dangerous to a woman's health, they should be removed.

Although it is not common, cysts can also be caused by endometriosis, cancer, or by dermoid cysts, which are small tumors that contain skin and skin derivatives. In these cases, removal of the cyst by a health care professional is recommended.

Reccurrence of cysts can be a symptom of hormonal imbalance. If you find yourself getting cysts regularly, stop taking birth control pills and discontinue hormone replacement therapy. Intense exercise can also bring on cysts by banging around the ovaries, which don't have much cushioning to support them.

Symptoms

A cyst is usually first discovered during a routine pelvic exam. If cysts are large or numerous, they can cause lower abdominal swelling, pain in the lower pelvic area, pain during intercourse, or irregular menses. If you experience any of these symptoms, bring them to the attention of your gynecologist.

Treatment

Natural medicine can be quite effective for treating smaller cysts, but larger cysts may require surgery. However, even if you must go the surgery route, consider the dietary and lifestyle changes suggested here; they will help prevent reccurrences.

The protocol for treating ovarian cysts focuses on regulating hormones, decreasing outside sources of estrogen, improving liver function, promoting prostaglandin production to reduce inflammation, improving lymphatic drainage, increasing circulation to the womb, and removing toxins from the body.

HERBAL THERAPY

Several herbs can be helpful in preventing and treating ovarian cysts.

Angelica (*Angelica archangelica, A. atropurpurea*). The root normalizes menstrual bleeding and inhibits blood platelet aggregation. It is an anti-inflammatory, astringent, diuretic, emmenagogue, tonic, and uterine stimulant. Avoid during pregnancy and in cases of heavy bleeding or diabetes. In rare cases, the root causes photosensitivity.

Black cohosh (*Actaea racemosa*). Black cohosh root soothes irritation and congestion of the cervix, uterus, and vagina. It is often recommended to relieve menstrual pain. It is an alterative, anti-inflammatory, antiseptic, antispasmodic, astringent, circulatory stimulant, emmenagogue, and vasodilator. Avoid during pregnancy, except in the final stages, and then only under the guidance of your health care provider. Avoid while nursing and in cases of high blood pressure or pressure in the inner eye. Consult with your health care provider before use. This herb is endangered in the wild; do not use wildcrafted supplies.

Blessed thistle (*Cnicus benedictus*). This herb strengthens the spleen and the liver. It is an alterative, antihemorrhagic, and emmenagogue.

Blue cohosh (*Caulophyllum thalictroides*). The root of blue cohosh can be used to relieve pain caused by ovarian cysts and Mittelschmerz (ovulation pain). It is anti-inflammatory, antispasmodic, diuretic, emmenagogic, oxytocic, and a uterine tonic. Avoid during pregnancy, except in the final stages, and then only under the guidance of your health care provider. Make sure the root is dried, not fresh. This herb is endangered in the wild, so do not use wildcrafted supplies.

Bupleurum (*Bupleurum chinense, B. falcatum*). Bupleurum root stabilizes menses and relieves liver stagnation. It is an alterative, analgesic, anti-inflammatory, chi tonic, choleretic, and tonic. Avoid in cases of fever, headache, or high blood pressure.

Celandine (*Chelidonium majus*). The herb helps detoxify the liver, supporting its ability to break down excess hormones. It is an alterative, anti-inflammatory, cholagogue, and diuretic. Use only in small doses; 2 or 3 drops of tincture three times daily is adequate. Consult with your health care provider before use, and avoid during pregnancy.

Chaparral (*Larrea tridentata*). The leaf helps reduce the size of growths associated with elevated estrogen levels. It is an alterative, antifungal, antioxidant, antiseptic, antitumor, antiparasitic, and immunostimulant. Avoid in cases of liver or kidney disease, including cirrhosis and hepatitis, and during pregnancy. Discontinue use if nausea, fatigue, fever, or jaundice occur. Do not use for more than a month at a time. Consult with your health care provider before use.

Chickweed (*Stellaria media*). The herb helps dissolve cysts in the body; it can be used to treat not only ovarian cysts but also breast cysts and fibroids. It is an alterative, anti-inflammatory, astringent, discutient, and vulnerary.

Codonopsis (*Codonopsis pilosula*). The root relieves stagnation in the pelvic area. It is an adaptogen, chi tonic, and nutritive.

Cramp bark (*Viburnum opulus*). Cramp bark relieves uterine pain. It is analgesic, anti-inflammatory, antispasmodic, astringent, diuretic, and a uterine sedative.

Dandelion (*Taraxacum officinale*). Dandelion root is a cholagogue and helps the liver break down excess estrogen.

Dong quai (*Angelica sinensis*). The root relieves blood stagnation in the pelvic area. It is alterative, anticoagulant, blood tonic, emmenagogic, and a uterine tonic. Avoid during pregnancy, except under the guidance of your health care provider. Do not use in cases of diarrhea, heavy menstrual flow, poor digestion, or bloating. Do not use in conjunction with blood-thinning medications such as ibuprofen.

False unicorn (*Chamaelirium luteum*). This root is both an antiseptic and a uterine tonic. It can be helpful in treating uterine cysts as well as amenorrhea, dysmenorrhea, endometriosis, infertility, leukorrhea, and uterine prolapse. The bitter taste of this herb can cause vomiting. Excessive amounts may cause kidney and stomach irritation, blurred vision, and hot flashes. Do not use without employing birth control during sex unless pregnancy is desired. Discontinue use during pregnancy. False unicorn is endangered in the wild; do not use wildcrafted supplies.

Figwort (*Scrophularia nodosa*). The herb and root help decongest the lymphatic system. Figwort is often recommended in treatments for polycystic ovarian disease and ovarian cysts. It is alterative, anodyne, antifungal, antiseptic, anti-inflammatory, demulcent, depurative, and vulnerary.

Fraxinus (*Fraxinus americana*). The bark is a circulatory stimulant that helps reduce uterine inflammation.

Ginger (*Zingiber officinale*). Gingerroot improves circulation to the reproductive system and reduces blood platelet aggregation. It is analgesic, anti-inflammatory, antioxidant, antiseptic, and anticoagulant. Avoid large doses in cases of acne and eczema. Discontinue use if heartburn results.

Goldenseal (*Hydrastis canadensis*). The root is a tonic to mucous membranes of the genitourinary tract. It is an alterative, anti-inflammatory, astringent, cholagogue, and deobstruent. Goldenseal is very bitter, and most people find it easiest to ingest in capsule form. The tea can be used as a douche. This herb is endangered in the wild; do not use wildcrafted supplies. Avoid during pregnancy.

Lady's mantle (*Alchemilla xanthochlora*). The herb promotes blood coagulation and tissue healing. It is helpful for reducing heavy bleeding caused by uterine cysts. It is anti-inflammatory, astringent, diuretic, emmenagogic, hemostatic, liver decongestant, and vulnerary.

Licorice (*Glycyrrhiza glabra, G. uralensis*). The root soothes irritated mucous membranes and inhibits prostaglandin production. It is anti-inflammatory. Avoid during pregnancy and in cases of edema, high blood pressure, or diabetes. Do not use in combination with digoxin drugs. Excessive use can cause sodium retention and potassium depletion.

Motherwort (*Leonurus cardiaca*). The herb inhibits blood platelet aggregation. It is often recommended for treating both breast and ovarian cysts. It is an astringent, circulatory stimulant, diuretic, emmenagogue, rejuvenative, and vasodilator. Avoid in cases of heavy menstrual bleeding and during pregnancy, except during the final stages, and then only under the supervision of your health care provider.

Oregon grape (*Mahonia aquifolium*). The root (including the root bark) improves liver function and helps dilate blood vessels. It is an anti-inflammatory, antiseptic, alterative, astringent, cholagogue, diuretic, and immunostimulant. Avoid during pregnancy, and do not exceed the recommended dosage.

Partridgeberry (*Mitchella repens*). The herb has a long tradition of use as a uterine normalizer. It is an alterative, astringent, emmenagogue, uterine stimulant, and uterine tonic. Dosages in excess of what is recommended can irritate the mucous membranes. This herb is endangered in the wild; do not use wildcrafted supplies.

Peony (*Paeonia lactiflora*). Peony root nourishes muscles, including those of the uterus, and improves blood flow to the reproductive organs. It is an alterative, anti-inflammatory, antiseptic, antispasmodic, astringent, blood tonic, emmenagogue, hepatotonic, immunostimulant, and vasodilator. Avoid during pregnancy and in cases of diarrhea.

Pipsissewa (*Chimaphila umbellata*). This herb improves all uterine disorders, including cysts. It is an alterative, anti-inflammatory, astringent, diuretic, and urinary antiseptic.

Pokeweed (*Phytolacca americana*). The root increases T-cell activity in the immune system. It is an alterative, anti-inflammatory, immunostimulant, and lymphatic decongestant. In large amounts, pokeweed root can be toxic. Take only 2 or 3 drops of the tincture daily; after one week, increase the dosage to 5 drops (2 drops in the morning, 3 drops at night). Drink copious amounts of water while you are taking pokeweed root. Consult with your health care provider before use.

Prickly ash (*Zanthoxylum americanum, Z. clava-herculis*). The bark cleanses the body, especially the lymphatic system. It is alterative, anodyne, antiseptic, antispasmodic, astringent, emmenagogic, and a circulatory stimulant. Avoid during pregnancy and in cases of stomach inflammation.

Red clover (*Trifolium pratense*). The blossom is an excellent lymphatic cleanser and can be helpful for clearing breast and ovarian cysts. It is alterative, anti-inflammatory, and antitumor.

Red raspberry (*Rubus idaeus*). Red raspberry leaf is a universal remedy for all women's health concerns. It is an alterative, antiseptic, antispasmodic, astringent, hemostatic, hormone regulator, nutritive, and uterine tonic.

Redroot (*Ceanothus americanus*). The root encourages the elimination of catabolic waste and breaks up congestion in the body. It is often recommended in treatments for cysts, dysmenorrhea, and lymphatic congestion. It is antispasmodic and astringent.

Sarsaparilla (*Smilax* spp.). The root is a blood and lymphatic cleanser. It helps purify the genitourinary tract by binding with toxins and carrying them from the body. It is an alterative, antispasmodic, diuretic, and rejuvenative.

Saw palmetto (*Serenoa repens*). The berry reduces ovarian enlargement and pain. It is a diuretic, nutritive, rejuvenative, and urinary antiseptic.

Trillium (*Trillium* spp.). Trillium root is an antispasmodic pain reliever that is often recommended in treatments for dysmenorrhea. It also can stanch uterine hemorrhage. It is an alterative, antiseptic, antispasmodic, astringent, emmenagogue, hemostatic, and a uterine tonic. Avoid during pregnancy, except under the guidance of your health care provider. This herb is endangered in the wild; do not use wildcrafted supplies.

Turmeric (*Curcuma longa, C. aromatica*). The root inhibits yeast overgrowth and prevents blood platelet aggregation. It is an alterative, anticoagulant, antifungal, anti-inflammatory, antioxidant, cholagogue, circulatory stimulant, emmenagogue, hepatotonic, and vulnerary.

Vervain (*Verbena hastata, V. officinalis*). The herb stimulates uterine activity and improves the body's assimilation of nutrients. It is an anticoagulant, anti-inflammatory, antitumor, astringent, cholagogue, diuretic, emmenagogue, hepatostimulant, vasoconstrictor, and vulnerary. Avoid during pregnancy.

Violet (*Viola odorata*). The leaf is often used in traditional Oriental medicine to treat cysts and abscesses. It also helps break up congestion in the lymphatic system. It is alterative, antifungal, antiseptic, demulcent, and diuretic. You can incorporate violets—flowers and all—into your diet; try tossing them into fresh salads. You can also use the leaves as a compress.

Vitex (*Vitex agnus-castus*). The berry inhibits excessive cellular growth in the ovaries. It is emmenagogic, phytoprogesteronic, and vulnerary.

Wild yam (*Dioscorea opposita, D. villosa*). This root can reduce inflammation, move congested chi, and relieve ovarian pain. It also helps normalize hormone production. It is an anti-inflammatory, antispasmodic, cholagogue, diuretic, nutritive, and uterine sedative. Avoid therapeutic doses during pregnancy, except under the guidance of your health care provider. The *Dioscorea villosa* species is endangered in the wild; do not use wild-crafted supplies.

Yarrow (*Achillea millefolium*). The herb increases circulation to the reproductive system. It is an anti-inflammatory, antiseptic, antispasmodic, astringent, cholagogue, circulatory stimulant, diuretic, hemostatic, and urinary antiseptic. Avoid during pregnancy, except under the guidance of your health care provider.

YONI SUPPOSITORY

Use a Radical Resistance Yoni Suppository (see page 260) for five nights in a row. Every morning, douche with a tea made from yellow dock root and myrrh resin. Take a two-day break, then repeat. Continue this cycle for a month.

NUTRITIONAL THERAPY

Any of the nutritional supplements recommended for cervical dysplasia will also be helpful for resolving ovarian cysts. See page 257 for more information.

CASTOR OIL COMPRESS

The application of castor oil is thought to stimulate prostaglandin and immune system activity. Soak a flannel cloth in castor oil and apply to the lower abdominal area, over the liver and ovaries. Cover with a sheet of plastic and a hot water bottle, and relax for ninety minutes. Apply the compress once daily for three days. Take a four-day break, then repeat the cycle.

AROMATHERAPY MASSAGE

The essential oils of clary sage, lavender, neroli, rose, and thuja (cedar leaf) can help disperse congestion. Make a massage oil from one of these essential oils, or a combination thereof, following the instructions in chapter 5, and use it to massage your abdominal area. You can also add 5 drops of essential oil to a bath.

ENDOMETRIOSIS

The endometrium is the mucous membrane that lines the uterus and is shed during menstruation. Endometriosis occurs when tissue similar to endometrial tissue starts growing outside the uterus, such as on the ovaries, the fallopian tubes, the ligaments outside the uterus, the abdomen, the bladder, and the intestines. In extreme cases, endometrial tissue has been found in the nasal passages, lungs, arms, legs, and brain. These endometrial growths sometimes respond, like the endometrium itself, to the body's hormonal cycle: they build up, break down, and bleed. Intense pain and cramping can result. If endometriosis progresses, the renegade endometrial tissue can strangle the fallopian tubes and cause infertility or increase the likelihood of ectopic pregnancy.

Symptoms of endometriosis range greatly, and its exact cause is unknown. Researchers believe there may be a genetic link or altered immune system function at its root, but more research is needed. Dioxin, a toxin found in herbicides, pesticides, and industrial waste, has proved to be a trigger for endometriosis. Women who bleed heavily, experience strong cramps, have short cycles, and had early menarche are more likely candidates for endometriosis. IUDs and tampons may be factors because they cause irritation and sometimes scarring in the uterine area. (In fact, tampons can themselves be a carrier of dioxin if not made from organic unbleached cotton.) And endometriosis is often accompanied by other conditions, such as candidiasis, lupus, eczema, asthma, and a range of immune system disorders, although the connections between the diseases has not yet been discovered.

For more information about the causes, symptoms, and treatments of endometriosis, contact the Endometriosis Association (see the resources section on page 479).

Symptoms

Classic symptoms of endometriosis include chronic pelvic pain, severe menstrual cramps, pain during intercourse, fatigue, inflammatory bowel syndrome, and allergies. However, symptoms vary greatly, and diagnosis is difficult. The only way to confirm endometriosis is with laparoscopy, a surgical procedure in which a small viewing tube is inserted into the abdomen, usually through a horizontal incision above the navel.

If you do have a laparoscopy, use homeopathic ARNICA to reduce swelling and homeopathic BELLIS to help the tissue heal. Use 30C potencies of both, and take 4 drops or 4 pellets under the tongue four times daily for several months, or as directed by a homeopath.

Treatment

In treating endometriosis, it's important to focus on five goals.

1. **Improve the health of the liver.** The liver breaks down hormones and filters out toxins that contribute to the disease.
2. **Build up the health of the blood.** Healthy blood supports good health, good energy, and good circulation.
3. **Dispel stagnation.** Stagnation in the liver interferes with the breakdown of excess hormones, and stagnation in the pelvic area contributes to the development of blockages and growths.
4. **Dry mucous membranes.** Endometriosis is considered to be a condition of excess moisture and lymphatic congestion. Drying out the mucous membranes helps reduce this congestion.
5. **Relieve pain.** Endometriosis can be extremely painful, and the pharmaceutical painkillers that are often recommended for it can stress or even harm the liver. Natural methods for relieving pain generally often won't eliminate it altogether, but they can reduce both the severity and duration of pain.

Though endometriosis can be difficult to cure completely, symptoms and pain can be greatly improved. Plan on spending eight months to a year on improving the condition. If treatment doesn't show immediate results, don't become discouraged. Pain may remain unresolved for the first couple of months as old clots and stagnation are released from the body.

High levels of estrogen stimulate the endometrium and outlying endometrial tissues to grow. Pregnancy produces high levels of progesterone, which overpowers estrogen. Therefore, some health care providers might suggest pregnancy as a treatment for endometriosis. This solution is of questionable value. First, it's temporary; when the pregnancy is over, the symptoms often return. And second, pain relief seems like an irresponsible reason to have a baby, unless you really want one.

SITZ BATHS

Alternating hot and cold sitz baths is a helpful hydrotherapy technique for increasing circulation to and clearing congestion in the pelvic area. See chapter 10 for instructions.

HERBAL THERAPY

Herbal therapy for endometriosis is gaining recognition in the medical community for its effectiveness. For best results, continue therapy for at least six months.

Alfalfa (*Medicago sativa*). The leaf aids in cellular detoxification. It is anti-inflammatory, diuretic, and nutritive.

Asparagus (*Asparagus officinalis, A. cochinchinensis*). Aparagus root supports and moistens yin, which, in turn, supports the endocrine system. It is a demulcent, diuretic, female tonic, nutritive, and sedative.

Black cohosh (*Actaea racemosa*). The root dries mucous membranes and helps regulate menses. It also improves circulation and relieves congestion in the cervix, uterus, and vagina. Black cohosh is often recommended for dysmenorrhea. It is an alterative, anti-inflammatory, antispasmodic, astringent, diuretic, emmenagogue, and muscle relaxant. Avoid during pregnancy, except in the final stages, and then only under the guidance of your health care provider. Avoid while nursing and in cases of high blood pressure or pressure in the inner eye. Consult with your health care provider before use. This herb is endangered in the wild; do not use wildcrafted supplies.

Blue cohosh (*Caulophyllum thalictroides*). The root relieves endometrial pain and helps regulate menses. It also dries mucous membranes. It is anti-inflammatory, antispasmodic, diuretic, emmenagogic, and a uterine tonic. Avoid during pregnancy, except in the final stages, and then only under the guidance of your health care provider. Make sure the root is dried, not fresh. This herb is endangered in the wild; do not use wildcrafted supplies.

Bupleurum (*Bupleurum chinense, B. falcatum*). Bupleurum root clears stagnation from the liver and blood. It helps normalize menses and can relieve pain. It is an alterative, anti-inflammatory, and muscle relaxant. Avoid in cases of fever, headache, or high blood pressure.

Burdock (*Arctium lappa*). The root cleanses glands and normalizes their function. It also improves the function of the organs of elimination, thereby reducing the load on the liver, and removes dampness. It is an alterative, anti-inflammatory, cholagogue, diuretic, laxative, and nutritive.

Chamomile (*Matricaria recutita*). Chamomile flower helps to detoxify the liver. It is often recommended in treatments for amenorrhea and dysmenorrhea. It is analgesic, anodyne, anti-inflammatory, antispasmodic, emmenagogic, and a mild sedative.

Cramp bark (*Viburnum opulus*). The bark relaxes muscles, relieving pain. It is an alterative, analgesic, anti-inflammatory, antispasmodic, diuretic, nervine, sedative, and uterine sedative.

Dandelion (*Taraxacum officinale*). The root clears congestion from the liver. It is a cholagogue, diuretic, and liver tonic.

Dong quai (*Angelica sinensis*). The root of dong quai clears stagnation from the blood and improves circulation. It also relieves congestion in pelvic tissue, helps regulate menses, and relaxes smooth muscles. It is an alterative, anticoagulant, antispasmodic, blood tonic, and uterine tonic. Avoid during pregnancy, except under the guidance of your health care provider. Do not use in cases of diarrhea, heavy menstrual flow, poor digestion, or bloating. Do not use in conjunction with blood-thinning medications such as ibuprofen.

Ginger (*Zingiber officinale*). The root improves circulation and helps relieve inflammation. It is often recommended for amenorrhea and dysmenorrhea. It is analgesic, anticoagulant, anti-inflammatory, and antispasmodic. Avoid large doses in cases of acne and eczema. Discontinue use if heartburn results.

Hibiscus (*Hibiscus sabdariffa*). The flower is anti-estrogenic, suppressing estrogen-induced growths in the uterus. It also helps regulate menses. It is an alterative, anti-inflammatory, antispasmodic, astringent, emmenagogue, and hemostatic.

Ho shou wu (*Polygonum multiflorum*). The root discourages blood clotting and helps reduce benign growths. It is an alterative, analgesic, antispasmodic, anti-inflammatory, and hepatotonic.

Jamaican dogwood (*Piscidia piscipula*). The bark is excellent for endometriosis affecting the fallopian tubes and pain that causes nausea. It is a potent pain-relieving agent, calming ovarian and uterine discomfort. It is also an anti-inflammatory and a sedative.

Lady's mantle (*Alchemilla xanthochlora*). The herb helps prevent excess menstrual bleeding and clears congestion from the liver. It promotes blood coagulation and healing of tissue, and is often recommended for dysmenorrhea and menorrhagia. It is anti-inflammatory, astringent, diuretic, emmenagogic, and hemostatic.

Licorice (*Glycyrrhiza glabra, G. uralensis*). Licorice root inhibits the production of the prostaglandins that contribute to irritation of the mucous membranes. It is anti-inflammatory, antispasmodic, demulcent, and phytoestrogenic. Avoid during pregnancy and in cases of edema, high blood pressure, or diabetes. Do not use in combination with digoxin drugs. Excessive use can cause sodium retention and potassium depletion.

Motherwort (*Leonurus cardiaca*). The herb relaxes vaginal muscles, thereby improving blood flow to the pelvic region and contributing to the breakdown and removal of endometrial tissue. It is often recommended for amenorrhea and dysmenorrhea. Motherwort is an antispasmodic, astringent, circulatory stimulant, emmenagogue, nervine, sedative, and uterine tonic. Avoid in cases of heavy bleeding and during pregnancy, except during the final stages, and then only under the supervision of your health care provider.

Myrrh (*Commiphora myrrha*). The resin clears stagnation from the blood and dries out mucous membranes. It is often recommended for amenorrhea and dysmenorrhea. It is an alterative, analgesic, antispasmodic, and emmenagogue. Avoid during pregnancy, and do not use for more than one month at a time.

Oregon grape (*Mahonia aquifolium*). The root strengthens the liver and helps curb excessive menstrual bleeding. It is alterative, anti-inflammatory, astringent, cholagogic, and diuretic. Avoid during pregnancy, and do not exceed the recommended dosage.

Partridgeberry (*Mitchella repens*). The herb relieves pelvic congestion, although dosages in excess of what is recommended can irritate the mucous membranes. Partridgeberry is an astringent and a uterine tonic. This herb is endangered in the wild, so do not use wildcrafted supplies.

Peony (*Paeonia lactiflora*). Peony root relieves cramps, relaxes uterine muscles, and improves blood flow to the uterus. It is an alterative, anti-inflammatory, antispasmodic, emmenagogue, hepatotonic, and uterine astringent. Avoid during pregnancy and in cases of diarrhea.

Prickly ash (*Zanthoxylum americanum, Z. clava-herculis*). The bark is warming to the abdominal region, thereby helping to clear congestion from the pelvic area. It is an alterative, anodyne, analgesic, antispasmodic, astringent, circulatory stimulant, emmenagogue, and glandular stimulant. Avoid during pregnancy and in cases of stomach inflammation.

Red clover (*Trifolium pratense*). A wonderful tonic for general health, red clover blossom also reduces blood clots. It is alterative, anodyne, anticoagulant, anti-inflammatory, antispasmodic, diuretic, nutritive, and phytoestrogenic.

Red raspberry (*Rubus idaeus*). The leaf helps prevent premenstrual spotting, decreases uterine swelling, and relieves muscle cramps. It is an alterative, antispasmodic, anodyne, astringent, demulcent, hemostatic, and uterine tonic.

Rehmannia (*Rehmannia glutinosa*). The root strengthens and purifies the liver and relieves abdominal pain. It is an alterative, anti-inflammatory, blood tonic, diuretic, hemostatic, and uterine tonic. Avoid in cases of loose stools, poor appetite, bloating, or a coated tongue.

Turmeric (*Curcuma longa, C. aromatica*). Compounds in turmeric root may compete with estrogen for receptor sites, reducing the production of hormones in the body. It can reduce blood clots and uterine tumors and is often recommended for amenorrhea and dysmenorrhea. It is an alterative, anticoagulant, anti-inflammatory, astringent, cholagogue, circulatory stimulant, emmenagogue, and hepatotonic.

Valerian (*Valeriana officinalis*). The root encourages smooth muscles to relax, relieving pain. It is an anodyne, antispasmodic, astringent, nervine, and sedative.

Vitex (*Vitex agnus-castus*). The berry reduces estrogen production and thus reduces endometrial growth. It helps normalize menstrual cycles and regulate the pituitary gland. It is antispasmodic, emmenagogic, and phytoprogesteronic.

White willow (*Salix alba*). The bark sedates the pelvis, repressing the perception of pain. It also reduces inflammation by inhibiting the production of prostaglandins. It is an alterative, analgesic, anodyne, anti-inflammatory, antispasmodic, and astringent.

Wild yam (*Dioscorea opposita, D. villosa*). The root reduces inflammation, clears congested chi, and calms painful cramps—particularly in the fallopian tubes. It contains phytosterols, which help normalize the body's production of hormones. It is anti-inflammatory, antispasmodic, cholagogic, diuretic, and nervine. Avoid therapeutic doses of wild yam root during pregnancy, except under the guidance of your health care provider. The *Dioscorea villosa* species is endangered in the wild; do not use wildcrafted supplies.

Yarrow (*Achillea millefolium*). The herb can curb the excess menstrual bleeding sometimes associated with endometriosis. It is an anti-inflammatory, antispasmodic, astringent, cholagogue, diuretic, emmenagogue, hemostatic, and uterine sedative. Avoid during pregnancy.

YONI SUPPOSITORY

Use the Radical Resistance Yoni Suppository described on page 260 for ten nights in a row. Take two days off, then repeat. Continue this cycle for a month.

CHINESE PATENT FORMULA

TO WAN. The Chinese patent formula TO WAN, also known as the REGULATE MENSES PILL, disperses blood stagnation and relieves cramping. In my experience, and that of my fellow herbalists, TO WAN has been effective in resolving many cases of endometriosis.

NUTRITIONAL THERAPY

Food is always the first choice in providing nutrients for the body. Turn to chapter 3 to identify natural sources of the nutrients listed below. But as you work on improving your diet, you may also wish to use supplements.

Vitamin B_6. Vitamin B_6 encourages progesterone production and supports the liver's ability to break down estrogen. Take 25 to 300 mg daily.

Choline and inositol. These two members of the vitamin B complex help the liver break down fats and fat-soluble hormones such as estrogen. Take 25 to 500 mg of each daily.

Vitamin C with bioflavonoids. Vitamin C, combined with bioflavonoids, supports the oxygenation of tissues, which reduces blockages and promotes tissue elasticity and capillary strength. Take 1,000 mg of vitamin C with 500 mg of bioflavonoids daily.

Vitamin E. Vitamin E can improve the body's use of oxygen and prevent the formation of scar tissue, thereby reducing the development of blockages. Take 100 to 1,200 IU daily.

Magnesium. Magnesium relaxes nerves, allowing chi to flow freely, and also encourages the relaxation of muscles, relieving pain. Take 500 to 750 mg daily.

Methionine. This amino acid, like choline and inositol, aids in the breakdown of fats and fat-soluble hormones. Take 500 mg daily. You won't find methionine listed in chapter 3; good natural sources include apples, Brazil nuts, Brussels sprouts, cabbage, cauliflower, chicken, chives, corn, cottage cheese, eggs, fish, garlic, lentils, milk, nuts, pineapple, rice, ricotta cheese, sesame seeds, soy foods, sunflower seeds, watercress, whole grains, and yogurt.

CASTOR OIL COMPRESS

Castor oil compresses improve circulation to the pelvic area, stimulate immune system activity, assist pain relief, and soften scar tissue. See page 267 for instructions on making and applying the compress.

HOMEOPATHIC REMEDIES

When endometriosis is accompanied by any of the conditions that are described below, try the suggested homeopathic remedy. The usual dosage is 4 pellets, or as many liquid drops as the package label recommends, taken under the tongue four times daily. Rather than swallowing the pellets whole, allow them to dissolve slowly.

APIS MELLIFICA. The pain feels similar to bee stings and is worse on the right side. The abdomen and uterus feel tender. The patient lacks thirst and produces scant urine.

ARSENICUM ALBUM. The ovarian area burns. The patient experiences early, heavy menses with throbbing pain. She feels restless and thirsty. Movement and cold worsen symptoms and cause fatigue.

AURUM MURIATICUM NATRONATUM. The endometriosis is chronic. The uterus is enlarged, and the vagina and cervix are ulcerated.

BELLADONNA. The pain comes on and disappears suddenly. Sensations of burning, clutching, and stitching occur. The patient feels tired but is unable to sleep. She may experience incontinence.

CANTHARIS. The ovaries are inflamed. The patient may have had gonorrhea.

CHAMOMILLA. The patient is irritable and oversensitive to the pain, which shoots down the thighs.

CIMICIFUGA RACEMOSA. The pain occurs just before the menses. The menses are irregular, accompanied by backache, and produce dark, profuse blood.

COLOCYNTHIS. The patient experiences intense emotions, especially vexation. Doubling over and the application of hard pressure lessens the pain.

DIOSCOREA. The pain is sharp and shoots out in multiple directions. The pain is worse when the patient is lying down or doubled over; it lessens when the patient is moving, stretched out, or bending backward.

GELSEMIUM. The uterus feels like it is being squeezed. The patient experiences dysmenorrhea and light menses. The pain affects the hips and back.

HELONIAS DIOICA. The menses are frequent and profuse. The patient feels swelling and burning in the endometrial region.

LACHESIS. The menses are light and painful. Soreness extends from the pelvic region to the chest. The ovaries are inflamed. The pain decreases during menstruation.

LYCOPODIUM. Sharp pain extends across the body in the pelvic area. The patient discharges blood from the genitals during bowel movements.

MAGNESIUM PHOSPHATE. The pain comes on suddenly and increases with cold, touch, and at night. Warmth and the application of pressure lessen pain.

MERCURIUS CORROSIVUS. The patient experiences pain similar to labor pain in the vagina and abdomen. There is a yellowish discharge from the vagina. The menses arrive early.

MERCURIUS VIVUS. The patient experiences abdominal pain, stinging pain in the ovaries, and heavy menses. There is a greenish bloody discharge from the vagina.

NUX VOMICA. The pain is worse in the early morning and when cold or pressure is applied. The pain lessens during menstruation, when heat is applied, and when pressure is applied to the head.

PULSATILLA. The menses are light. The patient has diarrhea before the onset of menstruation. There are cutting pains in the uterus, which is sensitive to touch. Intercourse is painful.

SEPIA. Menses is either excessively light or profuse and late or early. The patient experiences a sharp clutching or bearing-down pain.

SILICEA. The patient experiences bleeding between cycles and feels cold. There is an acrid, milky, leukorrhea-like discharge during urination.

VIBURNUM. The pain is more sudden and more severe before menstruation. The pain lessens when pressure is applied.

FLOWER ESSENCES

There are a couple of flower essences that can support the treatment of endometriosis. The usual dosage is 3 drops under the tongue or taken with a glass of water three or four times daily.

Blackberry. This essence stimulates the liver, boosts blood circulation, and improves hormonal function.

Star Tulip. Star Tulip helps people who seem to have a protective wall around their emotions to open up.

AROMATHERAPY

Try the following essential oils in massage oil, the bath, or inhalations. For instructions on preparing these treatments, turn to chapter 5.

- **Angelica**—disperses stagnation and is phytoestrogenic.
- **Chamomile**—relieves pain and inflammation.
- **Cypress**—disperses stagnation.
- **Geranium**—disperses stagnation.
- **Hyssop**—disperses stagnation.
- **Lavender**—relieves inflammation and calms the nerves.
- **Oregano**—disperses stagnation.
- **Rosemary**—improves circulation to the pelvic area.

FIBROCYSTIC BREAST CONDITIONS

Fibrocystic breast *disease,* a term sometimes still heard in the medical community to describe having lumps in the breast, is a misnomer. Every woman has had cysts or fibrous tissue in her breasts at one time or another; a fibrocystic condition, then, is normal, not a disease.

Some lumps in the breast are simple cysts, or fluid-filled sacs. Others are fibroadenomas, or benign tumors of glandular origin. Still others are simply dense areas of otherwise normal breast tissue. Only 10 to 15 percent of breast lumps are cancerous.

Most noncancerous breast lumps do not require medical treatment. If cysts are large, a surgeon can remove the fluid from them. If a lump is large enough to interfere with your ability to properly examine the tissue around it, your health care provider may recommend that you have it surgically removed.

Symptoms

Monthly breast exams will help you become familiar with the normal lumps of your breasts. These may grow or decrease in size through the evolution of the menstrual cycle. If you find a new lump in your breast, don't panic. Unless you have a family history of breast cancer—in which case you should bring the lump to the immediate attention of your health care provider—you may want to keep an eye on the lump for a couple of menstrual cycles. If it disappears or grows smaller during this time, it's probably not a cancerous growth. If it stays the same size or grows, have it evaluated by your health care provider. Nipple discharge, especially bloody, should be evaluated by a health care provider.

To prevent or reduce the size of noncancerous lumps in the breasts, consider the treatment suggestions that follow.

Treatment

The breasts have a high concentration of lymphatic tissue and lymph nodes. If lymph glands or lymph flow in the breasts is obstructed, inflammation and cysts can develop. Therefore, supporting the health of the breasts involves, in part, supporting proper lymphatic circulation. That's good news for our immune system, because the lymph system, which transports liquid lymph throughout the body, is a vital component of immune function. Lymph is filled with white blood cells called lymphocytes; some of these lymphocytes evolve into lymphoblasts, which are capable of recognizing and eliminating antigens.

It's also important to support the liver and the colon. The liver breaks down excess hormones in the body. If liver function is impaired, the resulting hormone overload can lead to the development of cysts in the breasts as well as many other maladies. The colon is the organ of elimination. If colon function is impaired, waste matter builds up in the body, imbuing it with toxins.

WEAR NATURAL-FIBER CLOTHING

Most women are conscious these days of the importance of wearing natural-fiber clothing to allow skin to breathe. Yet most bras are made with synthetic fibers, which means we encase our breasts with polyester foam fill and metal wires. These synthetic materials prevent sweat—a waste product—from flowing freely, trapping toxins in the breast region. Stop the madness! Wear bras that are made of cotton or another natural fiber (preferably organic). And go braless when possible (like as soon as you get home). Undershirts can be cool!

EXERCISE

Exercise boosts circulation in the lymph system and supports the elimination of metabolic wastes, helping to prevent cysts from developing. Good exercises for improving lymphatic drainage include jumping on a trampoline and walking while allowing the arms to swing freely.

Yoga postures that help alleviate sore cystic breasts include Laid-Back Camel, Corner Hang, and Twisted Angle. These postures can be learned in a yoga class or from books on yoga.

AVOID ANTIPERSPIRANTS

Commercial antiperspirants are designed to keep you from sweating. Many contain aluminum, which, when it comes in contact with the skin, causes an allergic-type reaction. The pores of the skin swell and close, preventing perspiration from escaping.

Now let's think about this. Perspiration is one of the means by which we excrete metabolic wastes. If we can't excrete metabolic wastes, they must be stored somewhere in the body. So when we apply antiperspirant to our armpits, the metabolic wastes in that area must find a storage location. What roomy, fleshy area is located just around the corner? That's right—our breasts.

Years ago, a wise older woman friend told me she would never use antiperspirants because she thought that they contributed to breast cancer. In my sixteen-year-old naïveté, I thought she was being ridiculous. A few weeks later, while at boarding school, I accidentally knocked a bottle of commercial antiperspirant behind my dresser, and it smashed on the floor. But then the bell rang, and I had to run off to class. Being a busy and messy kid, it was a few days before I got around to moving the dresser to clean up the mess behind it. I was amazed to see that the deodorant had hardened into a plasticlike sheet. Yikes! I never bought another commercial antiperspirant after that; I use instead only natural, aluminum-free deodorants.

DIET

If you have breast cysts, avoid coffee, tea, cola drinks, and chocolate. They contain caffeine, and most health care practitioners agree that caffeine in any form contributes to the development of breast cysts and pain. These products also contain methylxanthines, compounds that impair the enzymatic activity of cells, contributing to poor digestion and the development of blockages in the body. Even decaffeinated coffee contains methylxanthines.

Avoid hydrogenated oils, such as those found in fried foods and margarine, because they congest the liver. Minimize your intake of dairy products, which cause mucous congestion and often contain the residues of synthetic hormones that were used in raising the dairy animals. The one exception to this rule is plain yogurt; eat at least one serving every day to promote the growth of friendly microorganisms in the colon. Just be sure that the yogurt contains live bacteria cultures and was made from the milk of animals raised by organic methods and without hormone treatments.

To support healthy elimination, drink plenty of water. Juice made from an equal mix of carrots, beets, and celery can improve the functions of all the organs of elimination and provide the body with a great range of minerals. Try drinking a cup of it several times a week.

Include plenty of seaweeds in your diet as they help drain and disperse congestion and also support the endocrine system. If seaweed doesn't suit your palate, take a kelp supplement.

You should see results in two to six months.

HERBAL THERAPY

There are many herbs that can help reduce the size and occurrence of noncancerous breast lumps.

Agrimony (*Agrimonia eupatoria*). The herb inhibits blood platelet aggregation, which can be a factor in the development of cysts. It is an anti-inflammatory, astringent, diuretic, emmenagogue, and tonic. Avoid during pregnancy and in cases of constipation.

Astragalus (*Astragalus membranaceus*). The root stimulates immune system response and inhibits the development of free radicals. It is an adaptogen, antiviral, blood tonic, chi tonic, circulatory stimulant, immunostimulant, and vasodilator.

Black cohosh (*Actaea racemosa*). The root helps reduce pain in the breasts. It is alterative, anti-inflammatory, antiseptic, antispasmodic, astringent, circulatory stimulant, emmenagogue, and vasodilator. Avoid during pregnancy, except in the final stages, and then only under the guidance of your health care provider. Avoid while nursing and in cases of high blood pressure or pressure in the inner eye. Consult with your health care provider before use. This herb is endangered in the wild; do not use wildcrafted supplies.

Blessed thistle (*Cnicus benedictus*). The herb strengthens the spleen and the liver. It is an alterative, emmenagogue, and hemostatic.

Burdock (*Arctium lappa*). Burdock root supports proper functioning in the organs of elimination. It also relieves lymphatic congestion. It is alterative, antifungal, antiseptic, anti-inflammatory, antitumor, choleretic, demulcent, diuretic, laxative, nutritive, and rejuvenative.

Calendula (*Calendula officinalis*). The flower improves liver and lymphatic function. It reduces glandular swelling and improves peripheral circulation. It is an alterative, anti-inflammatory, astringent, and vulnerary.

Cleavers (*Galium aparine*). The herb is a lymphatic cleanser. It clears heat and relieves inflammation and pain in the breasts. It is an alterative, anti-inflammatory, antitumor, astringent, and vulnerary.

Dandelion (*Taraxacum officinale*). Dandelion root improves liver function and supports the elimination of toxins. It also relieves stagnation in the reproductive organs. It is antifungal, antitumor, cholagogic, and a Liver tonic.

Dong quai (*Angelica sinensis*). The root improves circulation and clears stagnation in the liver. It is an alterative, anticoagulant, and blood tonic. Avoid during pregnancy, except under the guidance of your health care provider. Do not use in cases of diarrhea, heavy menstrual flow, poor digestion, or bloating. Do not use in conjunction with blood-thinning medications such as ibuprofen.

Echinacea (*Echinacea purpurea, E. angustifolia*). The root stimulates T-cell production and macrophage activity in the immune system. It also improves peripheral blood circulation. It is alterative, antifungal, anti-inflammatory, antiseptic, antitumor, and depurative.

False unicorn (*Chamaelirium luteum*). The root normalizes estrogen production and helps reduce both the occurrence and size of breast cysts. It is often recommended as a reproductive tonic. The bitter taste of this herb can cause vomiting. Excessive amounts may cause kidney and stomach irritation, blurred vision, and hot flashes. Do not use without employing birth control during sex unless pregnancy is desired. Discontinue use during pregnancy. False unicorn is endangered in the wild, so do not use wildcrafted supplies.

Fringe tree (*Chionanthus virginicus*). Fringe tree bark improves liver function, clears circulatory obstructions, and reduces inflammation. It is an alterative and cholagogue.

Ginger (*Zingiber officinale*). The root improves circulation, helps clear stagnation, and encourages lymphatic cleansing. It is anti-inflammatory, antispasmodic, antioxidant, and anticoagulant. Avoid large doses in cases of acne and eczema. Discontinue use if heartburn results.

Goldenseal (*Hydrastis canadensis*). The root improves liver function. It is an alterative, anti-inflammatory, antiseptic, astringent, cholagogue, and vasoconstrictor. Goldenseal is very bitter, and most people find it easiest to ingest in capsule form. This herb is endangered in the wild; do not use wildcrafted supplies. Avoid during pregnancy.

Hawthorn (*Crataegus* spp.). The leaf, flower, and berry help break down fatty deposits in the body, including those that form lumps in the breasts. This herb is astringent, a circulatory stimulant, and a vasodilator.

Lady's mantle (*Alchemilla xanthochlora*). The herb is a hormone balancer. It reduces inflammation, clears heat, and relieves congestion in the liver. It is an astringent.

Licorice (*Glycyrrhiza glabra, G. uralensis*). Licorice root stimulates the immune system and inhibits the production of prostaglandin E2, which contributes to inflammation. It also soothes irritated mucous membranes. It is an anti-inflammatory, antiseptic, antitumor, chi tonic, demulcent, nutritive, and rejuvenative. Avoid during pregnancy and in cases of edema, high blood pressure, or diabetes. Do not use in combination with digoxin drugs. Excessive use can cause sodium retention and potassium depletion.

Nettle (*Urtica dioica, U. urens*). The leaf benefits all systems of the body. It is an alterative, astringent, cholagogue, circulatory stimulant, galactagogue, nutritive, and rubefacient. Contact with the fresh plant will irritate the skin; use only dried herb. Wear gloves when collecting.

Pau d'arco (*Tabebuia impetiginosa*). The bark increases red blood cell production, helps the body resist autoimmune diseases, and improves liver function. Pau d'arco can also reduce both the size and occurrence of tumors. It is alterative, antifungal, anti-inflammatory, antioxidant, antiseptic, antitumor, and immunostimulant.

Pokeweed (*Phytolacca americana*). The root improves lymphatic function and increases T-cell activity in the immune system. It is an alterative, anti-inflammatory, immunostimulant, and lymphatic decongestant. In large amounts, pokeweed root can be toxic. Take only 2 or 3 drops of the tincture daily; after one week, increase the dosage to 5 drops (2 drops in the morning, 3 drops at night). Drink copious amounts of water while you are taking pokeweed root. Consult with your health care provider before use.

Red clover (*Trifolium pratense*). The flower is an excellent lymphatic cleanser. It is alterative, anti-inflammatory, and antitumor.

Red raspberry (*Rubus idaeus*). The leaf helps normalize hormone production. It is an alterative, antiseptic, astringent, hemostatic, hormone regulator, nutritive, and yin tonic.

Sarsaparilla (*Smilax* spp.). The root is a blood and lymphatic cleanser. It contains compounds that bind with toxins and carry them from the body. It is an alterative and a rejuvenative.

Vervain (*Verbena hastata, V. officinalis*). The herb improves the body's assimilation of nutrients and helps reduce the size and occurrence of breast and ovarian cysts. It is an anticoagulant, anti-inflammatory, antitumor, astringent, cholagogue, diuretic, emmenagogue, hepatostimulant, vasoconstrictor, and vulnerary. Avoid during pregnancy.

Violet (*Viola odorata*). The leaf has long been used as treatment for cysts, breast cancer, lymphatic congestion, and mastitis. Eat as a salad herb and use topically as a poultice. It is alterative, antifungal, antiseptic, demulcent, and diuretic.

Wild yam (*Dioscorea opposita, D. villosa*). The root is a hormone balancer. It reduces inflammation and clears congested chi. It is an anti-inflammatory, cholagogue, diuretic, and nutritive. Avoid therapeutic doses during pregnancy, except under the guidance of your health care provider. The *Dioscorea villosa* species is endangered in the wild; do not use wild-crafted supplies.

Yellow dock (*Rumex crispus*). The root improves liver, kidney, and lymphatic function. It is an alterative, astringent, blood tonic, and cholagogue.

NUTRITIONAL THERAPY

Food should always be the first source of nutrients for the body. You may also wish to use supplements as you work on improving your diet. Supplements that can be helpful for fibrocystic breasts include the following:

Antioxidants. Antioxidants support the body's immune system. They are best absorbed through natural sources of the nutrients beta-carotene, vitamin C, vitamin E, selenium, and superoxide dismutase. Good sources of each are provided in chapter 3.

Essential fatty acids. EFAs can reduce pain and inflammation. Evening primrose oil, borage seed oil, and black currant seed oil are excellent sources; take 1 tablespoon daily. Purslane, sesame seeds, sunflower seeds, and walnuts are also good sources of EFAs; incorporate these foods into your diet, amounting to 3 tablespoons daily.

Potassium. Potassium encourages the body to get rid of excess fluid. Eat plenty of potassium-rich foods, such as apricots, avocados, bananas, beans, beets and beet greens, blackstrap molasses, brown rice, cantaloupe, carrots, currants, dates, figs, fish, grapes, green leafy vegetables, lentils, oranges, papaya, peaches, potatoes, pumpkin seeds, raisins, seafood, spinach, sunflower seeds, tomatoes, watermelon, and wheat germ. You might also consider supplementing with 99 to 300 mg of potassium daily.

Vitamin B complex. The B vitamins support the immune system. Take 50 mg daily, or incorporate natural sources into your diet, such as alfalfa, beans, brown rice, Brussels sprouts, eggs, green leafy vegetables, nuts, and peas.

Vitamin E. Vitamin E can help reduce the size and number of breast cysts. Take 400 IU daily. Look for a vitamin E supplement that also contains selenium; women prone to breast cysts have been found to have low levels of selenium in their blood.

HOMEOPATHIC REMEDIES

When fibrocystic breast conditions are accompanied by the conditions that are described below, try the suggested homeopathic remedy. The usual dosage is 4 pellets, or as many liquid drops as the package label recommends, taken under the tongue four times daily. Rather than swallowing the pellets whole, allow them to dissolve slowly.

BELLADONNA. The patient has a strong constitution. She is filled with energy but may lack creative outlets for it.

BRYONIA. The breasts are sore and swollen during the menses.

CONIUM. The breasts are tender and swollen just before menstruation. The patient experiences aching muscles and disturbing dreams.

LACHESIS. The patient is absentminded and has swollen, aching breasts.

PHYTOLACCA. The breasts are sore and lumpy. There are enlarged lymph nodes under the arms.

PULSATILLA. The breasts are swollen and tender.

SILICEA. The lumps in the breast are hard.

AROMATHERAPY MASSAGE

Massage the breasts daily to improve circulation and lymphatic drainage. For added benefit, use a massage oil infused with essential oils that support cleansing of the circulatory and lymphatic systems, such as cypress, geranium, juniper, lavender, rose, rose geranium, and/or rosemary. (See page 139 for instructions on making a massage oil.) Also try adding 7 to 10 drops of any of these essential oils to the bath. Be sure to soak your breasts in the tub while bathing.

LEUKORRHEA

Leukorrhea is a vaginal discharge containing mucus and pus that results from inflammation or congestion of the mucous glands of the vagina or cervix. Having a slight discharge before the menses and a thicker discharge around the time of ovulation is normal. A change in that pattern or a consistent abnormal discharge signals a possible infection—especially if the discharge is yellow, greenish, or foul smelling.

Causes of Leukorrhea

The causes of leukorrhea are many. Candidiasis can cause excessive vaginal discharge; if the discharge is accompanied by itchiness and burning, suspect a Candida infection and turn to page 248. If the discharge is greenish and foul smelling, trichomoniasis (*T. vaginalis*) is the most likely culprit; see page 416 for more details. If the discharge is thin and grayish, suspect bacterial vaginosis (caused by the bacterium *Hemophilus*). If the discharge contains blood, you may have chlamydia, and you should see your health care provider for a proper diagnosis.

In all other cases, if leukorrhea is not accompanied by other symptoms, you may wish to try the treatments suggested below. If treatment does not clear up the symptoms within two to three weeks, visit your gynecologist for a proper diagnosis.

Treatment

Treatments for leukorrhea focus on supporting the immune system and reducing inflammation and irritation of the mucous membranes.

DIET

Dairy products and wheat contribute to the production of excess mucus, so they should be minimized in the diet. The one exception to this rule is plain yogurt, which contains live bacteria cultures that support friendly vaginal microorganisms and combat yeast overgrowth. Eat at least one serving of plain, organic yogurt daily. Vegans can use almond or sesame yogurt.

HERBAL THERAPY

The following herbs can be very effective in clearing up leukorrhea.

Burdock (*Arctium lappa*). The root is alterative, antibacterial, and antifungal. It improves the function of all the organs of elimination.

Dandelion (*Taraxacum officinale*). The root is an antifungal, cholagogue, and diuretic. It supports the body's cleansing systems.

Echinacea (*Echinacea purpurea, E. angustifolia*). The root strengthens the immune system and stimulates white blood cell production. It is alterative, antibiotic, antifungal, antiseptic, and antiviral.

Garlic (*Allium sativum*). The bulb counteracts a wide range of infectious conditions. It is an alterative, antibiotic, antifungal, antioxidant, antiprotozoan, and immunostimulant. Some people are allergic to garlic. Excessive use can cause emotional irritability and irritation of the stomach and kidneys. Avoid therapeutic doses during pregnancy, and avoid during the first three months of nursing, as it can cause breast milk to become unpalatable for infants. Avoid taking garlic for one week before having surgery.

Myrrh (*Commiphora myrrha*). The resin helps normalize mucous membrane activity. It is an alterative, antifungal, antiseptic, decongestant, and emmenagogue. Avoid during pregnancy, and do not use for more than one month at a time.

Yellow dock (*Rumex crispus*). The root improves kidney, liver, lymph system, and colon function, thus aiding all of the body's natural cleansing processes. It is an alterative, antiseptic, and astringent.

DISINFECTANT DOUCHE

The disinfectant douche below is both germicidal and astringent. It can clear infection and dry mucous membranes, helping eliminate the leukorrheal discharge. Douche just twice daily; getting overzealous with this treatment can wash away friendly vaginal flora. Follow up with a plain yogurt suppository.

DISINFECTANT DOUCHE

This douche inhibits unfriendly microorganisms.

1 teaspoon bayberry root
2 teaspoons calendula flower
¼ teaspoon goldenseal root
1 teaspoon lady's mantle herb
1 teaspoon white oak bark
6 cups water

Combine all the herbs. Bring the water to a boil. Add all of the mixed herbs. Remove from heat, cover, and let steep for one hour. Strain the liquid from the herbs, and compost the spent herbs. Pour the infused liquid into a douche bag. Add 2 cups of water. Douche.

THERAPEUTIC BATH

Add to the bath 7 to 10 drops of the essential oil of eucalyptus, lavender, tea tree, or a combination thereof. These oils are both germicidal and astringent and can help clear up infection and congestion in mucous membranes.

PAINFUL INTERCOURSE

Pain during intercourse can manifest as a deep aching pain, a sudden sharp twinge, a burning sensation, itchiness, or simple discomfort. The possible causes are many and can include allergies (to soap, bath bubbles, latex, contraceptive gel, and so on), candidiasis, constipation, endometriosis, herpes, pelvic inflammatory disease, scar tissue, urinary tract infection, vaginal dryness, and venereal warts. Seek the advice of a gynecologist to determine the cause and the appropriate treatment.

PELVIC INFLAMMATORY DISEASE

Pelvic inflammatory disease (PID) has become one of the most common gynecological infections contracted by young women. It is a leading cause of infertility. It is usually caused by an infection, such as gonorrhea, chlamydia, or *E. coli,* that travels up from the vagina and infects the ovaries, uterine lining, or fallopian tubes. If untreated, PID can cause scarring of the reproductive organs, which in turn can lead to infertility or, if conception is achieved, ectopic pregnancy.

Symptoms

About one-third of the population suffering from PID experiences no symptoms. When symptoms are experienced, they range from mild to severe and can include vaginal bleeding, vaginal discharge, abdominal pain, fever, chills, nausea, painful intercourse, and pelvic tenderness.

Treatment

Allopathic medicine, which tends to make use of antibiotics, is generally best suited for treating PID. Natural medicine may be used to support the effect of the allopathic treatment and to strengthen the body.

If you've been diagnosed with PID, note that your sexual partner should receive the same treatment that you are undergoing, even if he or she exhibits no symptoms of an infection. Most cases of PID are caused by sexually transmitted diseases, and it won't help to cure you of the disease only to have you catch it again from your partner.

HERBAL THERAPY

The following herbs are potent activators of the body's immune and cleansing systems and can be helpful additions to your treatment protocol for PID.

Calendula (*Calendula officinalis*). The flower is a time-tested remedy against deep-seated infections of the body. It improves liver and lymphatic function as well as peripheral circulation. It is alterative, anti-inflammatory, antifungal, astringent, and vulnerary.

Cleavers (*Galium aparine*). The herb clears heat and reduces inflammation. It is alterative, anti-inflammatory, mildly antiseptic, and diuretic.

Echinacea (*Echinacea purpurea, E. angustifolia*). The root stimulates immune response, including T-cell production and macrophage activity. It also dilates peripheral blood vessels, thus increasing circulation to the genitourinary tract. It is an alterative, antibiotic, antifungal, anti-inflammatory, antiviral, immunostimulant, and vulnerary.

Garlic (*Allium sativum*). The bulb neutralizes a wide range of pathogens. It is alterative, antibiotic, antifungal, and immunostimulant. Some people are allergic to garlic. Excessive use can cause emotional irritability and irritation of the stomach and kidneys. Avoid therapeutic doses during pregnancy, and avoid during the first three months of nursing, as it can cause breast milk to become unpalatable for infants. Avoid garlic for one week before having surgery.

Goldenseal (*Hydrastis canadensis*). The root is effective against a wide range of pathogens. It is anti-inflammatory, astringent, cholagogic, deobstruent, hemostatic, oxytocic, and a vasoconstrictor. Goldenseal is very bitter, and most people find it easiest to ingest in capsule form. The tea can be used as a douche. This herb is endangered in the wild; do not use wildcrafted supplies. Avoid during pregnancy.

Myrrh (*Commiphora myrrha*). The resin normalizes mucous membrane activity and stimulates white blood cell production. It is an alterative, anti-inflammatory, antifungal, antiseptic, astringent, and vulnerary. Avoid during pregnancy, and do not use for more than one month at a time.

Parsley (*Petroselinum crispum*). The leaf is rich in chlorophyll, which builds blood and helps the body resist infection. It is an antioxidant, antiseptic, and diuretic. Avoid therapeutic doses during pregnancy and in cases of kidney inflammation.

Pokeweed (*Phytolacca americana*). The root increases T-cell activity in the immune system. It is an alterative, anti-inflammatory, immunostimulant, and lymphatic decongestant. In large amounts, pokeweed root can be toxic. Take only 2 or 3 drops of the tincture daily; after one week, increase the dosage to 5 drops (2 drops in the morning, 3 drops at night). Drink copious amounts of water while you are taking pokeweed root. Consult with your health care provider before use.

Thyme (*Thymus vulgaris*). The herb expels mucus and relieves congestion throughout the body. It is an antibiotic, antifungal, antiseptic, diaphoretic, emmenagogue, and vulnerary.

NUTRITIONAL THERAPY

A healthy diet is imperative to overcoming a deep-seated infection of the body. Vitamin C and antioxidants may be of particular help.

Antioxidants. Antioxidants help prevent cellular damage to the body and speed the healing process. Antioxidants are best absorbed through natural sources of the nutrients beta-carotene, vitamin C, vitamin E, selenium, and superoxide dismutase. Good sources of each are listed in chapter 3.

Vitamin C. Large doses of vitamin C help the body resist infection and stimulate white blood cell production. Take 1,000 mg three or four times daily. Also incorporate into the diet natural sources of vitamin C.

POULTICES AND COMPRESSES

Poultices and compresses placed over an affected area can help draw out infection and relieve both congestion and pain. Apply these healing poultices or compresses at a time when you can lie low, relax, and really focus on the healing process.

Castor oil compress. A castor oil compress improves circulation to the pelvic area, thus helping clear congestion, and softens scar tissue. See page 267 for instructions on making and applying a castor oil compress. Apply for three days in a row, then take four days off. Repeat this pattern for as long as necessary.

Chamomile tea poultice. A chamomile tea poultice applied over the abdominal area can relieve pain, reduce inflammation, and provide a mild antiseptic action. The herb's gentle healing compounds are absorbed through the skin and pass into the bloodstream at the site of infection. To make the poultice, bring a quart of water to a boil. Remove from heat, stir in 4 heaping teaspoons of chamomile flowers or 4 chamomile tea bags, cover, and let steep for twenty minutes. Then remove the tea bags or strain out the blossoms. Soak a clean cloth in the hot tea, wring out, and apply to the pelvic area. Cover with a dry towel to help hold in the heat. When the cloth cools, resoak it in the hot tea and reapply. When it cools again, resoak and reapply one more time, so that you've made three applications total. Repeat once daily for as long as necessary.

Clay poultice. Clay poultices can help draw toxins from the body. Use only dry, cosmetic-quality clay. In a glass bowl, mix together about ½ cup of clay powder with enough water to make a paste. Apply over the liver area. Leave on until it dries thoroughly, then rinse off. Repeat once daily for as long as necessary.

AROMATHERAPY

Daily sitz baths (see chapter 10) increase circulation to the pelvic area, clearing congestion and stimulating immune system activity. For germicidal action, add to the water some essential oil of geranium, lavender, rosemary, or a combination thereof.

Massaging the abdominal area with a massage oil that includes some of the aforementioned essential oils will also be helpful in banishing infection.

URINARY TRACT INFECTIONS

Urinary tract infections can affect the bladder (cystitis), the urethra (urethritis), or the kidneys (nephritis). They are usually caused by the bacterium *E. coli* traveling from the colon to the bladder and urethra. Although urinary tract infections can be treated effectively with natural medicine, some cases are caused by sexually transmitted disease, so it's wise to visit your health care provider for a diagnosis of the cause.

Symptoms

If you need to urinate frequently and feel a burning sensation when you do so, even if you don't produce much urine, you probably have cystitis. If vaginal discharge or lumps around the genitals and anus are also present, suspect urethritis. If back pain, fever, chills, or a bloody discharge are also present, suspect kidney infection, and contact your health care provider immediately.

Treatment

The holistic approach to treating urinary tract infections focuses on supporting the urinary system, reducing inflammation, and stimulating the immune system.

DIET

To soothe irritation in the urinary tract, include in your diet plenty of cooling foods, such as asparagus, barley, carrots, celery, corn, cucumbers, grapes, green leafy vegetables, lotus root, millet, mung beans, parsley, pomegranates, squash, strawberries, vegetable juices, water chestnuts, and watermelon (eat the seeds too).

Also include foods that strengthen the kidneys and bladder, including, black sesame seeds, black quinoa, sea vegetables, and sun cured olives. Avoid foods that irritate the urinary system, such as alcohol, artificial sweeteners, cheese, fried foods, juices, coffee, sodas, spicy food, tomatoes, and vinegar.

To keep the urinary system well flushed, drink at least eight tall glasses of water every day.

Unsweetened cranberry juice is an excellent remedy for urinary tract infections because it contains hippuric acid, which inhibits the adhesion of bacteria to the walls of the urinary tract. Blueberries, which are in the same family as cranberries, also contain compounds that help prevent bacteria from adhering to the walls of the urinary tract.

HERBAL THERAPY

Useful herbs for treating urinary tract infections include the following:

Buchu (*Agathosma betulina*). The leaf soothes and strengthens the urinary system. It is an antiseptic, diuretic, Kidney tonic, and urinary antiseptic. Avoid during pregnancy and while nursing.

Cleavers (*Galium aparine*). The herb clears heat and reduces inflammation. It can help relieve the urge to urinate constantly. It is an alterative, anti-inflammatory, mild antiseptic, and diuretic.

Cornsilk (*Zea mays*). Technically the stigma of the corn plant, corn silk soothes and regenerates irritated tissue. It can help relieve the urge to urinate constantly. It is alterative, antiseptic, diuretic, demulcent, and tonic.

Couchgrass (*Elymus repens*). The rhizome has a high mucilage content and can soothe renal (kidney) tissue. It is antiseptic, demulcent, diuretic, and tonic.

Flax (*Linum usitatissimum*). The seeds help relieve the symptoms of cystitis, particularly the burning sensation associated with urination. They are anti-inflammatory, demulcent, and nutritive. Try grinding the seeds in a blender and incorporating 3 tablespoons daily into salads, salad dressings, and other dishes.

Goldenrod (*Solidago* spp.). The herb cleanses the kidneys. It is anti-inflammatory, antioxidant, mildly antiseptic, astringent, diuretic, and tonic. Do not use in cases of hot inflammation, such as fever or high blood pressure.

Hibiscus (*Hibiscus sabdariffa*). The flower relieves the symptoms of cystitis. It is an alterative, mild antiseptic, anti-inflammatory, antispasmodic, demulcent, and diuretic.

Horsetail (*Equisetum arvense*). The herb soothes irritated tissue. It is an alterative, anti-inflammatory, genitourinary antiseptic and astringent, diuretic, and nutritive. Use horsetail that has been collected in spring.

Juniper (*Juniperus communis*). The berry stimulates the flow of urine. It is anti-inflammatory, antiseptic, antiviral, and diuretic. Avoid during pregnancy, during acute renal inflammation, and in cases of blood in the urine. Do not use for longer than one month at a stretch.

Marsh mallow (*Althaea officinalis*). The root nourishes Kidney yin and can soothe an irritated bladder. It is an alterative, demulcent, diuretic, nutritive, and rejuvenative.

Nettle (*Urtica dioica, U. urens*). The herb dries the dampness associated with some cases of urinary tract infection. It is an alterative, circulatory stimulant, diuretic, Kidney tonic, and nutritive. Contact with the fresh plant will irritate the skin. Use only dried herb. Wear gloves when collecting.

Oregon grape (*Mahonia aquifolium*). The root is a urinary antiseptic and is especially helpful in cases of chronic infections. It is an alterative, anti-inflammatory, antiseptic, diuretic, and tonic. Avoid during pregnancy, and do not exceed the recommended dosage.

Pipsissewa (*Chimaphila umbellata*). The herb is an anti-inflammatory, urinary antiseptic, astringent, diuretic, and tonic. It may give urine a greenish color.

Plantain (*Plantago major*). The leaf clears heat and soothes irritated tissue. It is an alterative, anti-inflammatory, antiseptic, antispasmodic, demulcent, diuretic, and refrigerant.

Usnea (*Usnea barbata*). The lichen counteracts bacterial infections. It is an antibiotic, antifungal, and immunostimulant.

Uva ursi (*Arctostaphylos uva-ursi*). The leaf contains arbutin, which the body converts to hydroquinone, which helps alkalize the urine. It is an antiseptic, astringent, bladder tonic, diuretic, and vulnerary. Avoid during pregnancy.

NUTRITIONAL THERAPY

Supplementation with vitamin C and vitamin E, in combination with the dietary measures suggested above, may bolster the body's defenses against urinary tract infections. Natural sources of these vitamins are listed in chapter 3.

Vitamin C helps prevent bacterial infection. Take 1,000 mg three or four times daily. Vitamin E can help prevent scarring of bladder tissues. Take 400 IU daily.

HOMEOPATHIC REMEDIES

When bladder infection is accompanied by any of the conditions that are described below, try the suggested homeopathic remedy. The usual dosage is 4 pellets, or as many liquid drops as the package label recommends, taken under the tongue four times daily. Rather than swallowing the pellets whole, allow them to dissolve slowly.

APIS MELLIFICA. Urination causes a burning, stinging sensation, and the vaginal area is itchy and swollen. The patient is nervous and unable to urinate fully; the last few drops of urine are particularly painful.

BERBERIS VULGARIS. The bladder infection starts to settle in the kidneys or lower back area. Motion aggravates the symptoms, and there may be a reddish color to the urine.

CANTHARIS. The patient feels a severe burning in the vaginal area and a constant urge to urinate, though only a few drops pass each time. She may feel agitated, and there may be blood in the urine.

EQUISETUM. The patient experiences a feeling of fullness in the bladder, even after urinating.

MERCURIUS CORROSIVUS. The burning is less intense but ever-present, as is the urge to urinate. The patient may experience bladder spasms and painful urination. Symptoms tend to worsen when outside temperatures fluctuate.

SARSAPARILLA. Urination is painful and causes stress.

SEPIA. The patient is pregnant and experiences bladder pressure rather than pain.

STAPHYSAGRIA. The symptoms are caused by "honeymoon cystitis" (more sex than you're accustomed to having). The patient may feel an ever-present burning sensation. This remedy is also helpful for a bladder infection induced by emotional stress.

PIPSISSEWA SITZ BATH

A sitz bath in an infusion of pipsissewa will help disinfect the pelvic area. Bring a quart of water to a boil, add a large handful of pipsissewa herb, cover, and let steep twenty minutes. Then strain and pour into the sitz bath. Add more water if necessary, and adjust the temperature so it is not too hot.

For extra antiseptic action, add 16 ounces of baking soda (a whole box) or 1 cup of apple cider vinegar to the water.

AROMATHERAPY

Gentle abdominal massage can increase circulation to the pelvic region, transmit caring touch, and, when combined with antiseptic essential oils, help the body resist or fight off infection. Use a massage oil infused with the essential oil of eucalyptus, lavender, lemon, or niaouli. These antiseptic oils can also be added to the bath. See chapter 5 for advice on these techniques.

UTERINE FIBROIDS

Uterine fibroids, also called leiomyomas, are benign tumors that grow outside, inside, or in the walls of the uterus, sometimes distorting its shape. They range in size from that of a pea to that of a full-term fetus, and they are more common in women who have not had children. They tend to grow slowly, and their growth seems to be stimulated by estrogen. (Because they are dependent on estrogen, fibroids usually decrease in size after menopause.)

Symptoms

Most cases of fibroids are free of symptoms. However, if fibroids are of sufficient size or number, they may cause heavy or prolonged periods, painful periods, bleeding between cycles, anemia, the urge to urinate frequently, pain during intercourse, backache, constipation, or abdominal enlargement.

Treatment

You may be able to reduce the size of fibroids with some of the natural therapies suggested below. However, in cases where fibroids are causing serious pain or profuse bleeding, surgery may be necessary.

Natural therapy for treating fibroids focuses on supporting three important systems.

- The liver, which breaks down excess estrogen in the body
- The kidneys, which relieve stagnation, thereby preventing the formation of masses in the body
- The blood, which prevents blockages

If you have fibroids, avoid birth control pills and hormone replacement therapy, both of which provide the body with synthetic estrogen.

DIET

First things first. If you're overweight and fibroids are giving you trouble, lose the extra pounds. Overweight women tend to secrete proportionately higher levels of estrogen, which stimulates fibroid growth.

Avoid meat, eggs, and dairy products that derive from animals treated with hormones. Incorporate fermented soy products, such as miso, into your diet, because fermented soy helps regulate estrogen levels in the body.

Eat violet leaves and chickweed in salads as much as possible, taking in their healing, cleansing, soothing energy.

HERBAL THERAPY

Herbs that help reduce the size of uterine fibroids include the following.

Angelica (*Angelica archangelica, A. atropurpurea*). The root regulates menstrual bleeding and inhibits blood platelet aggregation. It is an anti-inflammatory, astringent, diuretic, emmenagogue, tonic, and uterine stimulant. Avoid during pregnancy and in cases of heavy bleeding or diabetes. In rare cases, the root causes photosensitivity.

Astragalus (*Astragalus membranaceus*). The root stimulates the immune system and inhibits the formation of free radicals. It is an adaptogen, antiviral, blood tonic, chi tonic, circulatory stimulant, immunostimulant, and vasodilator.

Black cohosh (*Actaea racemosa*). This root helps relieve the pain of fibroids. It soothes irritation and relieves congestion in the cervix, uterus, and vagina. It is an alterative, anti-inflammatory, antiseptic, antispasmodic, astringent, circulatory stimulant, emmenagogue, and vasodilator. Avoid during pregnancy, except in the final stages, and then only under the guidance of your health care provider. Avoid while nursing and in cases of high blood pressure or pressure in the inner eye. Consult with your health care provider before use. This herb is endangered in the wild; do not use wildcrafted supplies.

Blessed thistle (*Cnicus benedictus*). The herb strengthens the spleen and the liver. It is an alterative, antihemorrhagic, and emmenagogue.

Blue cohosh (*Caulophyllum thalictroides*). The root reduces pain and spasms in the uterus. It is anti-inflammatory, antispasmodic, diuretic, emmenagogic, oxytocic, and a uterine tonic. Avoid during pregnancy, except in the final stages, and then only under the guidance of your health care provider. Make sure the root is dried, not fresh. This herb is endangered in the wild; do not use wildcrafted supplies.

Burdock (*Arctium lappa*). The root improves the functions of the organs of elimination, such as the liver, the lymph nodes, and the kidneys. It is alterative, antifungal, antiseptic, anti-inflammatory, antitumor, choleretic, demulcent, diuretic, laxative, nutritive, and rejuvenative.

Calendula (*Calendula officinalis*). The flower improves liver and lymphatic function as well as peripheral circulation. It is an alterative, anti-inflammatory, astringent, and vulnerary.

Celandine (*Chelidonium majus*). Celandine herb detoxifies the liver. It is an alterative, anodyne, anti-inflammatory, and cholagogue. Use only in small doses; 2 or 3 drops of tincture three times daily is adequate. Consult with your health care provider before use, and avoid during pregnancy.

Chamomile (*Matricaria recutita*). The flower can relieve pain in the uterus. It is an antispasmodic, anti-inflammatory, and emmenagogue.

Chaparral (*Larrea tridentata*). The herb helps reduce the size of uterine fibroids occurring with elevated estrogen levels. It is an alterative, antifungal, antioxidant, antiseptic, antitumor, and immunostimulant. Avoid in cases of liver or kidney disease, including cirrhosis or hepatitis, and during pregnancy. Discontinue use if nausea, fatigue, fever, or jaundice occurs. Do not use for more than a month at a time. Consult with your health care provider before use.

Cleavers (*Galium aparine*). The herb is a lymphatic cleanser. It clears heat and reduces inflammation. Cleavers is an alterative, antitumor, astringent, and vulnerary.

Collinsonia (*Collinsonia canadensis*). The root can shrink small fibroids that congest the uterus and cause chronic irritation. It relieves congestion in the pelvic area and helps remove masses from the reproductive organs. It is a diuretic and an emmenagogue.

Cotton root (*Gossypium hirsutum, G. herbaceum*). The root bark constricts blood vessels and is recommended for uterine fibroids accompanied by hemorrhage. It is antitumor, emmenagogic, nutritive, and a uterine tonic. Avoid during pregnancy and in cases of urogenital irritation. Large doses may cause nausea and vomiting.

Cramp bark (*Viburnum opulus*). The bark relaxes muscles, thereby relieving pain and cramping. It is anti-inflammatory, antispasmodic, astringent, nutritive, and a uterine sedative.

Dandelion (*Taraxacum officinale*). The root and leaf improve liver function, aid in the elimination of toxins, and reduce stagnation in the reproductive organs. Dandelion is antifungal, antitumor, cholagogic, and a Liver tonic.

Dan shen (*Salvia miltiorrhiza*). The root invigorates blood and breaks up congestion. It can relieve pain in the uterus.

False unicorn (*Chamaelirium luteum*). The root strengthens the genitourinary tract and helps balance estrogen levels. It is an antiseptic and a uterine tonic. The bitter taste of this herb can cause vomiting, and excessive amounts may cause kidney and stomach irritation, blurred vision, or hot flashes. Do not use without employing birth control during sex unless pregnancy is desired. Discontinue use during pregnancy. False unicorn is endangered in the wild, so do not use wildcrafted supplies.

Fraxinus (*Fraxinus americana*). The bark reduces the size of fibroids, particularly when they are in the earlier stages of development. It is a circulatory stimulant.

Fringe tree (*Chionanthus virginicus*). The bark removes obstructions, including fibroids, and clears heat from the liver. It also reduces inflammation. It is an alterative, cholagogue, and hepatic.

Ginger (*Zingiber officinale*). The root improves circulation and helps clear stagnant material from the pelvic region. It encourages lymphatic cleansing and reduces blood platelet aggregation. Ginger is an analgesic, anti-inflammatory, antioxidant, antiseptic, antispasmodic, and anticoagulant. Avoid large doses in cases of acne and eczema. Discontinue use if heartburn results.

Goldenseal (*Hydrastis canadensis*). The root reduces pelvic congestion, improves liver function, and reduces bleeding. It is anti-inflammatory, astringent, cholagogic, deobstruent, hemostatic, oxytocic, and a vasoconstrictor. Goldenseal is very bitter, and most people find it easiest to ingest in capsule form. The tea can be used as a douche. This herb is endangered in the wild; do not use wildcrafted supplies. Avoid during pregnancy.

Hawthorn (*Crataegus* spp.). The berry, flower, and leaf improve circulation and help break down fatty deposits in the body. Hawthorn is an astringent, circulatory stimulant, and a vasodilator.

Lady's mantle (*Alchemilla xanthochlora*). The herb normalizes hormone production, reduces heavy bleeding, promotes blood coagulation, and encourages tissue healing. It is anti-inflammatory, astringent, diuretic, emmenagogic, hemostatic, as well as a liver decongestant, uterine tonic, and vulnerary.

Motherwort (*Leonurus cardiaca*). The herb inhibits blood platelet aggregation and helps normalize hormone production. It is an astringent, circulatory stimulant, diuretic, emmenagogue, rejuvenative, uterine tonic, and vasodilator. Avoid in cases of heavy menstrual bleeding and during pregnancy, except during the final stages, and then only under the supervision of your health care provider.

Oregon grape (*Mahonia aquifolium*). The root improves liver function and circulation. It is an alterative, anti-inflammatory, antiseptic, astringent, cholagogue, diuretic, and immunostimulant. Avoid during pregnancy, and do not exceed the recommended dosage.

Partridgeberry (*Mitchella repens*). The herb helps relieve pelvic congestion. It is an alterative, astringent, emmenagogue, uterine stimulant, and uterine tonic. Dosages in excess of what's recommended can irritate the mucous membranes. This herb is endangered in the wild; do not use wild-crafted supplies.

Pipsissewa (*Chimaphila umbellata*). The herb improves liver and kidney function, cleansing the body and helping to eliminate fluids. It is an alterative, anti-inflammatory, astringent, diuretic, and urinary antiseptic.

Pokeweed (*Phytolacca americana*). Pokeweed root increases T-cell activity in the immune system. It is an alterative, anti-inflammatory, immunostimulant, and lymphatic decongestant. In large amounts, pokeweed root can be toxic. Take only 2 or 3 drops of the tincture daily; after one week, increase the dosage to 5 drops (2 drops in the morning, 3 drops at night). Drink copious amounts of water while you are taking pokeweed root. Consult with your health care provider before use.

Prickly ash (*Zanthoxylum americanum, Z. clava-herculis*). The bark improves circulation throughout the body. It is an alterative, anodyne, antiseptic, antispasmodic, astringent, emmenagogue, and circulatory stimulant. Avoid during pregnancy and in cases of stomach inflammation.

Red clover (*Trifolium pratense*). The herb and flower are excellent lymphatic cleansers. Red clover is alterative, anti-inflammatory, and antitumor.

Red raspberry (*Rubus idaeus*). The leaf tonifies the uterus and the cervix. It prevents hemorrhage and helps balance hormones. It is an alterative, antiseptic, astringent, hemostatic, hormone regulator, nutritive, and yin tonic.

Redroot (*Ceanothus americanus*). The root encourages the elimination of catabolic waste and breaks up congestion in the body. It is often recommended for treating cysts, dysmenorrhea, and lymphatic congestion. It is antispasmodic and astringent.

Sarsaparilla (*Smilax* spp.). The root contains compounds that help purify the genitourinary tract by binding with toxins and carrying them out of the body. It is an alterative, antispasmodic, diuretic, and rejuvenative.

Saw palmetto (*Serenoa repens*). The berry reduces ovarian enlargement and pain, which can contribute to impaired circulation and drainage in the uterus. It is a diuretic, nutritive, rejuvenative, reproductive tonic, and urinary antiseptic.

Trillium (*Trillium* spp.). The root helps control excessive bleeding associated with fibroids. It is an alterative, antihemorrhagic, antiseptic, antispasmodic, astringent, emmenagogue, and uterine tonic. Avoid during pregnancy, except under the guidance of your health care provider. This herb is endangered in the wild; do not use wildcrafted supplies.

Turmeric (*Curcuma longa, C. aromatica*). The root prevents blood platelet aggregation. It is an alterative, anticoagulant, antifungal, anti-inflammatory, antioxidant, cholagogue, circulatory stimulant, emmenagogue, hepatotonic, and vulnerary.

Vervain (*Verbena hastata, V. officinalis*). The herb stimulates uterine activity and improves the body's assimilation of nutrients. It is an anticoagulant, anti-inflammatory, antitumor, astringent, cholagogue, diuretic, emmenagogue, hepatostimulant, vasoconstrictor, and vulnerary. Avoid during pregnancy.

Vitex (*Vitex agnus-castus*). The berry helps normalize the production of hormones and inhibits excessive cellular growth in the reproductive organs. It is antispasmodic, emmenagogic, phytoprogesteronic, and vulnerary.

Wild yam (*Dioscorea opposita, D. villosa*). The root reduces inflammation, clears congested chi, and helps normalize hormones. It is an anti-inflammatory, antispasmodic, cholagogue, diuretic, nutritive, and uterine sedative. Avoid therapeutic doses during pregnancy, except under the guidance of your health care provider. The *Dioscorea villosa* species is endangered in the wild; do not use wildcrafted supplies.

Yarrow (*Achillea millefolium*). The herb increases circulation to the pelvic region and promotes liver detoxification. It is an anti-inflammatory, antiseptic, antispasmodic, astringent, cholagogue, circulatory stimulant, diuretic, hemostatic, and urinary antiseptic.

CHINESE PATENT FORMULA

The Chinese patent formula TO JING WAN helps regulate the menstrual cycle and break up stagnation in the blood. TANG KWEI GIN can help shrink fibroids.

NUTRITIONAL THERAPY

Several supplements can contribute to the healing of fibroids. Good sources of each can be found in chapter 3.

Vitamin B complex. Elevated estrogen levels can result from a B vitamin deficiency. Choline and inositol, both part of the vitamin B complex, help the liver break down fats and fat-soluble hormones such as estrogen. Take 50 to 300 mg of vitamin B complex daily.

Vitamin E. Vitamin E helps regulate bleeding and normalizes estrogen levels. Take 400 IU daily.

Iron. If fibroids cause heavy menstrual bleeding, use an herbal liquid iron supplement, available at most natural food stores. Follow the dosage guidelines given on the product label.

Methionine. This amino acid aids in the breakdown of fats and fat-soluble hormones. Take 500 mg daily.

SITZ BATHS

Alternate hot and cold sitz baths, as directed in chapter 10. This treatment increases circulation to the pelvic region, moving blockages and allowing reabsorption of extra tissue.

CASTOR OIL PACKS

To improve circulation to the pelvic area and soften scar tissue, apply castor oil packs to the abdominal region three times a week. See page 267 for instructions.

PELVIC EXERCISE

Practice exercises that move energy in the pelvis, such as the Cat Stretch (see page 122) and Kegels (see page 118).

AROMATHERAPY

Massage over the abdominal area with a blockage-dispelling oil infused with jasmine, lotus, rose, rose geranium, or a combination of these, can be very helpful for fibroids. (See page 139 for instructions on making an aromatherapy massage oil.) The essential oils can also be used in an aromatherapy diffuser.

ACUPUNCTURE

Acupuncture treatments can be very effective for moving blockages in the body, such as fibroids. Begin treatment as soon as the fibroids are discovered, because they are easier to eliminate when they are still small and have not yet tightly adhered to surrounding organs. To find an acupuncturist in your area, contact the American Association of Acupuncture and Oriental Medicine; see the resources section on page 479.

UTERINE PROLAPSE

Prolapse means an organ has "slipped down" from its normal position. Prolapse of the uterus can be caused by childbirth, constipation, obesity, and the normal forces of gravity. In most cases it is not a serious health condition and may resolve itself. If it doesn't, surgical repair is always an option. Ask your health care provider for advice on the method of treatment that is best suited for your condition.

Symptoms

Signs of uterine prolapse include a heavy feeling in the lower abdomen, painful intercourse, backache, incontinence, frequent or difficult urination, constipation, urinary tract infections, and vaginal discharge.

Treatment

Try natural remedies for six months to a year before resorting to surgery. You might end up not needing it, and you'll certainly improve your health in the meantime.

The holistic approach to treating uterine prolapse focuses on resting the body, strengthening the genitourinary system, and stimulating the body's healing response.

REST

The most important treatment for uterine prolapse is simply rest. Give your body a chance to heal itself. Make sure you get plenty of sleep, avoid heavy lifting, and don't stand on your feet for long periods at a time.

BODYWORK AND EXERCISE

Bodywork and exercise directed toward strengthening the pelvic area can help the uterus find its way back home. Locate a bodyworker who knows how to do uterine massage and visit him or her for weekly sessions. Practice pelvis-strengthening exercises such as those described in chapter 4, and do lots of Kegels. Try inverted yoga postures such as the shoulder stand or head stand, or spend thirty minutes or so every day lying on a slant board (available at many sports shops and by mail-order from Bodyslant; see the resources section on page 477). The Plough is also a beneficial yoga pose for uterine prolapse.

CAUTION

A few notes of caution: Do not undertake these exercises if you have recently given birth, because they might trigger further bleeding. And don't force yourself into a headstand without supervision unless you are already adept at doing them. Avoid inversion poses during menses.

HERBAL THERAPY

Herbs that can help the body lift the uterus back to its proper position include the following:

Black cohosh (*Actaea racemosa*). The root stimulates the flow of chi, which can provide the body with the strength to lift prolapsed internal organs. Black cohosh relieves congestion in the cervix, uterus, and vagina. It is an alterative, anti-inflammatory, astringent, circulatory stimulant, emmenagogue, and vasodilator. Avoid during pregnancy, except in the final stages, and then only under the guidance of your health care provider. Avoid while nursing and in cases of high blood pressure or pressure in the inner eye. Consult with your health care provider before use. This herb is endangered in the wild; do not use wildcrafted supplies.

Dong quai (*Angelica sinensis*). The root nourishes vaginal tissues and clears stagnation of blood in the pelvic area. It is an alterative, anticoagulant, blood tonic, emmenagogue, and uterine tonic. Avoid during pregnancy, except under the guidance of your health care provider. Do not use in cases of diarrhea, heavy menstrual flow, poor digestion, or bloating. Do not use in conjunction with blood-thinning medications such as ibuprofen.

False unicorn (*Chamaelirium luteum*). The root strengthens the genitourinary tract. It is an antiseptic and a uterine tonic. The bitter taste of this herb can cause vomiting, and excessive amounts may cause kidney and stomach irritation, blurred vision, or hot flashes. Do not use without employing birth control during sex unless pregnancy is desired; discontinue use during pregnancy. False unicorn is endangered in the wild, so do not use wildcrafted supplies.

Horsetail (*Equisetum arvense*). Horsetail herb encourages the healing of bones, tissue, and cartilage. It has a high silica content, which helps strengthen the body's connective tissues. It is also anti-inflammatory, astringent, hemostatic, nutritive, and vulnerary. Use horsetail that has been collected in spring.

Lady's mantle (*Alchemilla xanthochlora*). The herb promotes tissue healing. It is an anti-inflammatory, astringent, diuretic, emmenagogue, hemostatic, liver decongestant, and vulnerary.

Red raspberry (*Rubus idaeus*). Red raspberry leaf tonifies the uterus. It is also an astringent, a hormone regulator, Kidney tonic, nutritive, and yin tonic.

If prolapse occurs after menopause, lack of estrogen may be a factor. In this case, herbs with phytoestrogenic activity, such as hops, sage, and wild yam, can be helpful. See chapter 17 for more information.

VAGINAL SUPPOSITORY

The astringent herbal bolus made from the Tissue-Tonifying Yoni Suppository formula below supports the body's healing response and prevents infection.

TISSUE-TONIFYING YONI SUPPOSITORY

Supports the body's healing response and prevents infection.

5 parts powdered witch hazel bark

1 part powdered goldenseal root

Coconut oil

Combine the herbs with enough coconut oil to make a thick paste. Roll into a suppository shape the size of your pinkie, and store in a glass jar in the refrigerator. Insert it as high as possible in your vagina before going to bed. You may wish to wear a cotton menstrual pad to prevent the oil from dripping over the bed sheets.

HOMEOPATHIC SEPIA

Homeopathic SEPIA tightens tissues and may benefit women with uterine prolapse. The usual dosage is 4 pellets, or as many liquid drops as the package label recommends, taken under the tongue four times daily. Rather than swallowing the pellets whole, allow them to dissolve slowly.

AROMATHERAPY

Abdominal massage can strengthen the muscles, helping the body pull the uterus back where it belongs. Use a massage oil combined with an antiseptic essential oil, such as lemon or rosemary. (See chapter 5 for instructions for making an aromatherapy massage oil.) These oils can also be included in a bath.

SITZ BATHS

To improve circulation and move blockages in the pelvic region, take a cold sitz bath every day for thirty seconds. (See page 169.)

VAGINAL DRYNESS

Vaginal lubrication is often a woman's initial response to sexual excitement. Small drops of fluid secretions appear throughout the vaginal folds; as the excitement continues, the drops of moisture fuse to form a lubricating coat.

Lack of vaginal lubrication is not always a sign of lack of excitement. It may, instead, be a symptom of a deeper health problem.

Causes

According to Oriental medicine, a deficiency in vaginal lubrication is often an indication of Kidney yin or Liver deficiency. Menopause and hysterectomies often affect vaginal lubrication; the drop in estrogen production can leave the mucous membranes high and dry. Other factors that can contribute to vaginal dryness include yeast overgrowth, diabetes, overdouching, sexually transmitted disease, stress, overwork, and excessive exercise. Alcohol and marijuana can cause vaginal dryness, as can some common prescription drugs, including antihistamine-filled allergy medications, diuretics, and birth control pills.

Treatment

Natural therapy for vaginal dryness focuses on nourishing mucous membranes, strengthening vaginal tissue, and normalizing estrogen production. Most important, visualize your river flowing!

DIET

Drink copious amounts of fluids. Barley water is highly nourishing and emollient; cook 2 cups of lightly pearled barley in 10 cups of water for two hours, then strain and sweeten to taste. To strengthen mucous membranes, eat plenty of foods that are rich in beta-carotene, including dark green, leafy vegetables, winter squash, sweet potatoes, and spirulina. To nourish the Kidneys, which govern yin moisture in the body, incorporate black sesame seeds and black soybeans into your diet.

SITZ BATH

Take a sitz bath using emollient herbs such as comfrey leaf and marsh mallow root, which will soothe and protect your skin. Bring a quart of water to a boil, add a large handful of the herb of choice, cover, and let steep twenty minutes. Then strain and pour into the sitz bath. Add more water if necessary.

HERBAL THERAPY

The following herbs all help promote vaginal lubrication.

Black cohosh (*Actaea racemosa*). The root soothes vaginal irritation. It is an alterative, anti-inflammatory, circulatory stimulant, and muscle relaxant. Avoid during pregnancy, except in the final stages, and then only under the guidance of your health care provider. Avoid while nursing and in cases of high blood pressure or pressure in the inner eye. Consult with your health care provider before use. This herb is endangered in the wild; do not use wildcrafted supplies.

Fennel (*Foeniculum vulgare*). The seed contains phytoestrogens and soothes irritated mucous membranes. It is a smooth muscle relaxant.

Longan (*Euphoria longan*). The berry is moistening and helps build blood. It is a restorative.

Vitex (*Vitex agnus-castus*). Vitex berry is phytoprogesteronic.

HERBAL SUPPOSITORY

Use a moistening herbal suppository at night to encourage moisture in the vaginal mucous membranes.

YONI MOISTENING SUPPOSITORY

Encourages moisture in the vaginal mucous membranes.

1 ounce cocoa butter

1 tablespoon powdered dong quai root

1 tablespoon powdered licorice root

1 tablespoon powdered marsh mallow root or slippery elm bark

1 tablespoon powdered wild yam

2 tablespoons vitamin E oil

2 drops essential oil of rose (optional)

Melt the cocoa butter, then add the powdered herbs and vitamin E oil. Scent with 2 drops of rose essential oil, if desired. Roll into a suppository shape the size of your pinkie, and store in a glass jar in the refrigerator. Insert before bedtime.

NUTRITIONAL THERAPY

Several supplements may be of assistance in relieving vaginal dryness. In addition to supplements, add plenty of vitamin-rich foods to your diet. Good sources of the nutrients listed below can be found in chapter 3.

Essential fatty acids. EFAs soothe irritated tissue and have an anti-inflammatory effect. Hempseed and fish oils are excellent sources of EFAs; take 3 tablespoons daily (or 1 to 3 fish oil capsules).

Vitamin A. Vitamin A helps strengthen and soothe mucous membranes. It is best taken in the form of beta-carotene; try 25,000 to 50,000 IU of beta-carotene daily.

Vitamin C. Vitamin C supports collagen production, thereby improving tissue tone. Take 1,000 mg twice daily.

Vitamin E. Vitamin E helps moisten tissues and soothes inflammation. Take 400 IU daily. You can also apply the oil from a vitamin E capsule directly to vaginal tissues.

Zinc. Zinc helps strengthen the vaginal lining. Take 15 mg daily.

ACIDOPHILUS

Yeast overgrowth is often a contributing factor in vaginal dryness. An acidophilus capsule inserted into the vagina inhibits yeast overgrowth and can help produce lubrication. Make sure you are not using an enteric-coated capsule, which will not dissolve in the vagina. You can use acidophilus in this manner on a continuing basis for as long as you need to.

HOMEOPATHY

Homeopathic remedies that are traditionally used to ease vaginal dryness include LYCOPODIUM, NATRUM MURIATICUM, and BRYONIA.

LUBRICANTS

If you can't produce your own lubricant, import it! The ideal lubricant should not become sticky, should liquefy at body temperature, and should stay slick for long periods of time. In preparation for intercourse, you can always use a water-based lubricant or a glycerin suppository. Coconut oil is also an excellent lubricant, but it cannot be used with barrier methods of contraception because it degrades the quality of the barrier. Check out the resources section for sources of yummy natural lubricants.

VAGINISMUS

Vaginismus describes the occurrence of vaginal muscle spasms that close the vagina so tightly that intercourse is difficult or impossible. The cause of this condition has yet to be discovered, although psychological factors are certainly involved. It can be helpful to work with a therapist.

The best approach to overcoming vaginismus is to proceed slowly, backing off whenever psychological stress or muscle spasms set in. Try looking at your genitals in a mirror after a relaxing bath. Try to insert a lubricated finger into your vagina while lightly bearing down. Enter a little bit at a time. When you can do this effectively on your own, try it with a partner you trust. Practice Kegels.

When you feel you're ready for intercourse, use lubrication, and make sure that foreplay is both extensive and fun. If the tension of the situation—will it happen, or won't it?—starts to affect you, back off, and save the actual penetration for another time. There are plenty of ways to make love, after all! When you are ready for penetration, use plenty of lubrication.

VAGINITIS

Vaginitis is the general term for a nonspecific vaginal infection. Most cases of vaginitis are caused by overgrowth of bacteria that are normally present in the body; the bacterium *Hemophilus,* for example, is a common culprit. Hormonal changes, birth control pills, excessive douching, tears in or irritations to vaginal tissue, stress, and synthetic-fiber clothing may all be contributing factors.

Symptoms

Symptoms of vaginitis are varied and range from mild to severe. The most common are abnormal discharge, burning or itching in the vulva, burning or stinging upon urination, and the need to urinate frequently.

Treatment

Treatment for vaginitis entails stimulating the body's immune response and nourishing the mucous membranes.

HERBAL THERAPY

Herbs that can counteract a bacterial vaginal infection include the following:

Astragalus (*Astragalus membranaceus*). The root stimulates the body's immune response. It is adaptogenic, antiseptic, a circulatory stimulant, and a vasodilator.

Echinacea (*Echinacea purpurea, E. angustifolia*). The root stimulates the body's immune response. It is an alterative, antibiotic, antifungal, anti-inflammatory, antiviral, immunostimulant, and vulnerary.

Garlic (*Allium sativum*). The bulb neutralizes a wide range of pathogens. It is an alterative, antibiotic, antifungal, antiprotozoan, and immunostimulant. Some people are allergic to garlic. Excessive use can cause emotional irritability and irritation of the stomach and kidneys. Avoid therapeutic doses during pregnancy, and avoid during the first three months of nursing, as it can cause breast milk to become unpalatable for infants. Avoid for one week before having surgery.

Goldenseal (*Hydrastis canadensis*). The root helps dry up excessive discharge from mucous membranes, and it is an effective antibiotic against a wide range of pathogens. It is also alterative and anti-inflammatory.

Goldenseal is very bitter, and most people find it easiest to ingest in capsule form. Alternatively, the tea can be used as a douche. This herb is endangered in the wild, so do not use wildcrafted supplies. Avoid during pregnancy.

Isatis (*Isatis tinctoria*). The root is a strong antimicrobial, anti-inflammatory agent.

Myrrh (*Commiphora myrrha*). The resin normalizes mucous membrane activity and stimulates white blood cell production. It is an alterative, anti-inflammatory, antifungal, antiseptic, astringent, and vulnerary. Avoid during pregnancy, and do not use for more than one month at a time.

Oregon grape (*Mahonia aquifolium*). The root has antibacterial activity against a wide range of pathogens. It is an alterative, anti-inflammatory, antibiotic, febrifuge, and immunostimulant. Avoid during pregnancy, and do not exceed the recommended dosage.

SUPPOSITORIES

Suppositories of garlic, yogurt, or boric acid can all help conquer a bacterial infection. See page 250 for more information.

ANTISEPTIC BATH

A warm bath increases circulation to and moves blockages from the pelvic region. To help clear infection, add 1 cup of apple cider vinegar and 7 drops of tea tree or lavender essential oil to the bathwater.

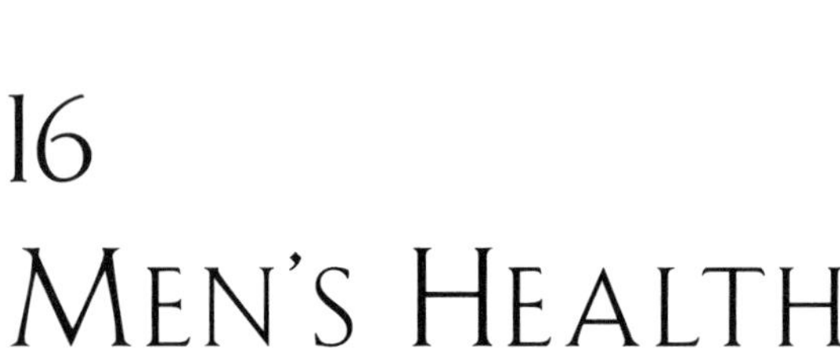

16
Men's Health

ON AVERAGE, MEN HAVE shorter lives than women. They also are more likely to have type A personalities, which foster stress and anxiety. And from boyhood to manhood, men are usually encouraged to be strong, both physically and emotionally. As a result, they tend to pay less attention to their health, ignoring signs and symptoms and avoiding medical care at all costs.

Men can greatly benefit from a healthy lifestyle, which prolongs life, reduces the physical effects of stress, and promotes overall good health. It also builds sexual energy and ability. When a man develops a health problem, a healthy lifestyle will both support and speed up his body's recovery process. Most important, a healthy lifestyle is a vital component of self-care. If medical care is a pesticide that keeps the human body free of "bugs," self-care is the river that waters and fertilizes the landscape of the body in harmony with the rhythms of nature. Furthermore, self-care allows a man independence, so that he himself can gauge the state of his health and decide whether a problem can be addressed at home or needs the expertise of a health care professional.

The healing techniques and remedies in this chapter focus on self-care as a first solution for sexual health problems. Men may also wish to consult with a health care provider with whom they feel comfortable communicating and working. Men over the age of forty, especially those with a family history of cancer, should consider having a yearly physical, including a rectal exam.

CLOTHING

Men need to remember that tight clothing can lead to reproductive problems. If I were a man, I would help bring sarongs, kilts, and yoga pants into fashion in the Western world. Make sure pants are loose enough; avoid tight belts and constricting underwear. If you wear a belt, placing the buckle to the side can avoid blocking energy that flows through the meridian of the navel.

TESTICULAR SELF-EXAM

Self-examinations, including testicular exams, are an integral part of self-care. Weekly testicular exams, begun at about age fifteen, take only about three minutes and can catch testicular cancer in its early stages, when it is still treatable, as well as many other reproductive dysfunctions. If you discover any irregularities, bring them to the attention of your health care provider.

1. Hold your scrotum in the palms of your hands. Gently roll each testicle between the thumb and forefingers of a hand, checking for lumps.
2. Probe the epididymis, a comma-shaped cord behind the testicles, for lumps. This is a site where many noncancerous reproductive problems occur.
3. Examine the vas deferens, which is right under the skin that runs up from the epididymis. It should feel firm and smooth and should move under the pressure of your fingers.

CIRCUMCISION AND FORESKIN HEALTH

Though many people would disagree, I believe that circumcision is an unnecessary, painful amputation that leaves the penis more vulnerable to disease than if left intact. We've been trained to think of a circumcised penis as "normal," when, in fact, it is quite abnormal. English-speaking countries began popularizing circumcision in the general population in the late 1800s in the hope that it would deter masturbation. (Didn't work, did it?) Today, the United States is the only country that still performs circumcision for reasons other than religious doctrine or medical necessity; about 80 percent of the planet's men are not circumcised.

Most of us would agree that the practice of removing the clitoris from a young girl qualifies as mutilation. What, then, is removal of the foreskin of an infant boy? The foreskin is a sensitive anatomical extension of the penis. It is rich in nerve endings and blood vessels, contains glands that produce antibacterial and antiviral proteins that help prevent infection, and protects a layer of emollient smegma that moisturizes the glans (the head of the penis), keeping it supple, warm, and free of bacteria.

The glans is designed to be an internal organ—protected by the foreskin—that emerges upon erection. Think of the foreskin as a protective hood, much like the eyelids. Its removal exposes the glans to friction (especially from rubbing against clothes) and takes away its moisturizing protection. The end result is that the penis becomes tougher and less sensitive.

Circumcision will not, as common myth would tell you, prevent cancer of the penis. This rare disease affects only 1 in 100,000 males, and it is most prevalent in elderly men. Should women cut off their breasts to prevent breast cancer?

Circumcision is a fifteen-minute operation; although it's usually quite safe, infection, scarring, and damage to the penis are all risks. And it's painful. Most babies scream during the procedure, and some even go into shock. A study done at Washington University School of Medicine showed that most infant boys would not nurse right after being circumcised, and those who did would not look into their mother's eyes. "Save the foreskins!" should be a bumpersticker.

It's my position that no one should have his or her genitals mutilated without his or her own informed consent. Should a male really want to be circumcised, he should be able to make that decision for himself when he reaches the age of eighteen. Research, then choose.

Cleaning under the Foreskin

Never retract the foreskin of an infant's penis to clean underneath it. Retracting the foreskin before it is ready can cause pain and bleeding and can contribute to infection and scarring. Furthermore, washing underneath the foreskin removes friendly flora that protect the penis against infection.

The foreskin will gradually separate from the glans during childhood. The exact age of separation differs from child to child, but it usually happens at the age of four. Once the foreskin has separated from the glans on its own, little boys can be taught to pull it back gently to clean the glans, wiping away any accumulated discharge.

Phimosis

Phimosis is a condition in which the orifice at the top of the foreskin is constricted, so that the foreskin cannot be retracted back over the glans. This is a normal condition in infants, but in rare cases it persists into adulthood. Gentle stretching of the foreskin, as well as topical creams available upon prescription from a physician, can encourage flexibility of the foreskin and, eventually, retractability.

The constriction of phimosis may be relieved by supplementation with vitamin C (500–1,000 mg three times daily) and zinc (25–50 mg daily), which improve skin elasticity. (Consult with your health care provider to determine proper dosages for children.)

Irritations and Infections of the Foreskin

If an uncircumcised infant, boy, or man develops irritation around the foreskin area, the following remedies should clear it up in about five days.

TOPICAL HERBAL APPLICATIONS

Three times daily, rinse the area with warm water, then apply one of the following:

- A few drops of calendula-infused oil, which has soothing, infection-fighting, and anti-inflammatory properties. It is available at most natural food stores and herb shops.
- 10 drops each of calendula tincture and echinacea tincture diluted in ⅓ cup of warm water. This remedy is a bit stronger than calendula-infused oil and can be used to treat a more stubborn irritation. It is drying rather than lubricating.
- A dusting of powdered goldenseal root and/or slippery elm

bark. Goldenseal fights infection and slippery elm soothes the inflammation.

- 1 tablespoon of cornstarch and 2 drops of lavender essential oil mixed in ¼ cup of warm water. After one to two minutes, wipe this mixture off with a soft cloth. Lavender essential oil is antiseptic, antifungal, and anti-inflammatory.

ANTISEPTIC BATH

Add ½ cup of apple cider vinegar and 5 drops of lavender essential oil to a full bath. If you're using a baby-sized bath, use only 3 drops of essential oil.

SUPPORT FOR THE IMMUNE SYSTEM

If an infection persists, take 1 dropperful each of echinacea, calendula, and marsh mallow root tinctures three times daily. You can mix the tinctures in a bit of juice or water to make them more palatable. (To calculate a child's dosage, see "Herbal Dosages" on page 244.)

CRYPTORCHIDISM

As a male fetus develops, the testes form in the abdominal area. Some time before birth, they drop from the body into the scrotum. Cryptorchidism is a condition in which the testes fail to descend into the scrotum. About 10 percent of newborn male infants are cryptorchid; although most cases will resolve within a few weeks, in rare cases the testes remain undescended. Increased hormone levels at puberty will usually encourage descent of the testes in cryptorchid boys, although some parents opt for hormone therapies or surgery. There is some evidence that parental exposure to xenoestrogens and pesticides may be a contributing factor to cryptorchidism.

Treatment: Encouraging the Descent

Cryptorchidism can impair sperm production and cause sterility if the testicles do not descend by puberty. For this reason, it is a good idea to try to resolve the problem during a boy's childhood. Physicians may suggest hormone therapy or surgery. The following techniques are more natural alternatives that you may wish to try first, before resorting to surgery.

PHYSICAL MANIPULATION

A urologist or trained health care provider can encourage the testes to drop through gentle manipulation, as long as there is no structural condition contributing to the problem. Consult with your health care provider to discuss this option.

MOXA

An acupuncturist may use moxa, which entails burning the herb mugwort (*Artemisia vulgaris*) and bringing the heat and aromatic smoke close to the scrotum. The moxa treatment increases circulation in the pelvic area, which can help move blockages and bring down the testes.

HERBAL THERAPY

An herbalist would recommend herbs that stimulate hormone production, such as fennel and saw palmetto. An adult dosage of these herbs is 1 dropperful of tincture three times daily. (To calculate a child's dosage, see "Herbal Dosages" on page 244.)

Fennel (*Foeniculum vulgare*). The seed contains phytosterols, which provide the body with raw material for creating its own hormones.

Saw palmetto (*Serenoa repens*). The berry is anabolic, meaning that it aids in the development of muscle tissue, thereby preventing atrophy of the genitals. It also contains phytosterols. It is a nutritive, stimulant, and tonic for the genitourinary system.

DELAYED EJACULATION

It is common for men to begin to experience delayed ejaculation as they age. However, it's also likely to be a symptom of drug or alcohol abuse, stress, anger, or lack of trust in a partner. Check in with yourself, and if you find that your lifestyle is contributing to this deficiency in your sexual chi, do what it takes to resolve the problem before other, more negative symptoms begin appearing.

For some older men, delayed ejaculation or the inability to ejaculate may be a permanent condition. This is not detrimental to health, so long as underlying health problems have been ruled out by a health care professional. In fact, making love without ejaculating can help build sexual chi.

EPIDIDYMITIS

The epididymis is a system of long, tangled ducts connected to the testes. It holds sperm until they mature and then feeds them to the vas deferens. Inflammation of the epididymis (called epididymitis) can be very painful. The cause of the inflammation cannot always be determined, although chlamydia and gonorrhea may be contributing factors. If you have epididymitis, it's a good idea to get checked for STDs.

Symptoms

Epididymitis manifests as pain in the scrotum. There is often a lump on the back of the testicles that is hot and tender to the touch. There may be a discharge from the penis or difficulty in urinating.

Treatment

Antibiotics are usually prescribed, but consider the following natural therapies. If you don't get results, get medical attention.

ELEVATION

Elevating an inflamed area helps reduce the swelling. Whenever you're able to take a few minutes to relax, lie down with a pillow under your bottom to elevate the scrotum. You could also try sleeping in this position.

COLD PACKS AND SITZ BATHS

Twice daily, alternate ice compresses on the testicles with hot sitz baths. This treatment can help clear the blockage. (For information on preparing a sitz bath, see page 169.)

HERBAL THERAPY

Herbal therapy for epididymitis focuses on stimulating the body's immune system and eliminating pathogens.

Echinacea (*Echinacea purpurea, E. angustifolia*). Echinacea root stimulates the immune system. It is also an alterative, antifungal, and antiseptic.

Goldenseal (*Hydrastis canadensis*). Goldenseal root is effective against a wide range of pathogens and is especially effective for inflammation of the mucous membranes. It is an alterative and an antibiotic. Goldenseal is very bitter, and most people find it easiest to ingest in capsule form. This herb is endangered in the wild; do not use wildcrafted supplies.

Usnea (*Usnea barbata*). This lichen stimulates the immune system and is effective against a wide range of pathogens. It is also an antibiotic and an antifungal.

ERECTILE DYSFUNCTION

In humans, erection requires both emotional and physical stimulation. Erection occurs when blood rushes in from the penile arteries, engorging the erectile tissue. Valves in the veins close down, limiting blood flow back to the body. The engorged penis expands to accommodate the extra blood, which amounts to sixteen times the amount of blood it normally contains. Nitric oxide, a short-lived gas, aids this process.

The penile arteries are tiny; their lumens, or cavities, are just slightly larger than the head of a pin. When blood flow to the penis is impeded—as may happen when circulation through the penile arteries is limited by blockages or muscle constriction due to tension—achieving and maintaining erection becomes difficult.

Identifying the Cause

Although aging is sometimes accompanied by the onset of erectile dysfunction, it is not itself the cause. Rather, as the raging hormonal tides of young adulthood subside to normal rhythms, erection becomes less a "default" state and more the result of healthy sexual impulses. A man, then, must be in good health, both physically and mentally, to achieve and maintain an erection.

It is estimated that about 80 percent of cases of erectile dysfunction are caused by physical dysfunction, with the other 20 percent resulting from psychological concerns. Distinguishing between a physical and a psychological dysfunction is not always easy, but two general guidelines should be considered:

- If the dysfunction gained hold slowly but progressively over time, with a gradual decrease in erectile ability, it is probably physical in nature.

If it appeared suddenly, with no gradual buildup of symptoms, it is probably psychological in nature.

- If the inability to achieve or maintain erection occurs in all situations, including masturbation, it is probably a physical problem. If it occurs only with a particular partner or in certain situations, it is probably a psychological problem.

Many men have tried this simple technique to see if they are having erections during sleep, an indication that the concern may be more psychological. Before bed, moisten a strip of four to six postage stamps and wrap it around the base of the lingam. Overlap the strip so it seals and forms a ring. Wear snug underwear and do this three nights in a row. If erections are occurring, the strip of stamps will tear somewhere, indicating that good blood flow to the genitals is still occurring.

Direct an eye at what's going on in your life or what was happening at the time the dysfunction began. Make a list of the situations in which erection is possible and impossible. If you can uncover a trigger or pattern, you're close to discovering the cause, and with it, the cure.

If you suspect that the dysfunction is physical in nature, visit your health care provider as soon as possible for a full examination. There are many diseases and health conditions that can contribute to erectile dysfunction, including atherosclerosis, diabetes, endocrine disorders, heart disease, high cholesterol, kidney disease, Leriche's disease, liver disease, Lou Gehrig's disease, multiple sclerosis, Parkinson's disease, penile dysfunctions, prostate disease, sickle-cell anemia, and vascular disease. Exposure to toxic substances, including radiation treatments for cancer, can also impair erectile function.

Treatment

It makes sense to try natural remedies, rather than drug therapy, as a first recourse. Natural therapies encourage your body to heal itself, and they generally have a wide-ranging healing effect, supporting many of the body's systems, rather than just those related to erection.

SEEK ALTERNATIVES TO PHARMACEUTICALS

Many medications, including antidepressants, antihistamines, antipsychotics, and tranquilizers, can adversely affect libido. Medications designed to reduce high blood pressure can be especially problematic, because erection depends upon the mechanics of raising blood pressure.

If you're taking any of the aforementioned medications, ask your health care provider if there are alternatives that do not have erectile dysfunction as a side effect. However, do not stop taking medication without first consulting with your health care provider. If you must continue to take these drugs, incorporate natural, health-supporting therapies such as massage, herbal supplements, nutritional supplements, and relaxation techniques to improve your overall health and, with luck, counteract the side effects of your medication.

TAKE A BREAK

A prohibition on intercourse and ejaculation for four to six weeks can do wonders for building sexual energy and pulling your head, heart, and health together. Sex therapists suggest sensate therapy: getting naked, touching, caressing, exploring, and communicating, all the while avoiding intercourse and ejaculation. If arousal and erection does occur, avoid ejaculation, focusing instead on building sexual chi, much like adding money to your savings account.

Spend more time on sensate therapy than you would having sex. Becoming more sexually active, rather than less, helps improve erectile function by boosting circulation to the genitals. It also helps couples revive feelings of sensuality and togetherness.

SUPPORT TESTOSTERONE LEVELS

Testosterone plays a large role in generating libido. It also facilitates erection, although the connection is not fully understood.

Stress and lack of exercise can diminish testosterone levels. Exercise itself is a good remedy for stress, so be sure to get plenty of it. However, be aware that very intense exercise decreases testosterone levels.

Elevated estrogen levels can interfere with testosterone activity, contributing to erectile dysfunction. Products from animals that have been treated with hormones to encourage growth and early maturation often contain estrogens; eating them can elevate your estrogen levels. Eat products only from animals that were raised without the "benefit" of hormones.

Testosterone levels are highest between 6 and 8 a.m. If you're having trouble with erectile dysfunction, try to time lovemaking sessions so that *they occur in the early morning.*

STOP SMOKING

Smokers are twice as likely as nonsmokers to develop erection problems. Smoking reduces lung capacity, sexual endurance, libido, and the intensity of orgasms. Nicotine, just one of many noxious cigarette ingredients, constricts the arteries and veins that supply blood to the penis and diminishes testosterone levels. It seems capable of causing erectile dysfunction all on its own.

STOP DRINKING

Men with erection difficulties should, at the very least, abstain from alcohol on the days they desire to make love. Alcohol is a depressant and can, at high levels, prevent arousal and erection. Drinking beer, in particular, contributes to elevated levels of prolactin, which can decrease testosterone levels.

MASSAGE

There are many simple types of massage that can stimulate hormone production, strengthen sexual chi, boost circulation to the penis, and help a man achieve and maintain an erection.

The meridians that support sexual potency run through the big toe. Try massaging the whole foot, focusing on the big toe, to encourage erectile ability.

In a Taoist exercise, the man sits in a hot bath and stimulates himself manually to the point of erection. When erect, he grasps his testicles and gently pulls down on them one hundred to two hundred times. A traditional Japanese technique is similar; men are advised to firmly but gently squeeze the testicles daily, once for every year of age.

Kegel exercises, of course, are also excellent therapy for erectile dysfunction, because they encourage blood flow in the genitals. See page 118 for instructions on how to perform Kegels. While you're there, check out the Deer exercise, which follows the section on Kegels.

Foreplay can itself consist of therapeutic massage. To stimulate circulation, a man's partner can stroke the penis from the base to the tip, massaging the frenulum and glans and squeezing and massaging the penis's shaft.

Form a ring with the forefinger and thumb around the area of the penis just below the frenulum; squeeze gently but firmly to prevent blood from flowing out of the penis. This can encourage erection and greatly build a man's confidence. Take care not to squeeze too tightly or for more than a couple of minutes.

NUTRITIONAL THERAPY

Clogged arteries can impair blood flow and nitric oxide to the genitals as well as everywhere else in the body! Cut out saturated fats, hydrogenated and partially hydrogenated oils, sugar, and cold foods and beverages. Cooked fatty foods can impair circulation, and sugar actually robs the body of nutrients, such as calcium and the B-complex vitamins, causing nutritional deficiencies and fatigue. Focus on eating foods that are rich in the following nutrients (see chapter 3 for good sources), or try supplementation. Extra virgin olive oil is recommended, as is the inclusion of raw nuts in the diet.

Arginine. The amino acid arginine is a precursor to nitric oxide, a compound that is responsible for vasodilation and, thus, plays a role in blood flow to the genitals. Creams that deliver arginine transdermally (through the skin) are now available; consult with your health care provider for advice on whether this treatment is right for you. Arginine is also available in tablets or powders, often in combination with other erection-enhancing compounds, which can be found at natural food stores and vitamin shops.

Protein. To improve erectile ability, be sure to eat adequate protein. Protein helps normalize physiological chemicals; without it, the body deteriorates. Lean organic meats, fish, avocados, nuts, and seeds are excellent sources of protein.

Zinc. Through indirect action, zinc stimulates testosterone production. Take 25 to 50 mg daily, or eat a handful of raw sunflower and pumpkin seeds every day.

HERBAL THERAPY

Herbs that can improve peripheral circulation and nourish the sexual chi include ashwagandha, catuaba, damiana, eleuthero, epimedium, fenugreek, ginseng, maca, milky oat seed, sarsaparilla, saw palmetto, tribulis, and yohimbe (read cautions on page 96). Any of these herbs would be appropriate for a man suffering from erectile dysfunction. Natural food stores will carry herbal supplements that contain combinations of these botanicals. Turn to the herbal compendium in chapter 2 for more information.

ORCHITIS

Orchitis is an inflammation of a testis. It can arise spontaneously, but it can also be a side effect of mumps, gonnorrhea, syphilis, or other infections. If you experience orchitis, see your health care provider for an examination to rule out these other causes.

Symptoms

Orchitis is usually accompanied by pain, swelling, and a heavy feeling in the testicles.

Treatment

Treatment for orchitis focuses on reducing the inflammation and clearing the infection from the testes.

ICE

Two or three times a day, lie down with a pillow under your buttocks and apply an ice compress to the testicles. The elevation and ice will work together to reduce inflammation.

HERBAL THERAPY

Herbs that help reduce inflammation and move stagnation in cases of orchitis include the following.

Chamomile (*Matricaria recutita*). The flower helps detoxify the liver, reduce inflammation, and move stagnation. It is an analgesic, anodyne, anti-inflammatory, antispasmodic, and a mild sedative.

Cleavers (*Galium aparine*). The herb clears heat and reduces inflammation. It is an alterative, anti-inflammatory, antitumor, and astringent as well as a lymphatic cleanser and vulnerary.

Cramp bark (*Viburnum opulus*). The bark relieves pain. It is an analgesic, anti-inflammatory, antispasmodic, astringent, and diuretic.

Dong quai (*Angelica sinensis*). The root clears stagnation from the blood, relieves congestion in pelvic tissue, and relaxes smooth muscles. It is an alterative, anticoagulant, antispasmodic, and blood tonic. Do not use in cases of diarrhea or poor digestion. Do not use in conjunction with blood-thinning medications such as ibuprofen.

Echinacea (*Echinacea purpurea, E. angustifolia*). The root stimulates the body's immune response. It is an alterative, antibiotic, antifungal, anti-inflammatory, antiviral, immunostimulant, and vulnerary.

PEYRONIE'S DISEASE

Also known as the "bent penis" syndrome, Peyronie's disease is a condition in which erection produces what's called a fibrous chordee, or downward bowing of the penis. In some cases, the bend is so severe that intercourse is not feasible. It is often the result of scarring or the development of fibrous plaque in the penis and considered to be due to stagnant Liver chi. Collect and consume cattail pollen. The pollen can be added to flax crackers and dehydrated.

For proper diagnosis, visit your health care provider. The penis may look normal when flaccid, so it's helpful to bring a photograph of what the penis looks like when erect (assuming that you might have a difficult time achieving erection in the doctor's office).

Treatment

Surgery is sometimes recommended for Peyronie's disease, but it may cause further damage. Natural therapies don't risk additional harm, so it makes sense to try them first.

First clean up your diet, eliminating hydrogenated oils, fried foods, excess red meat, and dairy products. These foods can contribute to arteriosclerosis, causing circulatory blockage and impairing blood flow throughout the body.

Some men suffering from Peyronie's disease have had positive results with vitamin E, which reduces scarring. Take 400 IU twice daily, or eat a handful of almonds, sunflower seeds, or pumpkin seeds daily. Vitamin E supplementation is most effective when undertaken within two years of the onset of the condition. Nattokinnase is an enzyme that can reduce inflammation. Dong quai can be taken internally by men as a tea or capsule to break up stagnation.

You might also try massaging the penis with castor oil, which can help break up scar tissue. Warm herbal soaks (think plantain, ginger, calendula) can also be done or even warm herbal wraps.

PRIAPISM

Priapism is a persistent abnormal erection. Though an erection that doesn't give up might sound like a man's (or woman's) dream come true, it can result in permanent impotence if not treated within a few hours.

Priapism is named for Priapus, the Greek and Roman god of male generative power, often depicted with a huge erect penis. It occurs when blood in the engorged penis is unable to drain back into the body; the blockage can be caused by high blood pressure medications, some antidepressants, some aphrodisiacs, blood disorders, anesthesia, or damage to the penis, brain, or spinal cord.

Symptoms

Priapism is characterized by a persistent erection accompanied by pain and tenderness. The erection often occurs without sexual desire.

Treatment

Get thee to a doctor! Apply an ice pack to the genitals until you receive medical attention; this will encourage the blood vessels to constrict. Your health care provider will probably give you medication—a shot or pill—to deflate the erection.

PROSTATE HEALTH

The prostate gland is composed of both muscular and glandular tissue. It's shaped much like a chestnut and surrounds the neck of the bladder and the urethra, which is the beginning of the urinary tract. The prostate secretes a milky fluid that makes up about 30 percent of the volume of semen; the fluid is alkaline, which makes the vaginal environment less acidic and, thus, less hostile to sperm.

Common Disorders of the Prostate

It is estimated that half of the men in the United States over the age of fifty will have prostate difficulty at some time. That staggering statistic may be, in part, a result of the placid Western lifestyle. In cultures where a high-fiber, low-red-meat diet and exercise are the norm, prostate problems are considered rare. Avoiding STD's can also help lower the risk to the prostate.

BENIGN PROSTATIC HYPERPLASIA

Benign prostatic hyperplasia (BPH), also known as prostatism or prostatic adenoma, is a nonmalignant abnormal enlargement of the prostate. It is characterized by the swelling of prostatic tissue, sometimes accompanied by the development of small nodes. The enlargement is thought to be triggered by increased production of the androgen *dihydrotestosterone* (DHT), a common phenomenon in men over the age of forty-five.

An enlarged prostate can constrict the urethra, resulting in the need to urinate frequently, the inability to empty the bladder completely, painful urination, and occasional dribbling of urine. It's generally not a serious health problem, although advanced cases can manifest as bladder infections, kidney problems, and sexual dysfunction. It does cause discomfort, however, and the disruption of sleep caused by having to get up three or four times a night to urinate can lead to general malaise.

There are many pharmaceutical treatments for this common disorder. Surgery is also sometimes recommended. However, natural therapies are often very effective at reducing the symptoms of BPH; given the risks associated with surgery and the sometimes-annoying side effects of pharmaceuticals, they are a wise choice for initial treatment. See page 329 for discussion of some natural remedies for prostate problems.

PROSTATITIS

Prostatitis is an inflammation of the prostate, usually due to a bacterial infection (but sometimes a viral one). It can cause fever, discharge, back pain upon defecating, and blood in the urine. It often afflicts men who abstained from sex for a long period of time and then overindulged.

When you exhibit symptoms of prostatitis, it is important to rule out several more serious infections that may be triggering the inflammation. Chlamydia and other venereal parasites are common causes. Sometimes prostatitis is not bacterial but a symptom of an autoimmune disorder or a glandular dysfunction. Consult with your health care provider for guidance.

Prostatitis usually responds readily to natural therapy. Cease sexual activity until the irritation has disappeared. Do eat lots of colorful fresh raw fruits and vegetables. Avoid caffeine, alcohol, and spicy foods, which can contribute to prostate irritation. Follow the guidelines for prostate health given below. Echinacea, pipsissewa, and zinc will be especially helpful in fighting off infection and supporting the prostate. If natural therapies do not clear the infection within ten days, seek the advice of your health care provider.

PROSTATE CANCER

In its early stages, prostate cancer exhibits symptoms similar to those of BPH: the need to urinate frequently, inability to empty the bladder completely, painful urination, and occasional dribbling of urine. In a more advanced stage, prostate cancer may also manifest as blood in the urine, fatigue, bone pain, and weight loss.

Most prostate cancers form on the side of the gland that faces the rectum. Prostate cancer appears to be most prevalent in men whose diets are high in animal fat, such as is found in meat, eggs, and dairy products.

Though surgery and chemotherapy are the usual treatments for prostate cancer, you may also wish to explore nutrition therapy, herbal medicine, and energetic healing under the guidance of your health care provider. Saw palmetto and pygeum may be of particular benefit.

The Prostate Exam

Any time you suspect you have a problem with your prostate, consult with your health care provider for a proper diagnosis. Early symptoms of prostate cancer can be similar to those of BPH, and a checkup with a competent urologist is needed to distinguish between the two. This will mean a rectal exam; for those of you who dread the procedure, remember that it is easier if you relax. The urologist will be able to determine the condition of the prostate from the way it feels.

Improving the Health of the Prostate

Natural therapies for supporting the health of the prostate focus on strengthening the prostate, improving the function of the liver and kidneys, cleansing the urinary and bowel systems, counteracting or reducing levels of DHT, and relieving inflammation.

NUTRITIONAL THERAPY

Avoid heated fats, including red meat. A high-fat diet leads to elevated cholesterol levels, which can impair prostate function and contribute to BPH. Also minimize coffee, alcohol, salt, and dairy products, which irritate the prostate gland. Beer contains hops, which contain phytosterol precursors to an estrogen called *estradiol,* which can contribute to an enlargment of the prostate. Focus on incorporating the following nutrients and supplements into your diet.

Acidophilus. An acidophilus supplement will help discourage unfriendly microorganisms from invading the prostate region. Try taking one or two capsules three times daily.

Amino acids. The amino acids alanine, glutamine, and glycine can help shrink an enlarged prostate gland. They can often be purchased in combination with beneficial herbs for reducing enlargement.

Bee pollen. Small amounts of bee pollen or flower pollen (which differs from bee pollen only in that it is collected directly from the flowers and saves the bees lots of work) can be helpful in treating prostatitis. It has anti-inflammatory properties and is antiandrogenic, meaning it helps to counteract some of the effects of excess DHT. Take 1 teaspoon or two 500 mg tablets twice daily. If you have a pollen allergy, start with just a couple of grains a day, increasing by one grain a day until you reach the recommended dosage.

Chia, flaxseed, and pumpkin seed. To soothe inflammation of the prostate, take 3 tablespoons of freshly ground flaxseed or pumpkin seed daily. Also take 50 mg of vitamin B_6 to help reduce the prostate's size.

Cranberries help prevent bacteria from adhering to the wall of the bladder, a common origin of bacteria in the prostate.

Estrogenic foods. Foods that have estrogen-like activity are considered beneficial, because they help reduce elevated testosterone levels. These include apples, barley, brown rice, carrots, cherries, soy products (fermented are best), olives, and yams. Omega-6 fatty acids increase prostate growth, whereas omega-3s inhibit it.

Fruits and vegetables, especially those that are deeply colored and rich in antioxidants, boost immunity. Eat at least one large green salad daily. Make your own dressing with olive oil.

High-fiber foods. A thin tissue separates the prostate from the rectum. Because a blockage in one system tends to back up nearby systems, avoiding constipation supports not only the colon but also the prostate. A diet that is rich in high-fiber foods such as fruits, vegetables, nuts, and seeds promotes normal elimination.

Natural diuretics. It is also important to keep the urinary system fully functional. When watermelon is in season, chew up the seeds—which are diuretic—to help clean out the urinary tract. Drink plenty of pure water to make the urine less acidic and irritating. Diluted pure cranberry and wheatgrass juice are also beneficial drinks; cranberry juice is antiseptic, and wheatgrass helps the body make better use of oxygen.

Seaweeds. Seaweeds such as kelp and kombu have a softening and draining effect on hardened masses in the body; they can help relieve cases of BPH and prostatitis.

Tomatoes contain the carotene lycopene, which helps slow the growth of tumors in men with prostate cancer. Slicing them and adding a drizzle of olive oil will make the lycopene more bioavailable.

Water. Stay hydrated to flush the prostate.

Vitamin E and selenium. As antioxidants that support cellular health, vitamin E and selenium also support prostate health. Take a 400 IU vitamin E/selenium formula daily. Also consider incorporating natural sources of vitamin E and selenium into your diet; see chapter 3 for more information.

Zinc. The prostate gland contains more zinc than any other part of the body; having plenty of zinc in the diet supports the health of the prostate. Zinc can help shrink an enlarged prostate and alleviate symptoms associated with it. Good sources of zinc include almonds, beans, eggs, nutritional yeast, oatmeal, oysters, pumpkin seeds, sunflower seeds, and tahini. Also consider supplementing with 50 mg of chelated zinc daily.

HERBAL THERAPY

Herbs that support and improve the health of the prostate include the following.

Buchu (*Agathosma betulina*). The leaf soothes and strengthens the urinary system and relieves muscle spasms. It is a diuretic, Kidney tonic, and urinary antiseptic.

Cleavers (*Galium aparine*). The herb soothes prostate inflammation. It is particularly helpful in cases where one feels the urge to urinate but is unable to do so. It clears heat and improves lymphatic function. It is an alterative, anti-inflammatory, antitumor, soothing diuretic, and vulnerary.

Corn silk (*Zea mays*). Corn silk helps relieve inflammation of the prostate and irritation or infection in the urinary tract. It relieves the urge to urinate frequently by soothing irritated tissues. It is an alterative, demulcent, diuretic, and tonic.

Couchgrass (*Elymus repens*). The rhizome is particularly helpful in treating prostatitis. Its mucilaginous nature helps it cool irritated mucous membranes. It is an antiseptic, demulcent, diuretic, and tonic.

Cubeb (*Piper cubeba*). The berry is used to treat infections of the genitourinary tract and can help relieve cases of prostatitis. It is an antiseptic and a diuretic. Avoid in cases of acute digestive or kidney irritation.

Echinacea (*Echinacea purpurea, E. angustifolia*). The root remedies infections of the urinary tract. It is an alterative, antifungal, anti-inflammatory, antiseptic, and vulnerary.

Fringe tree (*Chionanthus virginicus*). The root clears heat and reduces inflammation. It is an alterative, cholagogue, diuretic, and hepatic.

Goldenrod (*Solidago* spp.). The herb reduces inflammation, sedates urinary passages, promotes urination, prevents infection, and strengthens the bladder. It is an anti-inflammatory, antiseptic, astringent, diuretic, hepatic, and tonic. Do not use in cases of hot inflammation, such as fever or high blood pressure.

Gravel root (*Eupatorium purpureum*). The root helps break up accumulations, such as stones in the urinary system. It clears heat, reduces inflammation, and soothes irritated mucous membranes of the urinary tract. It is often recommended for prostatitis. It is astringent, diuretic, and tonic.

Horsetail (*Equisetum arvense*). The herb reduces benign prostatic enlargement. It is an alterative, antiseptic, anti-inflammatory, astringent, diuretic, and vulnerary. Use horsetail that has been collected in spring.

Hydrangea (*Hydrangea arborescens*). The root soothes irritated mucous membranes and sedates the urinary tract. It is a diuretic and a tonic.

Marsh mallow (*Althaea officinalis*). The root soothes inflammation; it is useful for treating prostatitis in particular. It is an alterative, demulcent, diuretic, immunostimulant, rejuvenative, vulnerary, and yin tonic.

Nettle (*Urtica dioica, U. urens*). The leaf and root improve the metabolism of the prostate gland and reduce benign prostatic hyperplasia. Nettle also treats bladder infection, cystitis, kidney inflammation, and stones. Nettle contains sterols—including beta-sitosterol, stigmasterol, and campesterol—that decrease DHT activity. It is an alterative, cholagogue, circulatory stimulant, diuretic, Kidney tonic, and nutritive. Contact with the fresh plant will irritate the skin. Use only dried herb. Wear gloves when collecting.

Oregon grape (*Mahonia aquifolium*). The root is an alterative, anti-inflammatory, antiseptic, astringent, cholagogue, diuretic, glandular tonic, and immunostimulant. Do not exceed the recommended dosage.

Parsley (*Petroselinum crispum*). The leaf and root help relieve pain during urination and help men to empty the bladder completely. Parsley is antioxidant, antiseptic, diuretic, and nutritive. Avoid therapeutic doses in cases of kidney inflammation.

Pipsissewa (*Chimaphila umbellata*). The herb contains hydroquinone, which has genitourinary antiseptic properties. It is an alterative, anti-inflammatory, urinary antiseptic, astringent, diuretic, and urinary sedative.

Pygeum (*Pygeum africanum*). The bark has a decongesting action that blocks cholesterol buildup in the prostate gland. It is also anti-inflammatory and can help shrink an enlarged prostate. It is often recommended for treating erectile dysfunction, prostate cancer, prostatic hyperplasia, chronic prostate inflammation, and urinary disorders. This herb is endangered in the wild; do not use wildcrafted supplies.

Saint John's wort (*Hypericum perforatum*). The herb dissolves obstructions and reduces swelling. It is an alterative, anti-inflammatory, antiseptic, cholagogue, and vulnerary. In rare cases this herb causes photosensitivity. Do not combine Saint John's wort with monoamine oxidase (MAO) inhibitors (chemical antidepressants) or selective serotonin reuptake inhibitors, such as Prozac.

Saw palmetto (*Serenoa repens*). The berry reduces inflammation, lessens pain, and relieves the need to urinate frequently. It also inhibits the conversion of testosterone to dihydrostestosterone (DHT). It enhances blood flow to the prostate and thus lowers the rate of cellular regeneration in the prostate gland. It is often recommended in treatments for prostatic hyperplasia and prostatitis. It is a diuretic, rejuvenative, urinary antiseptic, and tonic.

Uva ursi (*Arctostaphylos uva-ursi*). The leaf contains arbutin, which the body converts to hydroquinone, an antiseptic. It is a genitourinary antiseptic, astringent, Bladder tonic, demulcent, diuretic, and vasoconstrictor.

HOMEOPATHIC REMEDIES

There are several homeopathic remedies that can be used to improve prostate problems. If any of the descriptions below match the symptoms of your prostatic condition, try the suggested homeopathic remedy. The usual dosage is 4 pellets, or as many liquid drops as the package label recommends, taken under the tongue four times daily. Rather than swallowing the pellets whole, allow them to dissolve slowly.

ACONITUM NAPELLUS. The patient is suffering from the initial stage of prostatitis.

APIS MELLIFICA. The prostate is inflamed.

ARGENTUM METALLICUM. The patient is elderly and suffers from chronic prostate enlargement.

ARGENTUM NITRICUM. The patient is elderly and suffers from prostate enlargement with burning in the rectal anterior.

BARYTA CARBONICA. The patient is elderly and suffers from prostatic enlargement. He may experience a frequent urge to urinate and a burning sensation when he does so.

BELLADONNA. The patient suffers from throbbing prostatitis.

CANNABIS INDICA. The patient feels that he is sitting on a ball in the anal region.

CHIMAPHILA UMBELLATA. The patient experiences discomfort and the need to urinate frequently.

CONIUM. The patient has chronic prostatic enlargement and difficulty urinating, with the flow of urine starting and stopping.

FERRUM PICRICUM. The patient is elderly and suffers from prostate enlargement and inflammation.

LYCOPODIUM. The patient has an enlarged prostate and feels pressure in the perineum during urination.

PULSATILLA. The patient has prostate inflammation accompanied by increased sex drive and frequent erections.

SABAL SERRULATA. The patient has either chronic or acute prostate enlargement accompanied by burning or difficulty in urination.

SOLIDAGO VIRGAUREA. The patient has chronic prostate enlargement and obstructed urine flow.

SPONGIA TOSTA. The patient has prostate enlargement, and his testicles are red and swollen.

STAPHYSAGRIA. The patient experiences frequent urges to urinate but can produce only small amounts of urine, which burns.

SULFUR. Prostatic fluid escapes during urination or during bowel movements.

THUJA OCCIDENTALIS. The patient feels a constant urge to urinate but can produce only small amounts of urine. There is pain from the rectum to the bladder.

SITZ BATHS

To boost circulation and clear stagnation from the genital area, alternate hot and cold sitz baths, as directed in chapter 10.

Warm baths on their own will also have some benefit, relaxing the pelvic muscles and softening the prostate. In lieu of a bath, apply a hot water bottle to the perineal area (between the anus and scrotum).

EXERCISE

Various exercises can help improve circulation and clear congestion from the prostate. A slant board or inverted yoga posture such as the shoulder stand can help clear congestion. Kegel exercises are also helpful (see page 118).

When you get up in the morning and retire in the evenings, try this simple exercise. Lie on your back and bring the soles of your feet together. Extend your legs as far as you can while keeping the soles together, then bring them as close to your chest as possible, still keeping the soles together. Repeat ten times.

Of most importance, get adequate exercise. There's nothing better for improving circulation and supporting overall health. Try walking, swimming, or dancing, all of which are excellent, nonjarring forms of exercise.

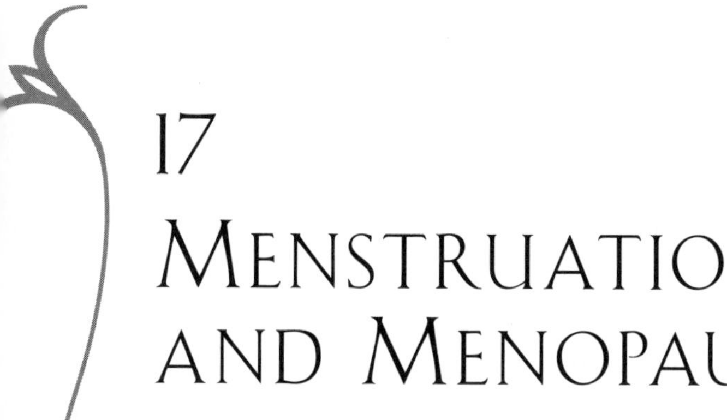

17
Menstruation and Menopause

MENSTRUATION AND MENOPAUSE are part of the natural rhythms of life. As such, they have their ups and downs. When you experience pain or other symptoms related to your menstrual cycle or menopause, try to nurture and care for yourself rather than placing the responsibility for your health in the hands of the medical establishment. Take back control of your own body. Go with the flow.

MENSTRUATION

The process of menstruation is driven by hormones released from the brain and from the organs of the reproductive system. A woman has two ovaries, and each contains millions of follicles—tiny balls of cells surrounding a germ cell, or egg. At the beginning of every cycle, the pituitary gland releases follicle-stimulating hormone (FSH), which stimulates the development of ten to twenty follicles. Usually only one of the follicles develops into a true ovum, or egg. The developing follicles secrete estrogen, which stimulates growth of the endometrium, the lining of the uterus. When the egg is released from the follicle, it is swept into one of the fallopian tubes; over the course of several days, it will travel along the fallopian tube to the uterus.

The leftover cells of the follicle, called the corpus luteum, now begin to secrete progesterone in addition to estrogen. The pituitary gland secretes luteinizing hormone (LH), which, in combination with the progesterone from the corpus luteum, stimulates tiny endometrial arteries to keep blood circulating through the endometrium.

If the egg becomes fertilized (which, in most cases, happens along its journey through the fallopian tubes), it implants in the endometrium and begins to grow, and a whole new round of hormonal production is set off. If the egg does not become fertilized, the corpus luteum is eventually absorbed into the ovaries, shutting off the supply of estrogen and progesterone and, consequently, shutting off the tiny arteries that feed the endometrium. The endometrium is starved of blood and eventually detaches from the uterus and is shed. We call that shedding process menstruation. The body then begins preparing for a new cycle by releasing FSH into the bloodstream. And so the cycle perpetuates, over and over.

Menstrual flow is composed of blood, endometrial tissue, and mucus. The unique odor of menstrual flow is caused by vaginal bacteria interacting with the blood. Blood loss averages between ¼ and ¾ of a cup. A loss of more or less than that can signal a larger health problem.

Menstruation can be a time of healing, rest, and regeneration. Many women experience it as a time of increased awareness. Unfortunately, many other women experience it as a time of great tension and pain; their bodies are unequipped to deal with the physical demands of menstruation, and their schedules don't permit them to slow down for a day or two. Imagine what it would feel like to be able to spend that first day of menstruation resting, meditating, pursuing quiet activity and inward thought. Glorious!

Research suggests that a woman's immune system is at peak strength during ovulation and begins to decline after the egg is released. It has been proposed that this decrease in strength keeps the immune system from attacking the fertilized egg. The wider implication is that surgery, vaccinations, and other medical procedures may be safest during the ovulation phase of a woman's cycle.

Whether or not you're able to gear down on the first day of menstruation, normalizing the menstrual cycle, regulating menses, eliminating cramps, and reducing premenstrual tension will help make the passage easier.

Feminine Hygiene Products

Until the 1920s, marketing feminine hygiene products was considered immoral. There were no commercial products available. Women had to make do on their own, and in my opinion, that may have been for the best.

In the 1930s, tampons became commercially available and wildly popular. For decades they were made primarily of cotton. In the early 1980s, four new, highly absorbent materials—carboxymethyl cellulose, polyacrylate rayon, viscose rayon, and polyester cellulose—were combined with the cotton to increase its absorption power. Soon after, toxic shock syndrome (TSS) became a household word.

Because cotton is not a food crop, there are no governmental restrictions on how many chemicals can be used in its production. As a result, most commercial brands of cotton tampons contain some pesticide residue. In addition, cotton is often bleached, which leaves it with a dioxin residue. So if you're going to use all-cotton tampons, I highly recommend that they be organic and unbleached.

ALTERNATIVES TO TAMPONS

Tampons can alter the balance of vaginal flora, can release irritating fibers into the vagina, and if they're used when flow is minimal, can make tiny tears in the vaginal wall. As a result, tampons can expose a woman to infection. In addition, tampons are themselves an internal blockage, which can impede the flow of energy. A woman using tampons may even experience exacerbated cramping as the menstrual flow backs up. This only makes cramps worse. Most of us recognize the environmental impact of thousands of plastic baby diapers in our landfills. We must consider also the impact of thousands of feminine hygiene products.

Reusable cloth menstrual pads are effective sanitary devices, comfortable, and, in the long run, less expensive than disposable tampons. Look for brands such as Glad Rags and Moon Pads. Consider that for what you might spend on pads within a year, you can use cloth and be set for life. You can find "lunar pads" at most health food stores or make them from pieces of absorbent flannel. Line your underwear with a pad, and replace it with a fresh one when necessary. Soak the used pads in a bucket of water to get rid of excess blood before running them through a washing machine. Pour the water from the bucket over the roots of a tree. Menstrual flow is, after all, the sacred blood intended to nourish a potential child. As a garden fertilizer, it's a lot closer to home than sheep's blood or cow's manure from animals you don't even know!

If you need to use an internal sanitary device from time to time (getting a massage, swimming, being in a pageant), consider a sea sponge, which is highly absorbent and reusable. Before each use, boil the sponge in water for five minutes. Then let air-dry. After each use, rinse the sponge well, soak it in apple cider vinegar, and rinse again. Dispose of the sponge after a few menses.

Also available are natural rubber or silicone menstrual cups, such as the Keeper, the Mooncup, and the Divacup. They're a more environmental alternative to tampons, but its best for the flow to go out.

Toxic Shock Syndrome

TSS is a life-threatening blood infection caused by the bacterium *Staphylococcus aureus*. Although researchers are not yet able to explain the connection between this Staph infection and tampons, we do know that using high-absorbency tampons, cervical caps, and other intrauterine birth control devices increases a woman's risk for developing TSS. The use of all-cotton tampons has not been linked to TSS.

Warning signs of TSS include:

- Sudden fever (usually over 102°F)
- Diarrhea
- Vomiting
- Faintness
- Rash

If you exhibit any of these symptoms while you are using a tampon, remove the tampon immediately. Seek medical help.

Because of the risk of TSS, tampon use should be restricted to brief periods when menstrual pads are impractical, such as while a woman is swimming, receiving a full-body massage, traveling, and so on. Avoid overnight use. Use only all-cotton tampons.

Premenstrual Syndrome

Premenstrual syndrome (PMS) is a major emotional and physical health concern for many women. It is sometimes referred to as premenstrual tension (PMT), and the terms are interchangeable. Common emotional symptoms include depression, crying spells, irritability, anger, agitation, and even a tendency toward increased absentmindedness and accidents. In severe cases, withdrawal and suicidal tendencies can emerge. In France, PMS has been accepted as grounds for a plea of temporary insanity. Common physical symptoms include water retention, weight gain, a feeling of heaviness in the abdomen, and tenderness in the breasts.

CAUSES OF PMS

PMS is usually linked to abnormally high levels of estrogen; women who suffer from PMS tend to have higher levels of estrogen in their blood five to ten days before menstruation than women who do not have PMS. Estrogen production is initiated at the onset of menstruation and continues to increase until the corpus luteum disappears. Once the follicle has ruptured and the egg has been released, the corpus luteum produces progesterone, which counteracts the effects of elevated estrogen levels. However, if progesterone levels are insufficient, then estrogen dominates and the symptoms of PMS are likely to intensify.

This is a simplified explanation of a complicated problem. There are a wide variety of hormone imbalances that contribute to PMS, and no single solution that works for every woman. While only a small percentage of women suffer from extreme PMS, many experience some of its symptoms, in varying degrees. If you suffer from extreme PMS, consult with your health care provider for diagnosis and appropriate treatment. If you experience only moderate symptoms, consider some of the natural therapies suggested below.

In traditional Oriental medicine, Liver stagnation is thought to be a major contributing factor to menstrual difficulties. The Liver governs the amount of menstrual flow and the regularity of the cycle. It also breaks down excess hormones, including estrogen. Therefore, treatments for PMS (as well as many other reproductive health concerns—including fibroids, cysts, hot flashes, prostate inflammation, and infertility) often focus on strengthening Liver function.

From a Western medical point of view, PMS can be broken into several categories, each with a particular set of symptoms and causes.

1. PMT-A is characterized by emotional difficulties, such as anxiety, mood swings, and tension. It is associated with elevated estrogen levels and decreased progesterone levels in the luteal phase of the cycle (post-ovulation).
2. PMT-B is characterized by breast soreness, bloating, and weight gain. It is associated with increased levels of aldosterone, an adrenal hormone that causes water and sodium retention. Increased levels of prolactin, a hormone released when the pituitary is stressed, can be a contributing factor to breast tenderness. Stagnation in the Liver often contributes to PMT-B.
3. PMT-C is characterized by food cravings, hypoglycemia, headache, and physical shakiness; in severe cases, it can result in fatigue, fainting, and heart palpitations. It is associated with blood sugar imbalances and, in some cases, low levels of prostaglandin.
4. PMT-D manifests as depression, lethargy, insomnia, crying, withdrawal, and forgetfulness. It is associated with increased levels of aldosterone and progesterone and low levels of estrogen. In extreme cases, PMT-D can stimulate suicidal tendencies and require psychiatric care.

Chart your cycle on a calendar so that you can see if there is a pattern to the changes you experience. For a diagnosis of PMS, you must experience the symptoms from one to fourteen days before your menses begin and then be free of symptoms for at least seven days after the menses end. On the chart, keep track of your emotional state, physical health, sexual energy, dreams, and diet. After a few cycles, you may discover some interesting correlations. Once you identify the patterns, you can use your energy in ways that support your body to best effect.

RELIEVING PMS

Some women would swear that PMS stands for "Please, more sweets." (Or perhaps "Putting Men through Shit," think some partners.) However, giving in to sugar cravings will only make mood swings more severe and more erratic. Avoid salty foods, which contribute to bloating and weight gain, and hydrogenated oils (found in fried foods, margarine, and shortening), which impair the liver's function and prevent it from breaking down excess estrogen. To satisfy cravings for salt, try eating raw nuts salted with Celtic sea salt, or sea vegetables. Air-popped popcorn is healthier than chips. To improve Liver and Kidney function, drink a lot of water with a squeeze of fresh lemon juice added to it. Also eat plenty of green leafy vegetables. In general, just eat healthier so your liver can do its job instead of getting bogged down with the hard-to-metabolize fats and sugars found in unhealthy foods.

Relaxation therapies can do wonders for PMS. Take aromatherapy baths. Get massages. Drink the "I Got the PMS Blues" tea described on page 355. Practice deep breathing. Play relaxation tapes. Take long walks. Undertake some sort of a creative pursuit, such as writing, drawing, or singing. Above all, do your best to nurture yourself during your "moon" time. Become more aware of the Moon and its phases; the full moon is said to stimulate FSH (follicle-stimulating hormones).

For advice on how to use any of the natural therapies suggested for PMS and the other menstrual dysfunctions discussed on the following pages, see "Natural Therapies for Healthy Menstruation" (page 346).

Dysmenorrhea

Dysmenorrhea is the term for difficult, painful menstruation. After ovulation, the uterine lining (endometrium) prepares itself for a fertilized egg. Tiny arteries feed it blood and embryo-nourishing substances. If fertilization does not occur, those tiny arteries shut down, and the lining starts to deteriorate. The arteries may spasm as the lining dies off. The cramping usually ceases sometime during menstruation, because the menstrual blood helps clean out the area.

CAUSES OF DYSMENORRHEA

Dysmenorrhea can be caused or exacerbated by a variety of hormonal and reproductive dysfunctions.

Constipation. Constipation can cause pressure on the uterus and contribute to cramping.

Inflammatory prostaglandins. Prostaglandins are hormonelike derivatives of unsaturated fatty acids that act as chemical messengers in the body.

There are several types. An overabundance of prostaglandin E1 is thought to contribute to premenstrual inflammation; its production can be controlled by evening primrose oil, zinc, and vitamin E.

Magnesium deficiency. A magnesium deficiency can cause cramping and spasms during menstruation. A poem that doesn't rhyme, but gets the message across is "If you have spasms. Think magnesium." (And, of course, green leafy vegetables are an excellent source.)

Calcium deficiency. Calcium is important not only for the bones and teeth but also for the muscles. Cramping and other symptoms of dysmenorrhea are similar to the symptoms of a calcium deficiency; maintaining adequate levels of calcium can prevent those symptoms from occurring.

Pelvic congestion. Dysmenorrhea can also be caused by ischemia (lack of blood flow) in the pelvic area. Pelvic ischemia is most common in young women who have not yet given birth. The herb blue cohosh can offer relief in this situation.

Tight clothes and tampons. Somehow the media has convinced women that during their periods, they should plug themselves up, wear tight white jeans, and go horseback riding! But when your body is trying to release menstrual blood, you'll certainly be more comfortable wearing looser clothing and sanitary pads, and going with the flow.

Spinal misalignment. If the spine is out of alignment, nerves may be pinched, causing cramping. Yoga, bodywork, and chiropractic adjustments can all be of service in this case.

RELIEVING DYSMENORRHEA

Physical tension or tightness can worsen dysmenorrhea, so do your best to stay warm and loose. Practice deep breathing (see page 124). Wear loose clothing. Stay warm. Avoid cold drinks and icy foods, which can cause muscle contractions. Apply a hot water bottle over the kidneys to relieve pain. A castor oil compress (see page 267) over the abdomen might also be helpful.

To prevent constipation, stick to a high-fiber diet. Be sure to include sources of omega-3 and omega-6 fatty acids, such as fish, flaxseed oil, and evening primrose oil, which can help control prostaglandin levels. Drink plenty of water. If you still need help, chew a handful of flaxseeds daily, or grind them up and sprinkle them on your food.

To reduce the occurrence and severity of cramps, eat plenty of foods that are rich in magnesium and calcium. While you're in the process of improving your diet, you may also wish to take magnesium and calcium supplements. See chapter 3 for more information on nutritional supplements.

The herbs black cohosh, chamomile, cinnamon, cramp bark, ginger, peppermint, red raspberry, and yarrow and the essential oils anise, carrot seed, clary sage, jasmine, and rose can all help relieve cramping.

Some women have found that crushing a bromelain tablet, mixing it with a bit of cocoa butter, and inserting it vaginally can help relieve severe cramps. Bromelain has an anti-inflammatory effect on the uterine tissues.

Leg lifts are a tremendously beneficial exercise for menstrual cramping. You may feel as though you couldn't possibly move an inch, but if you give it a try, you'll find that cramps become less severe. Massage of your Achilles tendons can also help.

Menorrhagia

Menorrhagia describes excessively long or excessively profuse bleeding during menstruation. Before attempting at-home treatment, consult with your health care provider; he or she will most likely give you a thorough examination to make sure that a cyst, tumor, or complication of pregnancy is not causing the bleeding.

CAUSES OF MENORRHAGIA

Menorrhagia is often a result of insufficient levels of progesterone; the tiny arteries that feed the endometrium aren't signaled to stop. In traditional Oriental medicine, excessive menstrual bleeding is thought to result from excess heat, deficient chi, or blood stagnation. Profuse dark clots of blood may indicate a Liver imbalance. Blood that is profuse and light red may indicate a Spleen imbalance (the Spleen governs the passage of blood through the channels of the body).

RELIEVING MENORRHAGIA

To stop alarmingly excessive bleeding, drink a glass of water to which you've added ⅛ teaspoon of cayenne pepper or the juice of a lemon. However, don't rely on this "Band-aid" approach. Pay attention and focus on correcting the imbalance causing the excess bleeding.

To compensate for blood loss, eat plenty of blood-building foods, such as beets and dark green leafy vegetables. To help normalize hormone production, eat plenty of cold-water fish, such as salmon, herring, sardines, and mackerel, and supplement with sources of essential fatty acids, such as flaxseed oil, evening primrose oil, and black currant seed oil. Nourish the thyroid gland, which helps regulate all the cycles of the body, by incorporating seaweeds into your diet. Iron-rich adzuki beans, lentils, and amaranth tea are excellent foods for women who bleed too much.

Herbs that can decrease the flow of blood include cinnamon, lady's mantle, nettle, red raspberry, shepherd's purse, uva ursi, and yarrow. Also consider supplementing with vitamin C (with bioflavonoids) to help strengthen your capillaries.

Amenorrhea

Amenorrhea is characterized by lack of menstruation in a woman who has experienced puberty but not yet menopause and who is not pregnant or lactating. It is not uncommon in women who exercise excessively, such as professional athletes; their bodies may focus less on estrogen production or reproduction.

CAUSES OF AMENORRHEA

There are many possible causes of amenorrhea, some of them quite serious. They include hormone imbalances, infertility, tumors, nutritional deficiencies, glandular dysfunctions, weight imbalances, exposure to environmental toxins, and stress. Some pharmaceutical medications can cause amenorrhea. Before attempting at-home treatment, consult with your health care provider. He or she will probably recommend a thorough physical examination to determine the cause and the appropriate treatment.

CORRECTING AMENORRHEA

In treating amenorrhea with natural therapies, it is imperative that you correct any nutritional deficiencies. Incorporate into your diet blood-building foods like beets, blueberries, parsley, raspberries, and nettles and iron-rich foods like apricots, blackstrap molasses, bran, carrots, chicken (dark meat), eggs, fish, green leafy vegetables, green peppers, Jerusalem artichokes, millet, miso, oatmeal, parsley, persimmons, prunes, pumpkin seeds, raisins, seaweeds, sesame seeds, squash, sunflower seeds, and turkey (dark meat).

Herbs that can help amenorrhea by building the blood and improving circulation to the pelvis include angelica, basil, blue cohosh, burdock, cinnamon, licorice, mugwort, nettle, and red raspberry.

Also consider supplementing with vitamin B complex, vitamin E, and a multimineral supplement to correct potential nutritional deficiencies.

Essential oils to use topically include clary sage, fennel, lavender, and rosemary. See chapter 5 for suggestions on how to use these oils.

Hot sitz baths can also help increase circulation to the reproductive organs. See page 169 for details.

Metrorrhagia

Metrorrhagia is the term used to describe menstrual bleeding that occurs at irregular intervals or outside the duration of normal menses. As with other menstrual dysfunctions, it can be a side effect of other, more serious health problems. Consult with your health care provider to rule out conditions such as endometriosis, fibroids, cancer, or cysts before beginning at-home treatment.

CAUSES OF METRORRHAGIA

In Oriental tradition, excessively early or late menses are said to be caused by a chi deficiency or by stagnation in the blood or Liver. If the menses are very light, coldness and deficiency are suspected.

From a Western perspective, menses that come early may be due to an insufficiency of either estrogen or progesterone. Menses that are delayed more than eight or nine days in the average twenty-eight-day cycle could be a symptom of a cyst, late ovulation, or lack of ovulation.

CORRECTING METRORRHAGIA

A common, often unrecognized factor in the regulation of menses is exposure to light. Light has a powerful effect on hormones, and aberrant patterns of light exposure can result in aberrant hormonal behavior. Too often we go to work in darkness, return home in darkness, spend our days under fluorescent lights, and spend our nights bathed in the artificial brightness of street lights, night-lights, and digital clocks. If you are suffering from metrorrhagia, try sleeping in total darkness—pull all the shades, close the door, and unplug all electrical appliances. And be sure to spend some time outdoors every day, enjoying natural, full-spectrum light.

Consider supplementing with vitamin C (with bioflavonoids) to strengthen the capillaries, iron to strengthen the blood, and vitamin K to improve the blood's clotting ability.

Herbs that can help regulate the menstrual cycle include dandelion root, false unicorn root, and vitex. If your menses tend to come too early, try rose hip and sage teas. If they tend to be delayed, try red raspberry leaf.

Essential oils that can be used topically to help regulate the menses include basil, clary sage, cypress, geranium, hops, nutmeg, oregano, parsley, peppermint, and savory.

NATURAL THERAPIES FOR HEALTHY MENSTRUATION

Natural therapies for normalizing and supporting the menstrual cycle focus on four main goals.

1. Building the blood and improving its circulation to help normalize the menstrual cycle.
2. Controlling blood sugar levels to reduce food cravings and minimize mood swings.
3. Regulating hormone production and metabolism to moderate emotional states and normalize the menstrual cycle. This includes strengthening the liver to support the expedient breakdown of excess hormones.
4. Relaxing the muscles helps reduce cramping and enables smoother menstrual flow.

Exercise

Women who exercise regularly are less likely to have menstrual difficulties than those who don't. Exercise improves circulation, strengthens the liver, and stimulates the production of "feel good" endorphins. Brisk walking and swimming are especially helpful for menstrual dysfunctions; they stimulate the body's systems without taxing the joints and muscles.

Diet

Keep blood sugar levels stable by eating small, frequent meals. And resist that sweet tooth; when we give in to sugar cravings, we're likely to get raving! Sugar raises glucose levels in the blood, making us feel temporarily energetic, but as soon as the sugar is burned up, we crash. Menstruation offers enough emotional difficulties on its own without the added pressure of a sugar-induced emotional roller coaster.

To normalize estrogen levels, incorporate into your diet cruciferous vegetables, such as broccoli, cabbage, and cauliflower. Soy is often promoted as a good source of phytoestrogens, which can help normalize the body's production of its own estrogen. However, soy can be difficult to digest and is a common allergen, and soy products are often manufactured from genetically modified soybeans. For these reasons, the best forms of soy are tempeh and miso (from organically grown, non-genetically-modified soybeans); they are fermented and easy to digest.

Eating less meat, or eating meat only from animals that were raised without hormone treatments, can also help. Many farm animals are fed estrogen-like drugs to promote earlier maturity and weight gain; traces of these hormones can be found in the meat from these animals. These synthetic hormones, some of which are known carcinogens, overburden the liver, interfering with its ability to break down our own hormones. Incomplete or delayed breakdown of hormones can cause systemic problems and a wide range of symptoms.

Cutting down on salt will help prevent water retention and bloating. To further the "no bloating" cause, eat foods that are naturally diuretic, such as artichokes, asparagus, watercress, and watermelon (including the seeds). Drinking more water will also help the body excrete sodium and excess fluids.

To build the blood, eat plenty of green leafy vegetables and seaweeds. Seaweeds can also help regulate erratic menstrual cycles, as can carrots.

Herbal Therapy

When reviewing the herbs that are beneficial for menstruation, keep in mind that those plants listed as phytoestrogenic are best used during the first phase of the cycle (from the first day of menstruation until ovulation). Plants with phytoprogesteronic activity are best used during the second phase of the cycle (from ovulation until the first day of menstruation).

Agrimony (*Agrimonia eupatoria*). The herb encourages the coagulation of blood, which can help reduce excessive menstrual flow. It also relieves cramps. It is an analgesic, anti-inflammatory, antispasmodic, astringent, diuretic, emmenagogue, hemostatic, and hepatic. Avoid during pregnancy and in cases of constipation.

Alfalfa (*Medicago sativa*). The leaf supports clotting of the blood, which can help women who bleed heavily during menstruation. It is also rich in nutrients that build the blood and is often recommended in treatments for anemia. It also relieves fatigue and normalizes estrogen production. It is anti-inflammatory, diuretic, nutritive, and phytoestrogenic.

Angelica (*Angelica archangelica, A. atropurpurea*). The root helps build blood, increase menstrual flow, and can normalize the menstrual cycle in women who tend to have delayed menses. It also relaxes the muscles and improves liver function. It's often recommended in treatments for amenorrhea, anemia, dysmenorrhea, migraine, and nausea. It is an anti-inflammatory, antispasmodic, diuretic, emmenagogue, nervine, phytoestrogen, tonic, and uterine stimulant. Avoid during pregnancy and in cases of heavy bleeding or diabetes. In rare cases, the root causes photosensitivity.

Anise (*Pimpinella anisum*). The seed relieves bloating, dysmenorrhea, and nausea. It may curb a sweet tooth. It is antispasmodic and phytoestrogenic.

Basil (*Ocimum basilicum*). The leaf can help calm anxiety and clear mental fogginess. It also increases circulation to the pelvic region. It is an antidepressant, antispasmodic, circulatory stimulant, and sedative.

Black cohosh (*Actaea racemosa*). The root can soothe irritation and break up congestion in the uterus, cervix, and vagina. It's often recommended in treatments for amenorrhea, dysmenorrhea, moodiness, and PMS. It is an alterative, anti-inflammatory, antispasmodic, astringent, diuretic, emmenagogue, phytoestrogen, muscle relaxant, nervine, and uterine stimulant. Avoid during pregnancy, except in the final stages, and then only under the guidance of your health care provider. Avoid while nursing and in cases of high blood pressure or pressure in the inner eye. Consult with your health care provider before use. This herb is endangered in the wild; do not use wildcrafted supplies.

Black haw (*Viburnum prunifolium*). The bark (including the bark of the root) helps relax the smooth muscles of the uterus. It's often recommended in treatments for amenorrhea, dysmenorrhea, and menorrhagia. It is an analgesic, antispasmodic, astringent, and uterine sedative.

Blessed thistle (*Cnicus benedictus*). The herb strengthens the spleen, liver, and reproductive system. It's often recommended for amenorrhea.

Blue cohosh (*Caulophyllum thalictroides*). The dried root can stimulate menstrual flow and relieves uterine inflammation and cramping due to insufficient blood flow. It's often recommended in treatments for dysmenorrhea and PMS. It is anti-inflammatory, antispasmodic, diuretic, emmenagogic, oxytocic, and a uterine stimulant. Avoid during pregnancy, except in the final stages, and then only under the guidance of your health care provider. Make sure the root is dried, not fresh. This herb is endangered in the wild; do not use wildcrafted supplies.

Bupleurum (*Bupleurum chinense, B. falcatum*). The root relieves pain and relaxes the muscles. It also boosts blood circulation and helps improve liver function. It is an alterative, anti-inflammatory, and tonic. Avoid in cases of fever, headache, or high blood pressure.

Burdock (*Arctium lappa*). The root is a great liver cleanser. It builds blood and can reduce tenderness in the breasts. It also helps dispel the irritability of PMS. It is alterative, anti-inflammatory, diuretic, nutritive, and rejuvenative.

Cayenne (*Capsicum annuum*). The fruit improves circulation and can also help decrease excessive menstrual flow. It is an alterative, astringent, and hemostatic. Avoid contact with eyes and mucous membranes. Avoid therapeutic doses during pregnancy and while nursing.

Chamomile (*Matricaria recutita*). The flower relieves cramps caused by stagnation in the pelvic region. It also has a potent effect on the psyche, calming anxiety, hysteria, and nervousness. It is often recommended in treatments for amenorrhea. It is an anti-inflammatory, antispasmodic, and analgesic. In rare cases, individuals exhibit an allergic response to this herb.

Cinnamon (*Cinnamomum cassia, C. verum*). The bark can reduce excessive menstrual bleeding. It is often recommended in treatments for dysmenorrhea, headache, and nausea. Avoid in cases of hemorrhoids, dry stools, bloody urine, or excess heat, such as fever and inflammation. It may exacerbate premature ejaculation. Avoid therapeutic dosages during pregnancy.

Codonopsis (*Codonopsis pilosula*). The root builds blood and tonifies the spleen. It can stabilize blood sugar levels, boost energy, and increase the time between menses. It is a chi tonic and nutritive.

Cotton root (*Gossypium hirsutum, G. herbaceum*). The root bark constricts blood vessels and is often recommended for menorrhagia that is caused by fibroids, as well as for dysmenorrhea, endometriosis, uterine fibroids, and uterine inflammation. It is emmenagogic, hemostatic, nutritive, oxytocic, and a uterine tonic. Avoid during pregnancy. Large doses may cause nausea and vomiting. Avoid in cases of urogenital irritation.

Cramp bark (*Viburnum opulus*). The bark relieves cramps, headache, and hysteria. It is an analgesic, anti-inflammatory, antispasmodic, astringent, diuretic, nervine, tonic, and uterine sedative.

Dandelion (*Taraxacum officinale*). The root is a cholagogue and Liver tonic; it improves liver function and can relieve tenderness in the breasts. The leaf is an alterative and diuretic; it can relieve edema and is often recommended in cases of anemia.

Dong quai (*Angelica sinensis*). The root helps regulate estrogenic activity. It improves circulation to the pelvis; increases menstrual flow, and can normalize the menstrual cycle in women who tend to have delayed menses. It is often recommended in treatments for amenorrhea, anemia, dysmenorrhea, and headache. It is an alterative, anticoagulant, antispasmodic, blood tonic, emmenagogue, muscle relaxant, and nervine. Avoid during pregnancy, except under the guidance of your health care provider. Do not use in cases of diarrhea, heavy menstrual flow, poor digestion, bloating, or in conjunction with blood-thinning medications such as ibuprofen.

False unicorn (*Chamaelirium luteum*). A uterine tonic, the rhizome increases circulation to the pelvic area. Diuretic and phytoestrogenic, it is often recommended for amenorrhea, cystitis, dysmenorrhea, endometriosis, hormone imbalance, infertility, leukorrhea, and uterine prolapse. The bitter taste can cause vomiting. Excessive amounts may cause kidney and stomach irritation, blurred vision, and hot flashes. Do not use without employing birth control during sex unless pregnancy is desired. Discontinue use during pregnancy. False unicorn is endangered in the wild; do not use wildcrafted supplies.

Fennel (*Foeniculum vulgare*). The seed increases menstrual flow and helps dispel liver congestion. It may curb an excessive desire for sweets. It is antispasmodic, diuretic, and phytoestrogenic.

Ginger (*Zingiber officinale*). The root improves circulation and relieves the type of cramps that improve with warmth. It is recommended when menses are delayed and produce scant dark blood. It is also helpful in cases of amenorrhea and nausea. It is an analgesic, anti-inflammatory, and anticoagulant. Avoid large doses in cases of acne and eczema. Discontinue use if heartburn results.

Hops (*Humulus lupulus*). The strobile calms anxiety and relieves cramping and headache. It can improve the temperament of those who have a quarrelsome nature. It is an anodyne, antispasmodic, diuretic, emmenagogue, muscle relaxant, nervine, phytoestrogen, sedative, and soporific. Avoid during pregnancy and in cases of depression. The fresh plant may cause dermatitis in some individuals.

Horsetail (*Equisetum arvense*). The herb helps prevent breakthrough bleeding (bleeding that occurs outside of the menstrual period) and excessive bleeding. It encourages blood coagulation, reduces edema, and relieves cramping. It is an alterative, anti-inflammatory, astringent, diuretic, hemostatic, and nutritive. Use horsetail that has been collected in spring.

Lady's mantle (*Alchemilla xanthochlora*). The herb relieves congestion in the liver and encourages blood coagulation. It is often recommended in treatments for excessive or irregular bleeding and dysmenorrhea. It is an anti-inflammatory, astringent, diuretic, emmenagogue, hemostatic, and tonic. Avoid during pregnancy, except in the final stages, at which point you should seek the guidance of your health care provider.

Licorice (*Glycyrrhiza glabra, G. uralensis*). The root normalizes ovulation and inhibits the production of prostaglandin E2. It is often recommended in treatments for amenorrhea caused by chi deficiency. It can help stabilize and calm the emotions. It is an anti-inflammatory, antispasmodic, chi tonic, and phytoestrogen. Avoid during pregnancy and in cases of edema, high blood pressure, or diabetes. Do not use in combination with digoxin drugs. Excessive use can cause sodium retention and potassium depletion.

Marijuana (*Cannabis sativa, C. indica*). Though cannabis has been used medicinally for thousands of years, it is currently illegal to grow or possess it in some parts of the world. Claims have been made that the herb can help relieve premenstrual anxiety and dysmenorrhea. It is an anti-inflammatory, analgesic, antispasmodic, muscle relaxant, and sedative.

Dry mouth and eyes are common side effects. Certain individuals may experience paranoia, perceptual disorders, and personality deviations. Do not drive while under the influence of marijuana. Excessive use can lower androgen production and, thus, libido. It can also lead to short-term memory loss. Avoid during pregnancy.

Meadowsweet (*Filipendula ulmaria*). The herb can help relieve the pain of cramps. It is analgesic, anti-inflammatory, antispasmodic, astringent, diuretic, progesteronic, and sedative. Avoid if you are allergic to salicylates.

Motherwort (*Leonurus cardiaca*). The herb dilates uterine blood vessels and thus eases pressure that can contribute to cramping. It is often recommended in treatments for amenorrhea, dysmenorrhea, and menses that are scanty when they begin. It is an antispasmodic, astringent, circulatory stimulant, muscle relaxant, emmenagogue, nervine, and vasodilator. Avoid in cases of heavy menstrual bleeding and during pregnancy, except during the final stages, and then only under the supervision of your health care provider.

Mugwort (*Artemisia vulgaris*). The herb is often recommended in treatments for amenorrhea and dysmenorrhea. It is an anti-inflammatory, antispasmodic, bitter tonic, emmenagogue, hemostatic, muscle relaxant, and uterine stimulant. Do not use for more than a month at a time. Avoid in cases of nervous system disorders and during pregnancy, except during labor, and then only under the supervision of your health care provider. Use only 5 drops of tincture or ¼ cup of tea no more than three times daily.

Nettle (*Urtica dioica, U. urens*). Nettle is a good herb to use for almost anything! It can reduce bloating, relieve tenderness in the breasts, prevent anemia, help control excessive menstrual bleeding, and clear stagnation from the liver or kidneys. It is an alterative, astringent, cholagogue, circulatory stimulant, diuretic, hemostatic, nutritive, and thyroid tonic. Contact with the fresh plant will irritate the skin. Use only dried herb. Wear gloves when collecting. Nettle may cause some irritation to the kidneys.

Oregon grape (*Mahonia aquifolium*). The root can relieve edema, clear liver stagnation, and correct menorrhagia. It is an alterative, anti-inflammatory, astringent, cholagogue, diuretic, hepatic, and thyroid stimulant. Avoid during pregnancy, and do not exceed the recommended dosage.

Parsley (*Petroselinum crispum*). The leaf helps regulate menstrual cycles. It can relieve tenderness in the breasts and edema and is often recommended in treatments for amenorrhea, anemia, and dysmenorrhea. It is an antispasmodic, diuretic, emmenagogue, nutritive, and sedative. Avoid therapeutic doses during pregnancy and in cases of kidney inflammation.

Partridgeberry (*Mitchella repens*). The herb is often recommended in treatments for amenorrhea and dysmenorrhea. It is an astringent, diuretic, emmenagogue, nervine, and uterine tonic. Dosages in excess of what is recommended can irritate the mucous membranes. This herb is endangered in the wild; do not use wildcrafted supplies.

Pennyroyal (*Hedeoma pulegioides, Mentha pulegium*). The herb can help counteract amenorrhea that is caused by blood stagnation. It is often recommended in treatments for dysmenorrhea, headache, and nausea. It is an antispasmodic, diuretic, emmenagogue, and uterine vasodilator. Avoid during pregnancy.

Peony (*Paeonia lactiflora*). The root helps bring menses closer together. It is often recommended in treatments for amenorrhea and dysmenorrhea. It is an alterative, anti-inflammatory, antispasmodic, blood tonic, diuretic, emmenagogue, hepatotonic, sedative, uterine astringent, vasodilator, and yin tonic. Avoid during pregnancy and in cases of diarrhea.

Peppermint (*Mentha piperita*). The leaf can relieve cramping, fatigue, headache, migraine, and nausea. It is an analgesic, anodyne, antispasmodic, cholagogue, diuretic, and vasodilator. It is among the safest of herbs, even for people who are very ill, with its only side effect being occasional heartburn.

Red clover (*Trifolium pratense*). The herb and flower build blood and can resolve blood clots. Red clover is alterative, anti-inflammatory, antispasmodic, diuretic, nutritive, and phytoestrogenic.

Red raspberry (*Rubus idaeus*). The leaf contains phytosterols. It strengthens the reproductive system and relaxes smooth muscles in the uterus. It is often recommended in treatments for amenorrhea, anemia, dysmenorrhea, and menorrhagia. It is an alterative, antispasmodic, astringent, hemostatic, hormone regulator, Kidney tonic, nutritive, and uterine tonic.

Rehmannia (*Rehmannia glutinosa*). The root tonifies and detoxifies the blood. It is often recommended in treatments for amenorrhea and menorrhagia. It is an alterative, diuretic, hemostatic, Kidney tonic, and Liver tonic. Avoid in cases of loose stools, poor appetite, bloating, or a coated tongue.

Rose (*Rosa* spp.). Rose hips contain vitamin C and bioflavonoids, which can strengthen capillaries and help relieve cramping. They are often recommended in treatments for menses that come too early and for deficient

Kidney chi. The hip is an astringent, diuretic, and hormone regulator.

Sage (*Salvia officinalis*). The leaf helps control excessive menstrual flow and delay menses that come too early. It can relieve cramping, depression, and migraines. It is an anti-inflammatory, antispasmodic, astringent, emmenagogue, hormone tonic, and phytoestrogen. Avoid therapeutic dosages in cases of vaginal dryness, during pregnancy, and while nursing.

Sarsaparilla (*Smilax* spp.). The root is both phytoprogesteronic and phytoestrogenic. It is often recommended in treatments for leukorrhea and ovarian cysts. It is an alterative, anti-inflammatory, antispasmodic, diuretic, and tonic.

Shepherd's purse (*Capsella bursa-pastoris*). The herb strengthens capillaries and is often used to control excessive menstrual bleeding and spotting between menses. It is an alterative, astringent, diuretic, hemostatic, and vasoconstrictor.

Skullcap (*Scutellaria lateriflora*). The herb helps draw menses further apart. It can also help dispel anger and anxiety. It is often recommended in treatments for dysmenorrhea and headache. It is an alterative, anodyne, anti-inflammatory, antispasmodic, astringent, diuretic, nervine, sedative, and yin tonic. Avoid during pregnancy.

Tribulus (*Tribulus terrestris*). The fruit helps draw menses further apart. It is often recommended in treatments for dysmenorrhea, headache, and leukorrhea. It is an alterative, analgesic, anodyne, antispasmodic, nervine, and tonic for the bones, Liver, and Kidneys.

Trillium (*Trillium* spp.). The root curbs excessive menstrual bleeding and helps relieve dysmenorrhea. It is an alterative, antispasmodic, astringent, emmenagogue, and uterine tonic. Avoid during pregnancy, except under the guidance of your health care provider. This herb is endangered in the wild; do not use wildcrafted supplies.

Uva ursi (*Arctostaphylos uva-ursi*). The leaf reduces blood flow to the pelvic area and can relieve edema. It is an astringent, diuretic, and vasoconstrictor. Avoid during pregnancy.

Vitex (*Vitex agnus-castus*). The berry helps regulate the menstrual cycle by normalizing the function of the pituitary gland. It helps control menses that are excessively profuse and too frequent, and it is often recommended in treatments for amenorrhea, breast tenderness, dysmenorrhea, metrorrhagia, and PMS. It also can dispel headaches and acne caused by menstruation. It is both phytoestrogenic and phytoprogesteronic.

White willow (*Salix alba*). The bark inhibits prostaglandin production, which reduces uterine inflammation. It can relieve headaches, migraines, and dysmenorrhea. It is alterative, analgesic, anodyne, anti-inflammatory, astringent, and phytoestrogenic. Avoid if you are allergic to salicylates.

Wild yam (*Dioscorea opposita, D. villosa*). The root relieves dysmenorrhea, ovarian pain, and glandular imbalances. It is an anti-inflammatory, antispasmodic, cholagogue, diuretic, nutritive, and phytoprogesterone. Avoid therapeutic doses during pregnancy, except under the guidance of your health care provider. The *Dioscorea villosa* species is endangered in the wild; do not use wildcrafted supplies.

Yarrow (*Achillea millefolium*). The herb reduces blood flow to the pelvic area. It is often recommended in treatments for amenorrhea, dysmenorrhea, and menorrhagia. It is an anti-inflammatory, antispasmodic, astringent, cholagogue, diuretic, hemostatic, and sedative.

Yellow dock (*Rumex crispus*). The root improves liver function. It is an alterative, astringent, blood tonic, cholagogue, and diuretic.

HEALING HERBAL TEAS FOR THE MENSTRUAL CYCLE

Warm herbal teas are a soothing balm to the body and the nervous system. Enjoy them 3 to 4 times daily, preferably with your feet up and a few minutes of deep relaxation.

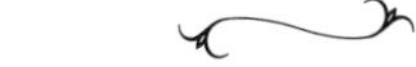

I Got the PMS Blues Tea

When your emotions are down, savor a cup of this sweet, uplifting, aromatic herbal tea.

1 quart water
½ teaspoon burdock root
½ teaspoon dandelion root
1 teaspoon basil herb
1 teaspoon fennel seed
1 teaspoon nettle leaf

Bring the water to a boil. Add the burdock and dandelion root, cover, and simmer for 20 minutes. Remove from heat and add the remaining herbs. Cover and let steep for 10 minutes. Strain. Store in the refrigerator. Drink 1 quart daily.

Cramps Begone Tea

When cramps make every move an effort, slow down and rest awhile. Sip this nourishing, relaxing, mineral-rich brew to calm the spasms.

1 quart water
1 teaspoon dandelion root
½ teaspoon cramp bark
1 teaspoon oatstraw
1 teaspoon chamomile blossom
1 teaspoon red raspberry leaf
1 teaspoon skullcap herb
½ teaspoon gingerroot
Honey (optional)

Bring the water to a boil. Add the dandelion root and cramp bark, cover, and simmer for 20 minutes. Remove from heat and add the remaining herbs. Cover and let steep for 10 minutes. Strain. Add honey to sweeten, if desired. Store in the refrigerator. Drink 1 quart daily.

Normalize the Flow Tea

If your menstrual bleeding is excessive, the blood-building, astringent, tonifying herbs in this formula will soon have you feeling like yourself again.

6 cups water
1 teaspoon vitex berries
1 teaspoon wild yam root
¼ teaspoon licorice root
2 teaspoons alfalfa herb
2 teaspoons nettle herb
2 teaspoons red raspberry leaf

Bring the water to a boil. Add the vitex berries, wild yam, and licorice root. Cover and simmer for 20 minutes. Remove from heat and add the remaining herbs. Cover and let steep for 10 minutes. Strain. Store in the refrigerator. Drink 1 quart daily.

Nutritional Therapy

Although the most effective way to maintain nutrition is by incorporating the foods your body needs into your diet, supplementation can also be helpful. See chapter 3 for good natural sources of the following nutrients.

Vitamin B complex. The B-complex vitamins offer great support to the liver. Vitamin B_6, in particular, can help prevent fluid retention and assist in the metabolism of estrogen. Choline helps prevent the buildup of fat, which can impair liver function. Take 50 mg of vitamin B complex daily.

Vitamin C. Vitamin C with bioflavonoids can help strengthen the capillaries. Bioflavonoids can also control estrogen levels. Take 1,000 mg of vitamin C with 500 mg of bioflavonoids three times daily.

Vitamin E. Vitamin E can help relieve tenderness in the breasts and control prostaglandin levels. Take 400 IU daily.

Magnesium. Magnesium is a natural diuretic; it can also help satisfy cravings for chocolate, relieve tenderness in the breasts, and control weight gain associated with PMS. It's a good idea to take magnesium and calcium together; it is usually recommended that you take half as much magnesium as you do calcium. Look for magnesium in a citrate form; it's easier to assimilate when citric acid is used as a carrier. Take 500 to 750 mg daily. An excess of magnesium may cause diarrhea.

Zinc. Zinc, like vitamin E, can help control prostaglandin levels, an overabundance of which can contribute to dysmenorrhea. Take 25 to 50 mg of chelated zinc daily.

Aromatherapy

Essential oils have a variety of healing applications for menstrual dysfunction, depending on the symptoms that need to be addressed. The oils recommended here can be used in massage, in the bath, and in inhalations. (See chapter 5 for more information on how to use the essential oils discussed below.)

To control emotional upheavals before and during the menses, try jasmine, lavender, and Roman chamomile essential oils.

To bring physical and emotional comfort during the menses, use basil, chamomile, clary sage, fennel, hyssop, juniper berry, lavender, marjoram, myrrh, peppermint, rose, and rosemary essential oils.

To relieve cramping, use anise, carrot seed, clary sage, jasmine, and rose essential oils.

To stimulate menstruation in cases of amenorrhea, try clary sage, fennel, lavender, and rosemary essential oils.

Homeopathic Remedies

When the symptoms of menstrual dysfunction match one of the descriptions below, try the suggested homeopathic remedy. The usual dosage is 4 pellets, or as many liquid drops as the package label recommends, taken under the tongue four times daily. Rather than swallowing the pellets whole, allow them to dissolve slowly.

ACONITUM NAPELLUS. The patient is experiencing amenorrhea or menorrhagia. She is cold, has a frail constitution, and is nervous. She may have an excessive fear of death.

ALETRIS FARINOSA. Menstruation is profuse, early, and filled with large blood clots. The patient feels weak from loss of fluids and has no appetite.

APIS MELLIFICA. The patient skips periods regularly, feels a stinging pain in the vagina, and exhibits cloudy thinking.

BELLADONNA. The patient has amenorrhea, dysmenorrhea with irregular cramping, or menorrhagia with profuse, foul-smelling, bright red blood. Urination and the pelvic area are painful, and the face is flushed. Symptoms are worsened by noise and excitement.

BRYONIA. The patient's breasts are tender for two or more weeks before menses. She has amenorrhea and may have frequent nosebleeds. Motion and rising suddenly worsen symptoms.

CALCAREA CARBONICA. The patient had delayed menarche (first menses), and her head sweats easily. She has a bloated abdomen and sore breasts. She has menorrhagia with copious, bright red blood. Symptoms are initiated by emotional shock.

CARBO VEGETABILIS. The patient has menorrhagia with long, early, copious bleeding.

CAULOPHYLLUM THALICTROIDES. The patient has dysmenorrhea and has suffered from intense cramps since puberty.

CHAMOMILLA. The patient has amenorrhea or cramps that are relieved by heat. She is stressed, impatient, and irritable about everything. One cheek may be red while the other is pale.

CIMICIFUGA RACEMOSA. The patient suffers from depression, cramps, pains that shoot down the hips, and headaches. The menses are profuse.

COCCULUS INDICUS. The patient has dysmenorrhea with nausea. She feels too weak to stand. Dark clots of blood appear in the menstrual flow.

COLOCYNTHIS. Menstruation is painful, but pressure applied to the area of pain brings relief. The patient is irritable.

DULCAMARA. The patient suffers from emotional ups and downs and tender, engorged breasts. She has amenorrhea caused by cold, damp conditions. She may have warts.

FERRUM METALLICUM. Menarche was delayed because of debility. The patient has puffy ankles and poor complexion. She suffers from menorrhagia that is early, profuse, and weakening. The menstrual flow is watery and pale.

HAMAMELIS VIRGINIANA. Menstruation is profuse.

IGNATIA. The menses are delayed because of emotional distress.

KALI CARBONICUM. The patient suffers from exhaustion and feels a pain in her left side. She is overweight and exhibits fear and anxiety. This remedy can also be used for amenorrhea if NATRUM MURIATICUM fails.

LACHESIS. The patient suffers from dysmenorrhea with severe headaches that abate as soon as menstrual flow begins. Wearing tight clothing worsens symptoms. This remedy may also be used for amenorrhea that is caused by fear, if menarche has not happened by eighteen years of age, and for menorrhagia with a heavy, painful flow containing dark blood clots.

LYCOPODIUM. The patient has vaginal dryness, bloating, and pain in the right ovary. She feels weepy, craves sweets, and suffers from premenstrual depression. Headaches may occur in the temples in late afternoon and early evening.

MAGNESIUM PHOSPHATE. The patient has dysmenorrhea. The pain is worse on the right side. Symptoms are worsened by cold and improved by warmth and bending over.

NATRUM MURIATICUM. The patient has PMS or amenorrhea. She craves salt, feels tired and weak, and suffers from bloating and fluid retention. She wants to be alone and cries.

PHOSPHORUS. The patient has metrorrhagia caused by fibroids.

PULSATILLA. The patient feels weepy and gentle. She faints easily. She suffers from migraines, backache, and diarrhea, and her endocrine system is unbalanced. Use this remedy for amenorrhea caused by wetness, dysmenorrhea accompanied by sore breasts, excessively delayed menarche, and menstrual irregularity caused by anger and overwork.

SABINA. The patient has early, long, and heavy periods. The menstrual flow may contain red blood clots, and cramping may be intense. She has menorrhagia; bleeding may occur without stopping until the next menses.

SENECIO AUREUS. The patient has amenorrhea that causes digestive upset.

SEPIA. The patient has amenorrhea; she discharges leukorrhea instead of menstrual flow. She has intense headaches and a delicate constitution. She may suffer from a general feeling that every action requires tremendous effort.

SILICEA. The patient suffers from general weakness. She is underdeveloped and has cold extremities. Her menses are excessively heavy, and her breasts are tender.

SULFUR. The patient has amenorrhea, and all other remedies have failed. She may also suffer from acne, itchy rashes, irritability, and forgetfulness. She may crave sweets and have headaches.

VIBURNUM OPULUS. The patient experiences sudden uterine pain, backache, and late, light menses. Symptoms worsen at night.

XANTHOXYLUM. The patient suffers from dysmenorrhea, with pain felt down the thighs. The menses are early and profuse. Menstrual flow is thick and blackish. Before menstruation, the patient develops a headache over her left eye. She has a nervous, frail constitution.

Flower Essences

Flower essences for women with menstrual difficulties include the following. The usual dosage is 3 drops under the tongue, or taken with a glass of water three or four times daily.

Evening Primrose. This essence helps balance hormone cycles and can be used in treatments for amenorrhea, dysmenorrhea, and metrorrhagia. It helps heal painful emotions picked up from our mothers.

Fairy Lantern. Fairy Lantern can help adolescent girls who are not developing physically or emotionally; the remedy can help them integrate better into the world and develop into responsible adults.

Impatiens. Impatiens can relieve nervous tension, calm emotional outbursts, and ease cramps.

Mugwort. This essence can help clear old, negative emotions and control hysterical, irrational behavior.

Pomegranate. Women who have a difficult time balancing their career and their family will find that this essence encourages creativity and a feeling of nurturing. It's especially helpful when psychological stress is affecting the reproductive system.

Star Tulip. Women who seem to have a protective wall around their emotions will find that Star Tulip helps them tune in to their inner voice and become more sensitive and receptive.

MENOPAUSE

Menopause is defined as the cessation of menstruation—derived from the Greek *men pausis,* meaning "month to end"—that happens as a natural part of a woman's life or as the result of a hysterectomy. It usually begins about forty years after menarche; if it occurs before the age of forty, it is considered premature. Menopause may pass through a woman's life very quickly or may persist for several years. When a woman has not had a period for thirteen months, it is time to celebrate her graduation from menopause and her entrance into the age of wise womanhood.

Of all the mammals, only humans experience menopause. Other mammals are capable of reproducing until they die. Perhaps this is part of the Great Plan, that women can be available to take care of their babies until they are all grown.

Though menopause may bring some discomfort, it is not an illness. It is, instead, a rite of passage. It is by no means the beginning of the end. After menopause, many women experience renewed energy, new creative potential, and self-empowerment. And they continue to live healthy, productive, joyous lives.

During perimenopause—the five to ten years preceding the end of the menses—the ovaries become sluggish and produce inconsistent amounts of hormones, which can cause menstrual cycles to become unpredictable. Anovulation (a menstrual cycle in which a woman fails to ovulate) becomes more common, even though thousands of immature follicles remain in the ovaries. Estrogen and progesterone levels vacillate, although the pituitary gland continues to produce follicle-stimulating hormone (FSH) and luteinizing hormone (LH). During menopause, estrogen levels fall to one-half to one-third of where they were premenopause, and progesterone levels fall to minute levels once ovulation no longer occurs.

Hormonal changes during perimenopause can have opposite menstrual results: very heavy bleeding and very light bleeding. These are early signs of menopause. Heavy bleeding (on par with menorrhagia) can occur when progesterone levels drop but estrogen levels do not. Although more common in African American women, heavy bleeding is not experienced by all women. Eventually estrogen levels drop as well, resulting in light bleeding and missed periods.

Most women experience the gradual cessation of menstruation, unless it occurs abruptly through surgery or other circumstances. Other signs of menopause may include hot flashes, vaginal dryness, and thinning vaginal walls; these are thought to be triggered by sudden drops in estrogen levels.

In the tradition of Oriental medicine, menopausal difficulties are often associated with a blood, Liver, or Kidney deficiency. If blood and yin fluids are imbalanced, night sweats, excessive menstrual bleeding, irritability, dizziness, headaches, and insomnia can occur. The Liver is responsible for breaking down and eliminating excess hormones; if the Liver is exhausted, depression, anger, restless sleep, and hot flashes can occur. The Kidneys govern sexual vitality and mental energy; when the Kidneys are deficient, lower back pain, decreased libido, and incontinence may result.

Menopause can be a good time to clear stored-up negative emotions. Are there people in your life to whom you owe an apology, a letter, flowers, or money? Is there someone you need to confront to clear your mind, such as a parent or an old lover? And if you've ever thought about recording your life and all the history of your family that you can remember, now is a good time to get started, while you're entering the introspective years of wise womanhood.

Enjoy this time of change and growth!

One of my favorite books about menopause is New Menopausal Years, The Wise Woman Way: Alternative Approaches for Women 30–90, *by Susun S. Weed (Ash Tree Publishing, 2001). If you're interested in learning more about menopause from a self-help, natural-healing standpoint, I wholeheartedly recommend this book as an excellent resource.*

Hot Flashes

Researchers have yet to pinpoint why menopausal women experience hot flashes, although they believe them to be linked to sudden drops in estrogen levels and elevated levels of FSH and LH. Hot flashes are characterized by a sudden feeling of intense warmth, often accompanied by heart palpitations, anxiety, faintness, flushing, headache, and sweating. On average, hot flashes last about three minutes, but they can persist for up to an hour.

When you're experiencing a hot flash, there's not much you can do but ride it out. If you're having hot flashes regularly, get prepared. Set a fan near your desk or wherever you spend most of your time. Drink plenty of cool beverages. Wear light clothing in layers so that you can strip down if you need to. Avoid hot and spicy foods, sugar, alcohol, and caffeine as they can all contribute to hot flashes. Deep slow breathing can help calm and cool a hot flash. Prepare an aromatic spritzer by mixing 8 ounces of water and 20 drops of peppermint essential oil; when you experience a hot flash, spritz this cooling mixture onto your face and neck (keep eyes and mouth closed). Furthermore, express your feelings. Bottled-up emotions can cause you to heat up and blow your top!

Hydrotherapy can also help with hot flashes. Fill a tub with cold water to a depth of six inches. Walk barefoot in the tub, pacing back and forth for about three minutes. Then dry your feet, put on shoes, and go for a short walk. You'll quickly feel cooled and energized.

Natural Therapies for Healthy Menopause

Natural therapies for encouraging health and minimizing discomfort during menopause focus on building blood, supporting the liver and kidneys, promoting vaginal elasticity, strengthening the bones, and normalizing estrogenic activity.

DIET

During menopause, eat plenty of foods that build blood and strengthen the liver, such as tart apples, beets, beet greens, black beans, black sesame seeds, fish, goji berries, green leafy vegetables, jujube dates, millet, mulberries, mung beans, pomegranates, string beans, walnuts, and yams. Also incorporate seaweeds into your diet; they're rich in minerals and help promote elasticity of the vaginal tissues.

Soy is rich in calcium, which helps build the bones, and isoflavone antioxidants, which can reduce hot flashes. However, soy can be difficult to digest for many people and is a common allergen. The best forms of soy are unpasteurized miso and tamari, which are fermented and easy to digest.

Dairy products are often touted for their calcium content. Because of the pasteurization process, we don't assimilate the calcium from milk and are better off getting it from the same place as the cows—greens. Eat plenty of green leafy vegetables, sesame seeds, tahini, and broccoli. Of all the dairy products, yogurt with probiotics is the most redeeming.

Minimize your intake of alcohol, sugar, caffeine, carbonated beverages, fried foods, and high-fat foods. When eaten in large quantities, they can worsen hot flashes.

EXERCISE

Weight-bearing exercise such as walking, jumping rope, dancing, or light weight lifting can help build bones, increase muscle mass, and control the tendency to gain weight. Be sure to stretch both before and after exercising to encourage flexibility along with strength.

To keep the reproductive organs in good tone, practice Kegel exercises daily. (See page 118 for instructions.)

HERBAL THERAPY

For best effect, an herbal protocol should be continued for at least three menstrual cycles. Some herbs may become your partners in health for years.

Alfalfa (*Medicago sativa*). The herb helps build blood and normalize estrogen levels. It is a diuretic, nutritive, phytoestrogen, and tonic. Avoid in cases of heavy menstrual bleeding.

Angelica (*Angelica archangelica, A. atropurpurea*). The root relieves muscle spasms and tension headaches. It has a gladdening effect on the emotional state. It is a diuretic, emmenagogue, nervine, phytoestrogen, and uterine stimulant. Avoid during pregnancy and in cases of heavy bleeding or diabetes. In rare cases, the root causes photosensitivity.

Asparagus (*Asparagus officinalis, A. cochinchinensis*). The root is particularly helpful for women who have had hysterectomies, because it helps relieve vaginal dryness. It also can improve libido and reduce irritability. It is an aphrodisiac, cardiotonic, demulcent, diuretic, nutritive, and Kidney tonic.

Black cohosh (*Actaea racemosa*). The root can soothe irritation of the cervix, uterus, and vagina; calm hysteria; and reduce FSH levels. It is often recommended in treatments for edema, hot flashes, and headaches. It is an antispasmodic, cardiotonic, emmenagogue, smooth muscle relaxant, phytoestrogen, and sedative. Avoid during pregnancy, except in the final stages, and then only under the guidance of your health care provider. Avoid while nursing and in cases of high blood pressure or pressure in the inner eye. Consult with your health care provider before use. This herb is endangered in the wild; do not use wildcrafted supplies.

Black haw (*Viburnum prunifolium*). The bark is a tonic and sedative for the reproductive organs and nervous system. It also can reduce heart palpitations. It is an antispasmodic, hypotensive, and sedative.

Blessed thistle (*Cnicus benedictus*). The herb strengthens the liver and reproductive organs. It is a bitter, meaning that it stimulates natural digestive secretions, and it is often recommended for menopausal women who have difficulty with digestion. It is an antidepressant, bitter tonic, and cholagogue.

Blue cohosh (*Caulophyllum thalictroides*). The root promotes estrogenic activity and can tonify a weak uterus. It is an anti-inflammatory, antispasmodic, diuretic, emmenagogue, and uterine tonic. Avoid during pregnancy, except in the final stages, and then only under the guidance of your health care provider. Make sure the root is dried, not fresh. This herb is endangered in the wild; do not use wildcrafted supplies.

Bupleurum (*Bupleurum chinense, B. falcatum*). The root supports liver function and promotes blood circulation. It can help dispel anger, grief, moodiness, and fatigue. It is an alterative, anti-inflammatory, chi tonic, choleretic, hepatic, muscle relaxant, and tonic. Avoid in cases of fever, headache, or high blood pressure.

Burdock (*Arctium lappa*). The root helps improve liver function, cleanse the kidneys, and relieve lymphatic congestion. It also tonifies the uterus. It can cool hot flashes and clear anger from the body. It is an alterative, aphrodisiac, diuretic, nutritive, phytoestrogen, and rejuvenative.

Chickweed (*Stellaria media*). The herb cools hot flashes and can help relieve vaginal dryness. It is an alterative, anti-inflammatory, demulcent, nutritive, and refrigerant.

Cramp bark (*Viburnum opulus*). The herb can calm heart palpitations. It is an anti-inflammatory, antispasmodic, cardiotonic, diuretic, nervine, sedative, uterine sedative, and tonic.

Dandelion (*Taraxacum officinale*). The root improves liver function;

the leaf improves kidney function. The leaf is also rich in potassium. The root and leaves are cholagogues, diuretics, and hypotensives.

Dong quai (*Angelica sinensis*). The root helps build blood and clear blood stagnation. It can relieve anxiety, depression, and hot flashes and help restore moisture to dry vaginal tissues. It is an alterative, anticoagulant, emmenagogue, and uterine tonic. Avoid during pregnancy, except under the guidance of your health care provider. Do not use in cases of diarrhea, heavy menstrual flow, poor digestion, or bloating. Do not use in conjunction with blood-thinning medications such as ibuprofen.

Elder (*Sambucus nigra, S. canadensis*). The flower helps the body regulate its temperature, discouraging hot flashes. The berry has a restorative effect for women who have had heavy menstrual bleeding. The flower and berry are alteratives, antispasmodics, and diuretics.

Eleuthero (*Eleutherococcus senticosus*). The root and root bark can cool hot flashes. It is often recommended in treatments for depression, high cholesterol, hypertension, infertility, and insomnia. As an adaptogen, it protects health during times of stress. It is also an anti-inflammatory, antispasmodic, aphrodisiac, cardiotonic, and chi tonic.

False unicorn (*Chamaelirium luteum*). The rhizome is a tonic for the reproductive organs and helps normalizes ovarian function. It is often recommended in treatments for hormonal imbalance. It is a diuretic and phytoestrogen. The bitter taste of this herb can cause vomiting. Excessive amounts may cause kidney and stomach irritation, blurred vision, and hot flashes. Do not use without employing birth control during sex unless pregnancy is desired. Discontinue use during pregnancy. False unicorn is endangered in the wild; do not use wildcrafted supplies.

Fennel (*Foeniculum vulgare*). The seed clears congestion from the liver and is a natural appetite suppressant. It has mild phytoestrogenic effect and is also antispasmodic and diuretic.

Fenugreek (*Trigonella foenum-graecum*). The seed boosts Kidney chi and contains phytosterols. It is an alterative, anti-inflammatory, aphrodisiac, demulcent, nutritive, rejuvenative, and restorative. Avoid during pregnancy. If you have diabetes, consult with your health care provider before use.

Ginger (*Zingiber officinale*). The root reduces the risk of stroke, invigorates the reproductive system, can inhibit blood clots, and lowers blood pressure. It is often recommended in treatments for amenorrhea, dysmenorrhea, and hypertension. It is an antioxidant, anticoagulant, and circulatory stimulant. Avoid large doses in cases of acne and eczema. Discontinue use if heartburn results.

Ginseng, American (*Panax quinquefolius*). The root can relieve both vaginal dryness and hot flashes. It is often recommended in treatments for adrenal deficiency and menorrhagia. It is an adaptogen, aphrodisiac, chi tonic, digestive tonic, rejuvenative, and restorative. Since ginseng can be energizing, avoid taking it within four hours of bedtime. Avoid during pregnancy. American ginseng is at risk of becoming endangered in the wild; use only cultivated—never wildcrafted—supplies.

Hawthorn (*Crataegus* spp.). The leaf, flower, and berry lower blood pressure and can relieve heart palpitations and insomnia. Hawthorn is high in flavonoids and functions as a cardiotonic, diuretic, hypotensive, and vasodilator. The flowers can also help cool hot flashes.

Ho shou wu (*Polygonum multiflorum*). The root tonifies the blood, liver, and kidneys and can help strengthen bones and muscles. It also calms the nerves. It is an alterative, antispasmodic, aphrodisiac, chi tonic, and rejuvenative.

Hops (*Humulus lupulus*). The strobiles can relieve heart palpitations, induce sleep, and calm feelings of anxiety, hysteria, and restlessness. Hops is an antispasmodic, phytoestrogen, emmenagogue, muscle relaxant, nervine, and soporific. Avoid during pregnancy and in cases of depression. The fresh plant may cause dermatitis in some individuals.

Horsetail (*Equisetum arvense*). The herb is a muscular and skeletal tonic that can help reverse bone loss. It is often recommended in treatments for menorrhagia. It is an alterative, anti-inflammatory, diuretic, hemostatic, and nutritive. Use horsetail that has been collected in spring.

Lady's mantle (*Alchemilla xanthochlora*). The herb promotes blood coagulation and tissue healing. It is often recommended in treatments for menorrhagia and for hot flashes that are accompanied by an itchy feeling. It also helps clear congestion from the liver. It is an anti-inflammatory, diuretic, emmenagogue, tonic, phytoprogesterone, and vulnerary.

Licorice (*Glycyrrhiza glabra, G. uralensis*). The root is phytoestrogenic and can improve adrenal function. It can be helpful after a hysterectomy. It is an adrenal tonic, anti-inflammatory, chi tonic, demulcent, nutritive, and rejuvenative. Avoid during pregnancy and in cases of edema, high blood pressure, or diabetes. Do not use in combination with digoxin drugs. Excessive use can cause sodium retention and potassium depletion.

Linden (*Tilea europaea, T. americana*). The leaf and flower cool hot flashes, calm anxiety, and relieve headache, insomnia, and stress. Linden is antispasmodic, choleretic, diuretic, hypotensive, nervine, sedative, and tonic.

Motherwort (*Leonurus cardiaca*). The herb cools and reduces the frequency of hot flashes and night sweats. It can relieve uterine pain associated with stress, cramps, feelings of emotional upheaval, and heart palpitations. It also clears stagnation from the blood and nourishes the mucous membranes of the vaginal walls. It is a heart and uterine tonic. Avoid in cases of heavy menstrual bleeding and during pregnancy, except during the final stages, and then only under the supervision of your health care provider.

Nettle (*Urtica dioica, U. urens*). The leaf is a muscular and skeletal tonic. It strengthens the kidneys and adrenals and can be used to clear chi stagnation from the liver and kidneys. It boosts the body's metabolism of fat and helps build blood. It can curb excessive menstrual bleeding. It is an astringent, circulatory stimulant, diuretic, nervine, nutritive, and thyroid tonic. Contact with the fresh plant will irritate the skin. Use only dried herb. Wear gloves when collecting.

Oat (*Avena sativa, A. fatua*). The spikelets and herb reduce the severity and frequency of night sweats and improve vaginal moisture. They nourish the nervous system and help strengthen the bones. They also strengthen the adrenals. Oat is an antidepressant, aphrodisiac, and a cerebral, endocrine, nutritive, rejuvenative, and uterine tonic.

Peony (*Paeonia lactiflora*). The root clears stagnation from the blood. It is often recommended in treatments for irregular menses, cramps, and emotional upheaval. It improves liver function and encourages elasticity of skin. It is a diuretic, emmenagogue, rejuvenative, sedative, and yin tonic. Avoid during pregnancy and in cases of diarrhea.

Poria (*Poria cocos*). The fungus is calming to the spirit and quieting to the heart. It is often recommended in treatments for anxiety, edema, headache, insomnia, or tachycardia. It is an antitumor, cardiotonic, chi tonic, diuretic, restorative, sedative, and tonic.

Red clover (*Trifolium pratense*). The herb is an excellent tonic for general health. It is alterative, antispasmodic, antitumor, diuretic, nutritive, phytoestrogenic, and vulnerary.

Red raspberry (*Rubus idaeus*). The leaf helps regulate the menses and cool hot flashes. It can relax smooth muscles in the uterus and is often recommended in treatments for anemia, cramps, heavy bleeding, and spotting. It is an astringent, adrenal tonic, Kidney tonic, nutritive, and uterine tonic.

Rose (*Rosa* spp.). Rose hips are rich in flavonoids and can strengthen the nails and hair. Rose is an antispasmodic, aphrodisiac, blood tonic, cholagogue, Kidney tonic, nutritive, and phytoestrogen.

Sage (*Salvia officinalis*). The leaf helps restore emotional balance and can relieve anxiety, hot flashes, migraines, and night sweats. It is an anaphrodisiac, antioxidant, antispasmodic, cerebral tonic, choleretic, nutritive, phytoestrogen, and rejuvenative. Avoid therapeutic dosages in cases of vaginal dryness, during pregnancy, and while nursing.

Sarsaparilla (*Smilax* spp.). The root has a mildly stimulating effect on endocrine activity. It also purifies the genitourinary tract and tonifies the reproductive organs. It is often recommended in treatments for hot flashes and after a hysterectomy. It is diuretic and nutritive.

Saw palmetto (*Serenoa repens*). The berry prevents atrophy of the reproductive organs. Use after a hysterectomy to help normalize the function of the remaining sexual organs. It is a mild aphrodisiac, diuretic, nutritive, rejuvenative, tonic, and urinary antiseptic.

Shepherd's purse (*Capsella bursa-pastoris*). The herb can control menstrual hemorrhage, minimize mid-cycle bleeding, and reduce varicose veins. It is an alterative, anti-inflammatory, astringent, hemostatic, hypotensive, urinary antiseptic, and vasoconstrictor.

Suma (*Pfaffia paniculata*). The root relieves fatigue and stress. It is often recommended in treatments for anemia. It is an adaptogen, aphrodisiac, chi tonic, demulcent, and nutritive.

Violet (*Viola odorata*). The leaf cools hot flashes and anger. It is an alterative, demulcent, diuretic, and nutritive.

Vitex (*Vitex agnus-castus*). The berry improves the activity of the corpus luteum. It encourages normalization of hormone levels and libido. It is often recommended in treatments for cysts, fibroids, depression, dysmenorrhea, hot flashes, menorrhagia, metrorrhagia, and vaginal dryness. It is phytoprogesteronic.

Wild yam (*Dioscorea opposita, D. villosa*). The rhizome clears chi congestion and can relieve dysmenorrhea. It is an anti-inflammatory, antispasmodic, aphrodisiac, cholagogue, diuretic, Kidney tonic, nutritive, and phytoprogesterone. Avoid therapeutic doses during pregnancy, except under the guidance of your health care provider. The *Dioscorea villosa* species is endangered in the wild; do not use wildcrafted supplies.

Witch hazel (*Hamamelis virginiana*). The bark and leaf contain flavonoids that help heal damaged blood vessels. Witch hazel is often recommended in treatments for dysmenorrhea, leukorrhea, menorrhagia, organ prolapse, and varicose veins. It is anti-inflammatory, astringent, hemostatic, sedative, and tonic.

Yarrow (*Achillea millefolium*). The herb can reduce excessive bleeding during menstruation. However, because it is a diaphoretic, it may intensify hot flashes and night sweats. It is also an anti-inflammatory, antispasmodic, bitter, cholagogue, circulatory stimulant, febrifuge, hemostatic, hypotensive, phytoprogesterone, and urinary antiseptic.

CHANGE-OF-LIFE TEAS

Herbal teas provide an easy, great-tasting way to balance the body and mind during menopause.

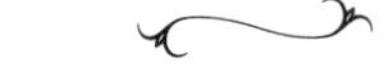

Hot Flash Stash Tea

These heat-relieving herbs will help your body keep its cool.

- 1 quart water
- 1 teaspoon dandelion root
- ½ teaspoon motherwort herb
- 1 teaspoon elder flower
- 1 teaspoon red raspberry leaf
- 1 teaspoon violet leaf
- Honey (optional)

Bring the water to a boil. Add the dandelion root, cover, and simmer for 20 minutes. Remove from heat and add the remaining herbs. Cover and let steep for 10 minutes. Strain. Sweeten with honey, if desired. Store in the refrigerator. Drink 1 quart daily.

Hormone-Balancing Tea

Instead of taking synthetic or animal-derived hormones to help your body through changing times, use the plant hormones (phytosterols) that Mother Nature provides so richly in her wild garden.

1 quart water
½ teaspoon vitex berries
½ teaspoon wild yam root
½ teaspoon dong quai root
½ teaspoon licorice root
1 teaspoon red clover blossoms
1 teaspoon alfalfa leaf

Bring the water to a boil. Add the vitex, wild yam, dong quai, and licorice. Cover and simmer for 20 minutes. Remove from heat and add the remaining herbs. Cover and let steep 10 minutes. Strain. Store in the refrigerator. Drink 1 quart daily.

Bone Health Tea

The health of our bones is bolstered by many practices, including weight-bearing exercises, eating calcium-rich foods, having strong kidneys, and avoiding mineral-depleting foods like sugar. The mineral-rich herbs in this formula, taken now, will yield healthy bones later.

1 quart water
1 teaspoon oatstraw
1 teaspoon horsetail herb
3 tablespoons nettle leaf
1 teaspoon alfalfa leaf
1 teaspoon red raspberry leaf
Honey (optional)

Bring the water to a boil. Remove from heat, stir in the herbs, cover, and let steep 10 minutes. Strain. Sweeten with honey, if desired. Store in the refrigerator. Drink 1 quart daily.

NUTRITIONAL THERAPY

Although women should be able to derive the nutrition they need from their daily diet, there are cases in which certain nutritional supplements can help ease a woman through "the change."

Vitamin A. If you suffer from vaginal dryness, consider supplementing with vitamin A, which nourishes the body's mucous membranes. Look for beta-carotene, which is the precursor to vitamin A; an overload of vitamin A can be toxic to the body, whereas an overload of beta-carotene is simply flushed out with other waste products. Take 10,000 IU of beta-carotene daily.

Vitamin B complex. Hot flashes increase a woman's need for B vitamins, which are lost in perspiration. The B-complex vitamins can also improve energy levels and reduce nervousness. Take 50 mg daily.

Vitamin C. Vitamin C clears heat, nourishes the adrenal glands, and supports collagen activity so that the skin remains elastic and supple. Look for a vitamin C supplement that also includes bioflavonoids, which have a chemical activity similar to that of estrogen. They can reduce excessive bleeding during menstruation, normalize menstrual cycles, relieve hot flashes, and increase vaginal lubrication. Take 1,000 mg of vitamin C with 500 mg of bioflavonoids.

Calcium and magnesium. These two nutrients are often bundled together into a single supplement. They work together to strengthen the bones, calm the emotions, and promote good sleep. If you're having trouble sleeping or if you have a family history of osteoporosis, I highly recommend that you consider this supplement. Take 1,000 mg of calcium and 500 mg of magnesium daily.

Vitamin E. Vitamin E can reduce hot flashes, restore emotional balance, and prevent vaginal dryness. Take 400 to 800 IU daily.

Iron. If menstrual bleeding is excessive, an iron supplement can help prevent anemia. Take 18 mg daily. Use only if needed.

DIM (Diinodolylmethane) and indole-3-carbinol made from crucifereous vegetables, especially broccoli, helps clear undesirable estrogens out of the body and can help relieve hot flashes.

Evening primrose oil. Evening primrose oil is rich in essential fatty acids. It can stimulate the production of estrogen and reduce excessive menstrual bleeding as well as hot flashes. If you can find evening primrose capsules, follow the dosage guidelines given on the package label.

Flaxseed oil. If your skin starts to become very dry during or after menopause, flaxseed can help. Take 3 tablespoons of freshly ground flaxseed daily. Chia seeds are also helpful.

CHINESE PATENT FORMULAS

There are several Chinese patent formulas that can be used to relieve discomfort and promote good health during menopause. Follow the dosage recommendations given on the package label.

BA WEI DI HUANG WAN. This is the famous EIGHT-FLAVOR REHMANNIA PILLS. It is particularly helpful for women who have deficient kidney yin that causes heat symptoms. It relieves nervous energy, night sweats, hot flashes, hot hands and feet, and insomnia and helps regulate hormone function and blood pressure.

DA BU YIN WAN. Also known as BIG TONIFY YIN PILLS, this formula helps relieve the heat effects of menopause, such as night sweats, hot flashes, and migraines.

ER XIAN TANG. Women who suffer from Kidney yin deficiency, hot flashes, night sweats, hot hands and feet, irritability, fatigue, depression, frequent urination, a burning sensation over the Kidneys, and insomnia will find relief with this formula.

GUI PI TANG. This formula, also known as RESTORE THE SPLEEN DECOCTION, can remedy excessive bleeding during the early stages of menopause. It also soothes the nerves.

TIAN WAN BU XIN WAN. Also known as CELESTIAL EMPEROR TONIFY HEART POWDER, this formula is helpful for calming emotional disturbances and relieving insomnia.

ZHI BAI DI HUANG WAN (OR ZHI BAI BA WEI WAN). This formula nourishes yin, tonifies the Kidneys, and can help prevent hot flashes, headaches, and irritability.

ZUO GUI WAN. This formula can benefit postmenopausal women who suffer from weak Kidneys, lack of libido, coldness, and lack of energy. It is also known as GATHERING/RETURNING TO THE LEFT PILLS.

HOMEOPATHIC REMEDIES

When the signs of menopause match one of the descriptions below, try the suggested homeopathic remedy. The usual dosage is 4 pellets, or as many liquid drops as the package label recommends, taken under the tongue four times daily. Rather than swallowing the pellets whole, allow them to dissolve slowly.

APIS MELLIFICA. The menses are suppressed, although the patient may feel as though they are about to begin. The patient feels apathetic and indifferent; she is fidgety, intolerant of heat and touch, and difficult to please. She may cry or scream suddenly. She suffers from edema and vaginal dryness.

BELLADONNA. Hot flashes suddenly come and go and are felt most on the face. The woman experiences intense flushing in which heat is given off by the skin. She exhibits red skin, profuse sweating, agitation, and restlessness and suffers from headache or pressure. Her menstrual flow contains bright red blood clots. Her vagina may be dry and too sensitive to touch.

BRYONIA. The vagina is dry and its walls are thinning. Stools are dry. The patient suffers from headache and irritability.

CALCAREA CARBONICA. The patient experiences hot flashes that cause her head to sweat. She feels cold easily, is pale, and tends toward flabbiness.

CANTHARIS. The vagina is raw and irritated and feels as though it is burning.

CINCHONA OFFICINALIS. The menses are profuse and painful. The patient is weepy, despondent, and sleepless. After menstruation, she is exhausted. Her skin is sensitive to touch. She may feel cold but perspire profusely. Warmth relieves the symptoms.

CROCUS SATIVUS. Menstrual flow is excessive and filled with blood clots, but it does not cause pain.

FERRUM METALLICUM. The patient experiences sudden hot flashes. She is in good health but tires easily.

GRAPHITES. The patient experiences facial flushing. She tends to gain weight and has nosebleeds.

IGNATIA. The patient is cultured or refined and also hypersensitive. She feels grief with anger; feeling angry gives her a headache. Her emotions are conflicting, and she bottles them up inside until she explodes. She sighs frequently. She may feel a lump in her throat.

IPECACUANHA. Menstrual flow is bright red. The patient suffers from continuous cramping, weakness, and occasional vomiting.

KALI CARBONICUM. Hot flashes are accompanied by backache and a feeling of weakness in the legs.

LECHERIES. The patient experiences daytime sweating and flushing. Hot flashes are often worse after going to bed and are accompanied by heart palpitations and headache. The patient is often filled with feelings of irritability, melancholy, gloom, hatred, jealousy, and resentment. She is hypersensitive and suffers from headaches, especially on the top of the head. She may speak rapidly and change subjects frequently. The symptoms are aggravated by heat and improved by cold.

LYCOPODIUM. The skin and vaginal membranes are very dry. The patient has poor self-esteem.

NATRUM MURIATICUM. The patient is emotionally vulnerable but doesn't express her feelings. She is teary, depressed, and exhausted. She has been disappointed by love and tends to hold on to resentments. She suffers from excessive menstrual flow, headache, and constipation. The vagina may be dry, painful, and irritated. This remedy is also useful for women whose menses have stopped after emotional trauma.

NUX VOMICA. The patient experiences hot flashes, night sweats, insomnia, and leg cramps. She is irritable and tends to find fault in others. She is also hypersensitive to noise and light.

PULSATILLA. The patient is moody but not aggressive. She craves approval, affection, and sympathy and fears rejection. Her moods are changeable. She becomes weepy when describing her symptoms. She experiences irregular menses and hot flashes, which may be followed by chills. This remedy is often most helpful for fair women with blue eyes and a gentle nature.

SABINA. The patient experiences intense cramps, weakness, and excessive menstrual flow that contains blood clots.

SANGUINARIA CANADENSIS. The patient's cheeks are red and burning. Her hands and feet are hot.

SECALE CORNUTUM. Menstrual flow is excessive but does not contain any blood clots. The patient suffers from severe cramping.

SEPIA. The patient experiences sudden flushes with sweating that leave her exhausted and weak. She experiences feelings of anger, gloom, depression, exhaustion, and irritability. She may be weepy and fidgety, except when talking about herself. She has a heavy feeling in her pelvis, lower back pain, and constipation. Menses are frequent, heavy, and painful. This remedy is often most helpful for women with a sallow complexion who enjoy dance and exercise.

SULFUR. The patient experiences hot flashes over her entire body, including her feet. She has a red face and flushes easily; her perspiration may have an offensive odor. The hot flashes are worse in the evening and after exertion. She is thirsty after night sweats. She may be forgetful, selfish, and untidy and reluctant to work. She may suffer from itchy dermatitis, coarseness of the skin, vaginal itching, and diarrhea. Menstrual flow is heavy, and the patient experiences weight loss and a craving for sweets.

VALERIANA. The patient suffers from facial flushing, sweating, and an inability to sleep.

FLOWER ESSENCES

Flower essences can also help a woman through the challenges of menopause. The usual dosage is 3 drops under the tongue, or taken with a glass of water, three or four times daily.

Alpine Lily. This essence helps restore a sense of self in women who feel disconnected from their femininity. Black cohosh root, used as tea, a tincture, or in capsules, is a good complement to this flower essence; it can help open blocked areas in the pelvis and release emotions relating to anger and violence.

Borage. Borage helps gladden the heart and can relieve feelings of despair and depression.

California Wild Rose. This essence can help invigorate and inspire those who feel exhausted and tend to focus on the past rather than the future.

Crab Apple. Crab Apple helps clear feelings of being polluted.

Fairy Lantern. Women who are obsessed with trying to look younger and are resisting menopause will find that this essence eases their emotional passage into wise womanhood.

Fuschia. Fuschia is often recommended in treatments for grief, sorrow, and sexual feelings that cause tension. It can help a woman comprehend repressed memories.

Hibiscus. This essence clears sexual blockages. It can be helpful for those who have lost sexual desire and feel emotionally dry. It is often recommended for women who have suffered sexual trauma.

Mallow. Mallow can relieve fears of aging.

Mimulus. Mimulus can relieve fears of a known origin and oversensitivity to crowds and noise.

Oak. Oak provides strength to those who need it to complete their mission in life.

Pomegranate. Pomegranate helps women channel procreative energy into new realms of creativity. It can clear emotional blockages in the realms of feminine creativity, career, and home life. It can relieve mental stress that leads to sexual dysfunction.

Scarlet Monkeyflower. This essence can help a woman understand the message of hot flashes.

Scleranthus. Scleranthus relieves mood swings and restlessness.

Walnut. Walnut is helpful for the woman who needs stability and has to let go of things that no longer serve her purpose.

Willow. Willow can relieve feelings of bitterness, resentment, and self-pity. It can encourage a woman to make a fresh start in life.

AROMATHERAPY

Essential oils have a variety of supportive, healing applications for menopause, depending on the particular side effects a woman is experiencing. The oils recommended can be used in massage, in the bath, in inhalations, and as spritzers. (See chapter 5 for more information on aromatherapy.) However, to avoid triggering a hot flash, take only cool baths, not hot ones.

To stimulate estrogenic activity and ease passage through menopause, use the essential oils of clary sage, sage, anise, fennel, angelica, coriander, cypress, and niaouli.

To relieve or prevent hot flashes, use the essential oils of basil, geranium, grapefruit, and thyme.

To counteract vaginal dryness and thinning vaginal walls, use the essential oils of clary sage and cypress. Clary sage can also help regulate the menses and lift depressed spirits.

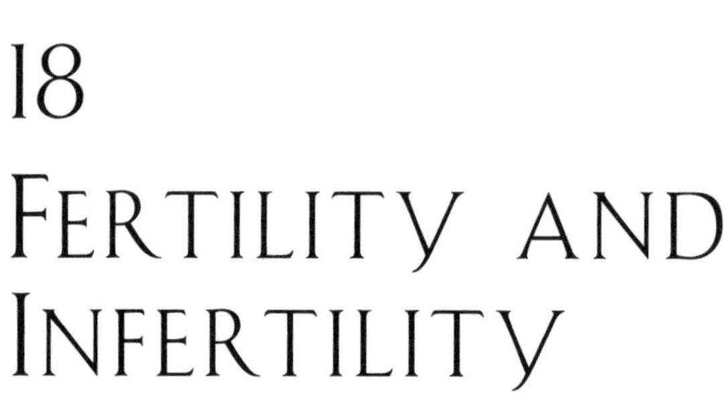

18 Fertility and Infertility

FERTILITY IS, IN ESSENCE, the ability to create and maintain a viable fetus. Although the human body is designed to procreate, conceiving a child is not as easy as it sounds. As we were all taught in our younger years, fertilization takes place only when a female egg (the ovum) fuses with a male sperm cell. The fertilized egg then finds its way into the uterus, where it is nurtured for approximately nine months, until birth. But there are a lot of very complicated processes that have to transpire correctly to set the stage for the meeting of ovum and sperm. And there are plenty of things that can knock the rendezvous off course.

Among the many reasons why a couple might have difficulty conceiving are the esoteric, which are no less powerful for being intangible. Consider this: The attempt to conceive a child is an invitation to a being, a soul, to come spend its life with you. If you were a child, is your house a place you would choose to live? If you spend all your time in front of the television, if you argue constantly with your spouse, if you have no regard for the health and beauty of the world, then the answer is probably no. Ask the being that you are trying to attract, "What qualities are you looking for in parents and a home?" Then be still. Listen. Create that reality.

WHY CAN'T WE CONCEIVE?

True infertility (or sterility, as it is technically defined for men) is an uncommon, though not rare, condition in which it is physically impossible to conceive a child. Most cases of what we call "infertility" are, instead, situations in which a person or couple is having difficulty conceiving. There's a rather large difference between the two. Fertility can be nurtured, after all, in numerous ways, ranging from pharmaceutical medications to surgery to (and preferably) natural therapies. If you're not infertile but just having trouble conceiving, you will, in most cases, be able to overcome the challenges presented to you and eventually achieve a full-term pregnancy.

For some people, fertility dysfunctions are biological in nature. Sometimes, but not always, it is possible to resolve them. Other people are living with, intentionally or unintentionally, environmental factors that interfere with their ability to conceive. In most cases, these detrimental factors can be eliminated and will not have lasting effects.

Biological Dysfunctions

The many biological dysfunctions that could interfere with fertility are too numerous to count, much less describe in this overview. Some of these problems are present from birth; they may even be insignificant enough, generally speaking, that the dysfunction is not noticed until the time comes when procreation is desired. Other problems result from damage to any of a number of reproduction-linked systems and organs.

Here we will focus on those biological dysfunctions that are most common and that can possibly be overcome or reversed.

ANTIBODIES

A woman can develop antibodies that act against a man's sperm; equally, a man can develop antibodies to his own sperm. If a woman is producing antibodies to a man's sperm, the man should wear a condom. When the woman is ovulating, discontinue use of the condom.

BLOCKAGES

Complete or partial blockage anywhere in the reproductive system can contribute to difficulty in conceiving. Blockages may be due to structural malformations, scarring, fibroids, endometriosis, blocked arteries, or even excess mucus. With proper diagnosis, many blockages can be cleared through the use of natural therapies or surgery.

HORMONE IMBALANCES

Hormones are like spark plugs, providing stimulus to drive both body and mind. Proper hormone function plays a major role in the reproductive cycle. If the endocrine (hormone-producing) system is not operating properly, ova may release sporadically or not at all, sperm count may be diminished, libido may disappear, and so on. In most cases, hormone production can be normalized through the use of natural therapies or pharmaceutical medications. (For more information, see appendix 1, "The Chemistry of Love," on page 460.)

HOSTILE CERVICAL MUCUS

If vaginal mucus is too acidic or too alkaline, it can be destructive to sperm. The pH of the vagina can largely be controlled through diet. Cutting back on sugars and carbohydrates can help.

> *Peak fertility in women arrives in their early twenties and begins to diminish thereafter, most rapidly from the mid-thirties. One in four women over the age of thirty will have some difficulty in conceiving. Men's fertility drops radically during their mid-forties.*

MENSTRUAL IRREGULARITY

Metrorrhagia (irregular menses) or amenorrhea (lack of menses) are symptoms of an imbalanced reproductive system. They also make it difficult to predict when or if ovulation is occurring.

Chapter 17 describes natural therapies that can help normalize menses.

THYROID DYSFUNCTION

The thyroid is an endocrine gland that secretes a number of hormones, including thyroxin, without which ovulation cannot occur. A healthy thyroid gland is essential for egg development and sperm production. Low thyroid function can contribute to lethargy and reduced testosterone levels. To support the health of the thyroid, add plenty of sea vegetables to your diet, and drink pure water instead of fluoridated tap water.

WEIGHT PROBLEMS

For women, being extremely overweight or underweight can inhibit ovulation. (Not much is known about the effects of weight on reproduction for men.) When weight levels normalize, menstrual cycles and ovulation often become more regular. Obesity, in particular, is linked to elevated levels of estrogen, which can interfere with menstruation. However, some body fat—between 17 and 21 percent—is necessary for hormone production.

If you suffer from weight problems, consult with your health care provider, who may be able to recommend a nutritionist. In general, to gain weight, eat more nuts and seeds. To lose weight, eat more fruits and vegetables.

ENVIRONMENTAL STRESSORS

Environmental factors that can contribute to difficulty in conceiving are all those toxins and physiologically active substances that we ingest or absorb—purposefully or unknowingly—in our daily lives. Most do not have lasting effects; once exposure to them is eliminated, their effects quickly or gradually disappear.

ALCOHOL

Excessive alcohol depresses testosterone levels in men, which can lead to erectile dysfunction, reduced testicle size, and decreased libido. For women, studies show that even moderate alcohol intake can be a factor in ovulatory infertility. Hops, found in beer, can interfere with FSH production and therefore be a factor in low sperm counts.

CONTRACEPTION

Birth control pills can cause blood stagnation in the reproductive organs, which can impede conception. Some women experience amenorrhea after they discontinue use of birth control pills; menses begin to normalize over time.

ENVIRONMENTAL TOXINS

Low sperm count is a progressive trend in modern times. Today's average sperm count is almost 40 percent lower than it was in the 1920s. Although biological problems could be a factor, I'm inclined to believe that the radical decrease in average sperm count is primarily linked to environmental causes. Some experts believe that herbicide and pesticide residues in the food we eat, the water we drink, and the land we live on may be factors. This theory makes sense to me—these substances are, after all, designed to destroy life. According to traditional Oriental medicine, low sperm count can be caused by a yin deficiency in the Kidneys. The Western and Oriental theories complement each other; the organs of the kidneys and liver serve as filters for metabolic wastes, and the toxic residues we absorb eventually pass through them, which could contribute to Oriental medicine's definitions of Kidney and Liver dysfunctions.

To lessen your exposure to environmental toxins, live organically. Use nontoxic cleaning products, wear organic-fiber clothing, and stop using pesticides and herbicides on your landscape. Eat low on the food chain, focusing the diet on organic vegetables, fruits, nuts, seeds, and whole grains. Avoid anti-fertility foods such as cottonseed oil, which contains a compound called gossypol, known to decrease sperm production.

ELECTROMAGNETIC ENERGY

Fields of electromagnetic energy surround the flow of electric current. Excessive exposure to electromagnetic energy is associated with an increased risk of cancer, a weakened immune system, and hormone dysfunctions, including fertility problems.

Electromagnetic energy can be difficult to avoid. Try to minimize contact with household electrical appliances, microwaves, electric blankets, water beds (which are warmed by electric heaters), computer monitors without protective screens, x-rays, and power lines. Most important, minimize their proximity to your sleeping area.

EXCESSIVE EXERCISE

Though exercise is wonderful for overall health and vigor, too much of it can tax the body to the point that conception is impossible. Excessive exercise can decrease progesterone levels that can prevent an embryo from implanting. Endurance training can lower testosterone levels in men, lowering libido and sperm count. Instead of running, biking, or weight lifting to exhaustion, practice—in moderation—exercises that facilitate fertility. See chapter 4 for suggestions.

"PROFESSIONAL" GEAR

Toxic residues and yin deficiencies aren't the only modern-day causes of low sperm count. For optimal sperm production, the testes must be at a temperature between 94 and 96 degrees Fahrenheit, which is just less than body temperature. Therefore, the testicles are suspended from the body in the scrotum; being slightly removed from the torso allows them to remain at a slightly cooler temperature. However, the amenities of civilization that are part and parcel of having a professional life—including synthetic-fiber clothing and office jobs that require men to sit all day long—can raise the temperature of the testes and reduce sperm production. If you ride a bicycle a lot, consider switching from a solid seat to one that has an oval opening built into the saddle to prevent sperm from getting overheated. Even heated car seats may reduce sperm.

If you're having trouble with low sperm count, take cool showers instead of hot baths. Wear boxer shorts instead of briefs. Avoid synthetic-fiber fabrics. And do your best to get up and move around as much as possible.

PHARMACEUTICAL MEDICATIONS

Many drugs, particularly ulcer medications, antibiotics, high blood pressure meds, and calcium channel blockers, can lower sperm count, diminish libido, contribute to erectile dysfunction, and negatively effect fertility in countless other ways.

If you're taking a pharmaceutical medication that has an adverse effect on fertility, ask your health care provider if there are alternatives. However, do not stop taking medication without first consulting with your health care provider. If you must continue to take these drugs, also undertake some of the natural, fertility-supporting therapies such as those suggested later in this chapter; with luck, they will counteract the side effects of your medication.

SMOKING

Smoking has a tremendously potent effect on fertility. Unfortunately, that effect is strictly negative. Female smokers have a 40 percent higher rate of infertility than nonsmokers, and 33 percent of male smokers have reduced sperm motility. Cigarettes also diminish the production of testosterone, leading to a wide range of erectile and sperm production dysfunctions.

STRESS

Stress has an effect on just about all aspects of health, including fertility. Consider meditation, prayer, biofeedback, guided imagery, relaxing music, or yoga to help you let go of your tensions.

TIPS FOR FERTILE LOVEMAKING

There are a thousand and one sure-fire, guaranteed-to-work, folkloric "cures" for conceiving. Some of them are quite insightful; others are just plain strange. I prefer to stick with common sense.

- *Build up sexual chi. A man should avoid ejaculation for a week before ovulation to "save up" sexual energy.*
- *Make sure you're both ready. Traditional Oriental medicine suggests that having intercourse when you are extremely angry, grieved, frightened, or intoxicated can increase the risk of a stillborn child.*
- *Urinate before, not after. The woman should urinate before intercourse so that she won't need to urinate immediately afterward. Urinating afterward can wash away some sperm and disrupt the movement of sperm toward the ovum.*
- *Avoid artificial lubricants. Lubricants can interfere with sperm motility, lessening chances of conception.*
- *Take time for foreplay. It is not imperative for a woman to have an orgasm for conception to occur, yet she should be stimulated enough to produce some vaginal mucus. Take some time with foreplay to ensure that the woman is aroused.*
- *Stick with the classic position. The best position for conception is the missionary position.*
- *Elevate. After union, the woman should lie on her back with her knees elevated to her chest for at least twenty minutes. Use a pillow or two to elevate her hips. (The very adept yogini is able to stand on her head after intercourse, but unless you're an expert at yoga, I wouldn't recommend trying it.)*

What is most important is that you're making love at the right time. If the woman is not ovulating, the odds of fertilization plummet. To find out how to monitor your ovulation cycle, *see page 233.*

Natural Therapies for Nurturing Fertility

Natural therapies for nurturing fertility focus on supporting overall health, strengthening the reproductive system, normalizing hormone production, dissolving blockages, clearing heat and congestion, encouraging libido, and nourishing the liver and kidneys.

DIET

I am always delighted when a couple hoping to conceive want to build their own bodies with good nutrition. Nutrition is the foremost contributor to a healthy baby, as well as a powerful factor in fertility.

The foods that support fertility also support overall good health and vigorous libido. A diet that focuses on the "sex tonic" foods would work wonders for supporting fertility. See chapter 1 for details.

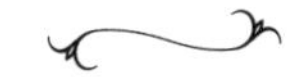

Fertility Shake

This is a super shake that can be shared by a couple trying to conceive. It boosts energy and is rich in protein, zinc, and vitamin E.

- 1½ cups fresh raw almond/pine nut/sunflower seed/or pumpkin seed milk
- 1 ripe banana
- 2 tablespoons raw pumpkin seeds, soaked overnight and rinsed
- 2 tablespoons raw sunflower seeds, soaked overnight and rinsed
- 1 tablespoon raw honey
- 1 tablespoon raw tahini
- 1 tablespoon maca powder

Combine all the ingredients in a blender and process. Share the mixture with your beloved, first making a toast to each other and to new life.

NUTRITIONAL THERAPY

Although real food should be the main source of nutrients, various supplements may be of service in supporting fertility.

Arginine. This amino acid enhances blood flow to the genitals and is essential for the production of sperm; it promotes normal sperm count and motility. Arginine may aggravate existing herpes conditions and should be used only after other nutritional approaches have been tried. Take 500 to 2,000 mg daily.

Beta-carotene. The precursor to vitamin A, beta-carotene supports the production of estrogens and androgens. A beta-carotene deficiency can be a factor in low sperm production. Take 15,000 IU daily.

Carnitine. This amino acid can help improve sperm motility and a man's endurance. Take 1,000 to 2,000 mg daily.

Chlorophyll. Chlorophyll, the "green blood of plants," helps detoxify the liver, build the blood, and regulate the menses. It is available at health food stores in capsule form or as a liquid. Use as directed on the package label. And remember that dark green leafy vegetables are a great source of chlorophyll in all-natural packaging. Eat at least one serving a day, and drink a fresh green vegetable juice several times a week.

Vitamin B complex. The B vitamins can raise progesterone levels, relieve erectile dysfunction, and remedy estrogen-related biochemical problems. Folic acid, in particular, helps prevent some types of birth defects, while vitamin B_{12} may elevate sperm count and help correct anemia. Look for a 50 to 100 mg B-complex supplement that contains about 300 mcg of vitamin B_{12}. A woman trying to conceive should also take 800 mg daily of folic acid.

Vitamin C. Vitamin C can increase sperm count, help to protect sperm against free-radical damage, and prevent sperm from clumping together. Excessive amounts of vitamin C have been known to bring on menses, however, so avoid exceeding the recommended dosage during pregnancy. Take 3,000 mg daily.

Vitamin E. Tocopherol, the scientific name for vitamin E, comes from the Greek *tokos* and *phero,* meaning "to bear offspring." A vitamin E deficiency can cause infertility in both men and women and may be a factor in the tendency to miscarry in women. According to various studies, vitamin E enhances sperms' ability to penetrate an egg; a deficiency can contribute to sluggish sperm. This antioxidant vitamin is deficient in many Western diets. Selenium improves the activity of vitamin E and is often combined with it in supplement formulas. Take 400 to 600 IU of vitamin E daily, in combination with 50 to 200 mcg of selenium.

Zinc. Zinc is a component of sperm, seminal fluid, and vaginal mucus. It is essential for the growth and maturation of the gonads and can help increase the number and motility of sperm. Men with azoospermia (absence of living sperm) and oligospermia (low sperm count) have benefited from supplementation with zinc. Zinc helps protect the prostate gland and is needed for testosterone production. Take 50 mg of chelated zinc daily.

Once you are pregnant for sure and rejoicing, you should begin taking a good natural prenatal vitamin. And actually, prenatal vitamins often contain all the nutrients that are helpful in the pre-pregnancy state, too, so you might consider taking them for at least three months before you try to conceive.

HERBAL THERAPY

The herbs generally recommended for boosting fertility are among the most potent activators of whole-body health. Once you choose and undertake an herbal regimen, you'll find that both your energy and health improve.

If you become pregnant, discontinue using herbs, except under the guidance of your health care provider. To aid fertility, try the following:

Alfalfa (*Medicago sativa*). The herb is one of the most nutrient-rich herbs on Earth. It is nutritive, phytoestrogenic, and tonic.

Alisma (*Alisma orientale*). The rhizome is a Kidney tonic that benefits libido and fertility for both sexes.

Angelica (*Angelica archangelica, A. atropurpurea*). The root helps regulate the menstrual cycle. It is usually taken from the time of ovulation to the time of menses. It is a tonic and a uterine stimulant. Avoid during pregnancy and in cases of heavy bleeding or diabetes. In rare cases, the root causes photosensitivity.

Ashwagandha (*Withania somnifera*). The root helps increase sperm count and is an excellent reproductive tonic for men. It is an adaptogen, aphrodisiac, hormone regulator, nutritive, rejuvenative, and uterine sedative.

Asparagus (*Asparagus officinalis, A. cochinchinensis*). The root is an ovarian tonic that supports estrogen activity. It is also an aphrodisiac, cardiotonic, demulcent, galactagogue, nutritive, rejuvenative, and Kidney tonic.

Astragalus (*Astragalus membranaceus*). The root helps increase sperm count and motility. It is an adaptogen, adrenal tonic, blood tonic, and chi tonic.

Damiana (*Turnera aphrodisiaca, T. diffusa*). The leaf improves sexual vitality by allowing nerve messages to spread more expansively through the body. It is an aphrodisiac and yang tonic. Avoid in cases of high blood pressure, urinary tract infections, kidney disease, or liver disease. Damiana is not recommended for use by pregnant women or nursing mothers, so discontinue when you know you are pregnant.

Dandelion (*Taraxacum officinale*). The root helps decongest the liver, aiding the breakdown of hormones.

Dong quai (*Angelica sinensis*). The root helps normalize menses. As a blood tonic, it builds the blood and improves circulation in the pelvic region. It is also a uterine tonic and yin tonic. Avoid during pregnancy, except under the guidance of your health care provider. Do not use in cases of diarrhea, heavy menstrual flow, poor digestion, or bloating. Do not use in conjunction with blood-thinning medications such as ibuprofen.

False unicorn (*Chamaelirium luteum*). The root is an alkaline tonic for the uterus, ovaries, and reproductive system. As one of my teachers once said, "It's the next best thing to sperm for getting you pregnant." The bitter taste of this herb can cause vomiting. Excessive amounts may cause kidney and stomach irritation, blurred vision, and hot flashes. Do not use without employing birth control during sex unless pregnancy is desired. Discontinue use during pregnancy. False unicorn is endangered in the wild; do not use wildcrafted supplies.

Fenugreek (*Trigonella foenum-graecum*). The seed tonifies the uterus and the kidneys. It is an aphrodisiac, rejuvenative, restorative, and yang tonic. Avoid during pregnancy. If you have diabetes, consult with your health care provider before use.

Ginkgo (*Ginkgo biloba*). The leaf has long been used to increase sperm count. It is an antioxidant, cerebral tonic, circulatory stimulant, Kidney tonic, and rejuvenative.

Ginseng, Chinese (*Panax ginseng*). The root nourishes the entire being. It is often recommended as a treatment for erectile dysfunction and low sperm count. It is an adaptogen, aphrodisiac, chi tonic, rejuvenative, restorative, and tonic. Avoid in cases of excess heat, such as inflammation, fever, and high blood pressure. Since ginseng can be energizing, avoid taking it within four hours of bedtime. Avoid once pregnancy is confirmed.

Ho shou wu (*Polygonum multiflorum*). The root is used to increase sperm count in men and fertility in women. It is an aphrodisiac, chi tonic, Liver tonic, rejuvenative, and yin tonic.

Licorice (*Glycyrrhiza glabra, U. uralensis*). The root helps normalize the ovulation cycle. It contains phytosterols, the raw material for hormone production. It is an adrenal tonic, chi tonic, nutritive, and rejuvenative. Avoid once pregnancy is confirmed and in cases of edema, high blood pressure, or diabetes. Do not use in combination with digoxin drugs. Excessive use can cause sodium retention and potassium depletion.

Nettle (*Urtica dioica, U. urens*). The leaf strengthens the kidneys and the adrenals. It is rich in both minerals and chlorophyll. It is a thyroid tonic and a cholagogue. This is a great herb for use during pregnancy; talk with your health care provider about its benefits. Contact with the fresh plant will irritate the skin, so wear gloves when collecting. Use only dried herb.

Oat (*Avena sativa, A. fatua*). The herb and spikelets help relieve exhaustion and stress, nourish the nerves, and make tactile sensations more pleasurable. Oat is an aphrodisiac, endocrine tonic, nutritive, rejuvenative, and uterine tonic.

Poria (*Poria cocos*). The fungus strengthens the kidneys. It is a chi tonic, restorative, and tonic.

Red clover (*Trifolium pratense*). The blossom is very alkaline and can help correct overly acidic vaginal conditions that prevent sperm from reaching the uterus. It is nutritive and phytoestrogenic.

Red raspberry (*Rubus idaeus*). The leaf helps regulate hormones. It is a Kidney tonic, nutritive, prostate tonic, uterine tonic, and yin tonic. This is a great herb for use during pregnancy; talk with your health care provider about its benefits.

Rehmannia (*Rehmannia glutinosa*). The root strengthens the kidneys and liver. It is a blood tonic, rejuvenative, and yin tonic. Avoid in cases of loose stools, poor appetite, bloating, or a coated tongue.

Sarsaparilla (*Smilax* spp.). The root contains phytosterols, the raw material of hormone production. It helps cleanse toxins from the reproductive system, and it is often recommended in treatments for erectile dysfunction, infertility, and ovarian cysts. It is an aphrodisiac, rejuvenative, and tonic.

Saw palmetto (*Serenoa repens*). The berry relieves inflammation and blockage in the genitourinary tract. It helps increase sperm count and is often recommended in treatments for erectile dysfunction, infertility, premature ejaculation, and prostatitis. It is an aphrodisiac, nutritive, rejuvenative, and tonic.

Schizandra (*Schisandra chinensis*). The berry is a whole body tonic and is often recommended in treatments for sexual debility. It is also an adaptogen, aphrodisiac, Kidney and Liver tonic, rejuvenative, and restorative.

Siberian ginseng (*Eleutherococcus senticosus*). The root is an anti-stress tonic for men and women. It is an adaptogen, aphrodisiac, and chi tonic.

Vitex (*Vitex agnus-castus*). The berry helps normalize hormone production and stimulates ovulation. Vitex can be used during the first trimester of pregnancy to maintain the corpus luteum in women with a history of miscarriage before the twelfth week.

Wild yam (*Dioscorea opposita, D. villosa*). The root helps clear congested chi. It is an aphrodisiac and nutritive. Avoid therapeutic doses once pregnancy is confirmed, except under the guidance of your health care provider. The *Dioscorea villosa* species is endangered in the wild; do not use wildcrafted supplies.

CHINESE PATENT FORMULAS

There are a number of patent formulas from traditional Chinese medicine that can be used to nurture fertility.

JIN KUI SHEN QI WAN (GOLDENBOOK TEA PILLS). Use to counteract low sexual vitality accompanied by lower back pain and cold extremities.

NU KE BA ZHEN WAN (EIGHT PRECIOUS HERBS). This chi and blood tonic works equally well for men and women. It is often recommended to regulate menses and to relieve fatigue.

ZHONG GUO SHOU WU ZHI. Use this formula to nourish the Liver, support the Kidneys, and invigorate the blood.

There are many other Chinese patent formulas available for many specific conditions. Consult with a practitioner of Oriental medicine to find the formula best suited to your needs.

HOMEOPATHIC REMEDIES

When an inability to conceive is accompanied by the conditions described below, use the suggested homeopathic remedy. The usual dosage is 4 pellets, or as many liquid drops as the package label recommends, taken under the tongue four times daily. Rather than swallowing the pellets whole, allow them to dissolve slowly.

AGNUS CASTUS. The patient experiences general weakness, low sex drive, and vaginal discharge.

ALETRIS FARINOSA. The uterus is weak.

AURUM MURIATICUM NATRONATUM. The patient experiences ovarian swelling or has undescended testicles.

BARYTA CARBONICA. The patient experiences general weakness, accompanied by premature ejaculation or immature ovarian function. He or she might also suffer from low hormone output and lymphatic blockage.

BORAX. Sexual desire and vitality are diminished.

CHININUM SULPHURICUM. Sexual desire is diminished and the patient is not able to produce sperm.

CONIUM. If the patient is a woman, the breasts feel hard and tender. If the patient is a man, he suffers from erectile dysfunction and is not able to produce sperm.

FERRUM METALLICUM. The patient experiences low sex drive, amenorrhea, and pain or decreased sensitivity during intercourse.

GRAPHITES. The patient has an aversion to sex and a history of sexual abuse. If the patient is male, he is unable to ejaculate.

IODUM. The patient feels pain and tenderness in the right ovary or the testicles.

KALI BROMATUM. There is atrophy in the ovaries.

LYCOPODIUM. If the patient is male, he experiences impotence or premature ejaculation. If the patient is female, the right ovary was previously inflamed.

NUX VOMICA. The patient has a history of painful, irregular periods. She experiences leukorrhea, constipation, and irritability.

PHOSPHORICUM ACIDUM. Fertility is diminished after an extended illness. If the patient is male, he experiences impotence, weak testicular function, and weak erections.

PHOSPHORUS. The patient feels no desire for sex and tends to overuse salt.

PITUITRINUM. The patient experiences vertigo, an inability to concentrate, and feelings of confusion.

PLATINA. The genital region is extremely sensitive. The left ovary may be tender. The patient is often prideful. He or she has a high sex drive but is unable to conceive.

SABAL SERRULATA. The genitals are atrophied.

SABINA. The patient experiences recurrent miscarriage at eleven weeks.

SEPIA. Intercourse is painful, and there is yellowish leukorrhea. The patient experiences abdominal pain, constipation, painful intercourse, and irregular menses. In men, sex drive is diminished.

SILICEA. The uterus and fallopian tubes are weak and the patient lacks physical stamina.

FLOWER ESSENCES

Flower essences to improve fertility include the following. The usual dosage is 3 drops under the tongue or taken with a glass of water three or four times daily.

Bells of Ireland. This flower essence encourages fertility in men and women.

Blackberry. Blackberry can counteract barrenness in women; it stimulates body rhythms.

Fig. Couples will find that Fig flower essence helps them develop trust.

Jasmine. This essence has a moderate effect on male fertility by stimulating sperm production.

Mallow. Mallow improves virility.

Mugwort. Mugwort is recommended as a treatment for male infertility.

Pomegranate. This essence can help women develop a sense of nurturing and can increase fertility.

Squash. Squash improves hormonal balance and helps rejuvenate sexual organs.

Watermelon. Watermelon encourages fertility in women and potency in men.

AROMATHERAPY

Essential oils that can be used to nurture fertility in massage, bathing, and inhalations include angelica, anise, basil, clary sage, cumin, fennel, geranium, jasmine, lemon balm, neroli, and rose. See chapter 5 for more information on these oils and their applications. Avoid these essential oils once you are pregnant.

REFLEXOLOGY

To stimulate fertility, try rubbing the Kidney point in a circular motion for three minutes a day. This reflexology point is located at the center of the ball of the foot. Also work on the area of the Achilles heel, which correlates to the reproductive organs.

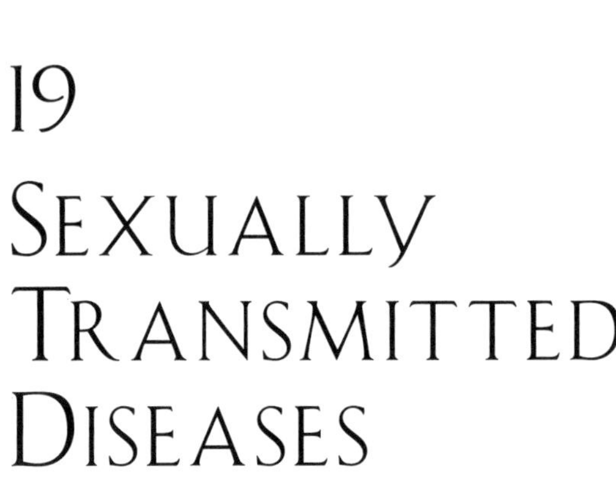

19 Sexually Transmitted Diseases

SEXUALLY TRANSMITTED DISEASES ARE the number one scourge of humankind. They have most likely been around since humans first started having sex—that is, as long as we have been in existence. They should not be taken lightly. They must be guarded against (see chapter 14), watched for, and treated appropriately.

In the United States alone, there are more than twelve million new cases of sexually transmitted diseases (STDs) diagnosed every year. They range from crabs—a type of pubic lice that causes no more harm than a terrible itchiness—to chlamydia, which can cause serious reproductive dysfunctions, to AIDS, which can be fatal. Some STDs can be treated effectively with natural therapies, but others require the strength and aggressiveness of allopathic medicine. When allopathic medicine is used, natural therapies can serve as a complement, helping the body rebound from the effects of the treatment and supporting overall good health.

I do believe that exposing one's genitals briefly to a private sun and air bath (starting at five minutes and working up to ten minutes) is a helpful technique that is antibacterial, immune strengthening, and helpful for preventing and treating health conditions "where the sun don't shine." Too much sun would be detrimental, but if you can create a time of safety and privacy, try to engage in this healthful practice.

You cannot tell from outward appearance whether a potential lover is likely to have an STD. STDs occur in people of all genders, all ethnicities, all sexual orientations, and all social classes. Even those seemingly clean-cut, carefully groomed, vibrantly healthy heartthrobs decked out in the latest chic clothing may be carriers of disease. You never know, and for that reason, it's important to ask a potential new lover whether he or she has been tested for STDs. You, too, must be tested on a regular basis for as long as you are engaging in sexual activity with multiple partners.

If you have an STD, it takes courage to talk to a potential sexual partner about it. However, it's important that you do. Keeping silent about an STD can lead to a situation in which your partner unknowingly puts himself or herself at risk of contracting the disease. If you're not responsible about discussing an STD, you may be responsible for giving it to a lover.

Having an STD does not equate to the end of your sex life; it does mean that you and your partner will have to take extra precautions to avoid sharing the disease. Tell your partner how you contracted the disease, how you felt, and how you are now dealing with it. Offer support literature (available from Planned Parenthood Federation of America and the STD and AIDS Hotline; see the resources section), and ask for understanding.

Transmission of an STD is usually dependent on skin contact or the exchange of bodily fluids. Some STDs are borne only in the blood; others can be transmitted through mucus and saliva in addition to blood. Some, like crabs, can get around on their own, though these organisms generally cannot travel more than a few inches. It's important to know how the different types of STDs can be transmitted. While you need to be careful not to put yourself at risk, you don't want to wear a Level 4 biohazard suit, so to speak, when you come into contact with an infected person. That sort of paranoia shows ignorance, and it makes the infected person feel like a social pariah, which doesn't do much to help him or her adjust to new parameters for sexual activity.

As the old saying goes, the path to wisdom is knowledge. I hope this chapter will start you off in the right direction.

STD can stand for "savor the disease," as catching one is a major wake-up call. The soul's messages through STDs is to invite you to investigate sexuality—what it truly means for you. "Savor the disease" means to embrace it as an opportunity to know yourself more deeply by honoring the message. STDs are a souvenir of love—rather than trying to "get over it," go "through it."

—Personal communication with the late Jeannine Parvati Baker, author of *Hygieia: A Woman's Herbal, Conscious Conception,* and *Prenatal Yoga and Natural Childbirth*

HERBAL DOSAGES

You'll find many recommendations for herbal therapy in this chapter. Unless stated otherwise, the therapeutic adult dosage for a recommended herb is:

- *1 cup of tea three times daily;*
- *1 or 2 capsules three times daily; or*
- *1 dropperful of tincture three times daily.*

CHLAMYDIA AND NONGONOCOCCAL URETHRITIS

Chlamydia is an infection caused by the parasitic bacterium *Chlamydia trachomatis;* in men, a chlamydial infection causes nongonococcal urethritis (infection of the urethra). Chlamydial infection is currently the most common sexually transmitted disease in the United States.

Most infected women and about half of infected men are asymptomatic; that is, they don't exhibit any symptoms of chlamydial infection. For this reason, the disease often goes undetected—and untreated—for years.

When symptoms do make an appearance, they manifest in men as a yellowish or whitish penile discharge, tenderness in the genitals, a need to urinate frequently, burning or painful urination, and redness at the tip of the penis. Women may notice a need to urinate frequently, yellow or greenish vaginal discharge, cramping, and occasional bleeding after intercourse. These symptoms are similar to those of gonorrhea, and chlamydia is often misdiagnosed as gonorrhea. Unfortunately, the treatment for gonorrhea does not have any effect on the *Chlamydia* bacteria.

A chlamydial infection can have very serious consequences. In women it can cause inflammation of the cervix (cervicitis) and pelvic inflammatory disease, which can lead to fertility dysfunctions. Pregnant women with chlamydia have an increased risk of miscarriage; their babies often suffer from a chlamydial eye infection, which can lead to blindness, as well as ear, lung, and genital infections. In men it can cause inflammation of the epididymis (epididymitis), which also can lead to fertility dysfunctions.

Given that most cases of chlamydial infection do not exhibit symptoms, it is wise to get tested for the disease whenever you've engaged in at-risk behavior—unprotected sexual activity with a new partner or in a nonmonogamous relationship. Your gynecologist can perform the test.

Transmission

Chlamydia can be spread through sexual contact involving the genitals, anus, or mouth. Taking birth control pills, which can deplete friendly vaginal bacteria, cause vitamin and mineral deficiencies, and unbalance hormone levels, can make women more susceptible to the infection.

Treatment

Given the severity of the possible consequences, chlamydial infection demands aggressive treatment. The most effective treatment is antibiotics. If you are committed to natural therapies, try one of the herbs described below, then get retested. If the infection has not disappeared, I strongly recommend that you begin a course of antibiotics. Otherwise, you risk compromising your fertility.

HERBAL THERAPY

Three herbs have particularly potent antibiotic activity against the *Chlamydia* bacteria.

Echinacea (*Echinacea purpurea, E. angustifolia*). The root has a powerfully stimulating effect on the immune system, activating T cells, interferons, and macrophages. It is also an alterative, antifungal, and antiseptic.

Goldenseal (*Hydrastis canadensis*). The root is active against a wide range of pathogens and is especially effective for relieving inflammation of the mucous membranes. It is an alterative and antibiotic. Goldenseal is very bitter, and most people find it easiest to ingest in capsule form. Avoid during pregnancy. This herb is endangered in the wild; do not use wildcrafted products.

Usnea (*Usnea barbata*). Like goldenseal root, usnea lichen is active against a wide range of pathogens. It is an antibiotic, antifungal, and immunostimulant.

PROBIOTICS

When you must take antibiotics, add to your diet fermented foods such as Rejuvelac, kombucha, plain active yogurt, unpasteurized sauerkraut, apple cider vinegar, miso, and tamari. These foods support and replenish the friendly bacteria in the body.

After a course of antibiotic therapy, begin a course of acidophilus therapy to restore the friendly bacteria that are necessary for digestion, elimination, and healthy reproductive organs. Take one or two capsules three times daily for three to four months.

CRABS

Crabs, also known as pubic lice, are creepy-crawly creatures (*Pthirus pubis*) that live in pubic hair and feed on human blood. They multiply rapidly by laying eggs (nits) at the roots of the pubic hair. They cause intense itching and irritation in the pubic area. They are not a serious health risk, but they can be an indicator that your sexual activity has put you at risk of contracting STDs.

Crabs are difficult to see; you'll most likely notice the itching first. Adult lice appear as very small black or rust-colored flecks; the nits look like tiny, shiny ovals clinging to the base of the hairs. A magnifying glass can help you identify what you're looking at.

Transmission

Crabs are usually spread from intimate contact. Intercourse can allow crabs to wander from one pubis to another; oral sex can allow them to infest the scalp, eyebrows, and chest hair. However, even naked people sitting on the couch together or sharing towels can transfer them, as can many other activities. Like head lice, they can also infest clothing and bed sheets; sleeping in a lice-infested bed puts you at risk of waking up with crabs.

Treatment

Natural therapies can be as effective as allopathic medicine for ridding the body of these parasites. The therapies focus on killing the lice, getting rid of nits, and making the body an inhospitable environment for lice. Note that the telltale itching can persist for several days, even after lice are dead.

THE SHAMPOO TREATMENT

Find a lice-treatment shampoo, which is formulated to kill crabs and other types of lice, at your local herb shop or health food store. They will contain substances like tea tree oil, eucalyptus, olive oil, and vinegar. (If you can't find the right shampoo at these outlets, you can find a medicated version at your local pharmacy.) Follow the instructions on the product label. After the shampoo treatment, work through your pubic hair with a fine-toothed comb to remove dead crabs and eggs. Then disinfect the combs by placing them in boiling water for ten minutes.

The lice shampoo will kill lice but not nits. Repeat the treatment in seven to ten days to get rid of any lice that may have hatched from eggs that survived the washing and combing.

Wash all clothing, bedding, and towels in hot water followed by a full hot cycle in a dryer. Dry clean all clothes and bedding that can't be washed, or pack them away in a plastic trash bag for two weeks; without access to human blood, the lice will starve and die. Vacuum all furniture. Scrub the house from top to bottom. Practice obsessive hygiene!

DIET

Garlic deters not only vampires but crabs as well. Take two 500 mg garlic capsules three times daily for a month. Seaweed can have a similar effect on your blood, imbuing it with a salty flavor that seems to repel crabs.

Crabs, like other parasites, seem to prey on weakness. A healthy liver and healthy blood is key to making your body inhospitable to critters looking for an easy ride. Bugs don't want to taste your blood when you eat planty of raw garlic (or use capsules) and get alkaline. Consume plenty of raw carrots, beets, burdock, dandelion greens, and kale, and drink teas made from blood-purifying plants, such as cleavers herb, dandelion root, echinacea root, and red clover blossoms.

SALT RUB

Dampen your pubic hair, then apply a handful of salt mixed with just enough water that it will stick. Leave on for thirty minutes. Then shower.

AROMATHERAPY HEAT TREATMENT

Heat tends to discourage crabs from sticking around; they'll leave a person overheated by fever or exercise. To replicate that effect, spend some time in a sauna. Crabs won't survive 120 degrees Fahrenheit for more than five minutes. After this heat treatment, apply a few drops of undiluted tea tree or lavender essential oil to the infested areas of the skin. (Both tea tree and lavender have a potent antiparasitic effect.)

Avoid this treatment if you are pregnant.

HOMEOPATHIC STAPHYSAGRIA

The homeopathic remedy STAPHYSAGRIA deters both crabs and head lice. Take 4 pellets, or as many liquid drops as the package label recommends, under the tongue four times daily for ten days. Take ten days off, then repeat the treatment for ten more days.

CRAB APPLE

The Bach Flower Essence Crab Apple can help you recover emotionally from the lice infestation. It restores feelings of beauty in a person who feels physically and mentally unclean. Take 3 drops under the tongue or with a glass of water three or four times daily.

Without saying: Practice Hysterical Hygiene. Use water, soap, vaccum, sunshine, dryers, and whatever other cleaning technologies you have. Then do it again ten days later. Everyone affected needs to get treated. Radiate your health aura. You are a stronger and more conscious creature than any nit. Outwit the nit.

GENITAL (VENEREAL) WARTS

Warts are caused by human papillomavirus (HPV), a group of over seventy viruses. The viruses are contagious, and the warts can be spread via sexual contact. On women the warts can appear on the vulva, the labia, inside the vagina, and on the cervix. On men they appear on the shaft of the penis, under the foreskin, and on the scrotum. They also can appear on the anus and in the mouth and throat.

External genital warts manifest as small, hard bumps; they are similar in appearance to regular warts. If left untreated, they grow, taking on a cauliflower-like appearance. Warts on the cervix are more properly called lesions. Cervical lesions have been linked to cervical cancer; likewise, rectal warts have been linked to rectal cancer. Cervical lesions are not visible to the naked eye and are usually discovered by Pap smear.

External warts may be too small to see with the untrained eye. They are generally painless, but if irritated, they can burn or itch. If you suspect that you have warts, try soaking the genitals in a 5 to 10 percent vinegar solution. After about six minutes, any warts will turn white, making them easily visible.

Genital warts take from one to nine months after exposure to appear. They may go away on their own or grow aggressively. They can be especially aggressive during pregnancy.

Transmission

Genital warts can be contracted through oral, vaginal, or anal contact with an infected person. Condoms can offer some protection against the spread of the disease. People with a suppressed immune system—such as HIV-infected persons—are at a higher risk for contracting the infection. Taking birth control pills, which can deplete friendly vaginal bacteria, cause vitamin and mineral deficiencies, and unbalance hormone levels, can make women more susceptible to the infection.

Treatment

There is no known cure for HPV. Upon diagnosis, it is important to remove existing warts to prevent the growth and transmission of the disease. Try the natural therapies described below. If the natural therapies do not cause the warts to disappear, then the more aggressive allopathic treatment is necessary.

In allopathic medicine, genital warts are usually painted with a caustic chemical that burns them away. The most common wart-removing chemical treatment is podophyllin, which is made from the root of mayapple (*Podophyllum peltatum*). Podophyllin can irritate the skin; you can protect the surrounding tissue by applying a calendula-comfrey salve. (You can often find calendula-comfrey salve in natural food stores and herb shops, or you can make your own following Cascade Anderson Geller's instructions on page 99.) Your gynecologist or urologist may also recommend cryotherapy (freezing them off), laser surgery, or surgical excision.

Removing the warts will not eliminate the infection. New warts may appear at some point in the future, and they, too, will have to be removed. The following natural therapies can deter the growth and occurrence of warts.

TOPICAL APPLICATIONS

Topical applications for removing genital warts include the following:

- Papaya sap
- Milky white sap from dandelion stems
- Garlic-infused oil
- Celandine juice
- Fresh elderberry juice
- Juice from the inner side of the pods of fresh broad beans
- Lemon juice
- Thuja (cedar leaf) essential oil

Be persistent. Apply these compounds three times daily for as long as it takes.

HERBAL THERAPY

Herbal therapy for genital warts focuses on attacking the virus, stimulating the immune system, strengthening the liver, and reducing inflammation. Many of the herbs are also thought to have antitumor properties, which can help prevent the warts from progressing to cancerous growths.

Burdock (*Arctium lappa*). The root is an alterative, antiseptic, antifungal, anti-inflammatory, and antitumor.

Cleavers (*Galium aparine*). The herb is an alterative, anti-inflammatory, antitumor, and lymphatic cleanser.

Dandelion (*Taraxacum officinale*). The root is an antifungal and cholagogue.

Echinacea (*Echinacea purpurea, E. angustifolia*). The root strengthens the immune system. It is an alterative, antiseptic, antifungal, anti-inflammatory, antitumor, and antiviral.

Nettle (*Urtica dioica, U. urens*). The herb is an alterative, cholagogue, and circulatory stimulant. Contact with the fresh plant will irritate the skin. Use only dried herb. Wear gloves when collecting.

Peppermint (*Mentha piperita*). The herb is an antiseptic, antiviral, and cholagogue.

NUTRITIONAL THERAPY

Supplements that can be useful for eliminating warts and preventing them from returning include the following:

Antioxidants. Antioxidants support the body's immune system. They are best absorbed through natural sources of the nutrients beta-carotene, vitamin C, vitamin E, selenium, and superoxide dismutase. Good sources of each of these are listed in chapter 3.

Lysine. The amino acid lysine can inhibit viral replication and seems to have a strong effect on HPV. Try taking 500 mg daily.

HOMEOPATHIC REMEDIES

When the development of genital warts matches one of the descriptions below, try the suggested homeopathic remedy. The usual dosage is 4 pellets, or as many liquid drops as the package label recommends, taken under the tongue four times daily. Rather than swallowing the pellets whole, allow them to dissolve slowly.

CALCAREA CARBONICA. The warts are smooth, soft, and round; they may be inflamed.

CALENDULA OFFICINALIS. The warts occur in the vaginal membranes, outside the uterus.

LYCOPODIUM. The warts are split and surrounded by an areola.

NATRUM MURIATICUM. The warts are old and cause a cutting pain.

NITRICUM ACIDUM. The warts are jagged, large, and in the genitoanal area. They may ooze, emit a fetid odor, or bleed upon washing.

PHOSPHORICUM ACIDUM. The warts are on the glans. They are indented and rugged.

SABINA. The warts are on the prepuce. They bleed easily and may produce feelings of numbness or a burning sensation.

SEPIA. The warts are on the margin of the prepuce. They feel horny in the center and are accompanied by a burning pain and inflammation.

STAPHYSAGRIA. The warts are figlike in appearance.

SULFUR. The warts are horny.

THUJA OCCIDENTALIS. This is the most common homeopathic remedy for genital warts. It is especially beneficial in cases where the warts are broad and conical, split easily, and appear in the genitoanal area and, in men, on the glans.

ESSENTIAL OIL TREATMENTS

A variety of essential oils with antimicrobial properties can be applied topically to warts to shrink or eliminate them. These oils include bergamot, cedar leaf, cinnamon, eucalyptus, lemon, niaouli, patchouli, tea tree, or a combination thereof. Combine these oils with an equal measure of olive oil and apply with a cotton swab to the wart. Take care to keep the solution on the wart; avoid painting the skin around the area as best you can.

SITZ BATHS

Hot and cold sitz baths increase circulation to the pelvic region, thereby helping the immune system combat the warts. See chapter 10 for instructions. Spend three minutes in hot water and one minute in cold water. Alternate, always commencing with hot and ending with cold.

GONORRHEA

Commonly known as "the clap," gonorrhea is caused by the bacterium *Neisseria gonorrhoeae*. It is the second most common sexually transmitted disease in the United States.

It is not uncommon for a gonorrheal infection to exhibit no symptoms. When symptoms do manifest, they show up about a week after exposure in men and about two weeks after exposure in women. Symptoms in men include frequent and painful urination, lower abdominal pain, and a greenish or gray discharge from the penis. Women may also suffer from painful urination as well as a greenish yellow discharge, inflammation of the cervix, and bleeding between menstrual periods.

If left untreated, gonorrhea can lead to chronic pain, tubal pregnancy, pelvic inflammatory disease, and damage to the testicles and the prostate. In rare cases, gonorrhea can spread to the heart, brain, and joints.

If you suspect that you have gonorrhea, visit your gynecologist or urologist for a complete examination.

Transmission

The bacteria cannot survive outside the body for more than a few seconds. It is transmitted via direct contact with an infected person during vaginal, anal, or oral sex.

Pregnant women can pass the disease to their newborns, where it can manifest as an acute eye inflammation known as gonococcal conjunctivitis, an ear infection, or a lung infection.

Treatment

Antibiotics are the standard treatment; different strains of the disease have become resistant to different antibiotics, so you may not find relief with the first prescription.

While you are taking antibiotics, add to your diet fermented foods such as plain yogurt and unpasteurized sauerkraut, apple cider vinegar, miso, and tamari. These foods support and replenish the friendly bacteria in the body.

After a course of antibiotic therapy, begin a course of acidophilus therapy to restore the friendly bacteria that are necessary for digestion, elimination, and healthy reproductive organs. Take 1 or 2 capsules three times daily for three to four months.

Gonorrhea is infamous for its high rate of recurrence, so follow-up visits are essential to be sure the infection has cleared.

HERPES

Herpes is a relative of chicken pox, Epstein-Barr virus, mononucleosis, and shingles. There are more than five types of herpesvirus; yet only herpes simplex I and herpes simplex II are considered sexually transmitted diseases. Herpes simplex I, or oral herpes, occurs usually on or around the lips and nose. It's sometimes referred to as cold sores or fever blisters. Herpes simplex II, or genital herpes, occurs usually on the labia, vulva, vaginal membranes, cervix, prepuce, glans, shaft of the penis, anus, rectum, buttocks, and thighs. There is a growing lack of distinction between the symptoms of these two types of viruses, however, because oral-genital contact has allowed some crossover.

Many people infected with herpes do not know that they have it, because the disease is often asymptomatic, meaning it produces no symptoms. The virus is highly contagious; it is estimated that one-sixth to one-third of the population in the United States aged fifteen to seventy-five is infected with genital herpes.

When symptoms do occur, they manifest as blisters on and around the genitals. The blisters may be accompanied by itching, pain, and fever. The blisters then burst and become oozing ulcers or lesions. The lesions will eventually crust over and heal.

It usually takes from two to twenty-eight days after exposure to the virus for an initial outbreak to occur. Stage I, called the prodromal or early-warning stage, can produce a localized numbing, tingling, burning, or itching sensation. Some infected persons also experience flu-like symptoms, including fatigue and swelling of the lymph nodes in the neck or groin area, which indicates that the body is working hard to deal with an infection. During stage II, a single blister or a cluster of blisters will appear. These blisters, also called vesicles, are small and grayish. Eventually they burst, leaving red, raw ulcerations. During stage III, the blisters may develop a yellowish crust before drying up and disappearing. The total attack may last anywhere from four days to a month.

After the symptoms of primary infection fade, the virus retreats to nerve cells deep within the body, where it lies dormant. When reactivated (see "Herpes Triggers," on page 407), it initiates a new outbreak of herpes lesions.

There are now sensitive and accurate blood tests available to diagnose herpes. To confirm a diagnosis of herpes topically, the blisters must be present. Your health care provider will use a cotton swab to collect serum from a lesion. The serum is examined for viral infection under a microscope. Other lesion-producing conditions that are sometimes confused with herpes include impetigo, fungal infections, syphilis, abrasions, boils, and some allergic reactions. The microscopic examination of the serum is necessary to distinguish one from the other.

Transmission

Herpes is most contagious during its active stages. The rate of transmission when no symptoms are present is less than 1 percent.

The virus can enter the body when an existing lesion comes in contact with the mucous membranes of the mouth or genitals. The transference may take place between an infected person and an uninfected person or between different sites on an infected person.

Direct contact is the most common means of transmission, but the herpesvirus can survive for brief periods of time outside the body. That means that towels, cigarettes, sex toys, eating utensils, and other items that may pick up fluid from an oozing herpes lesion can carry the disease. To avoid transmitting the disease, practice safe sex using barrier methods. (See chapter 14.) Do not engage in sexual contact during an outbreak of herpes lesions.

Wash your hands after touching the lesions and also first thing in the morning, in case you inadvertently touched them during the night. Wear cotton underwear and pajamas while sleeping to help prevent yourself from touching the lesions.

Never touch your eyes after touching a lesion. If the cornea becomes infected with the herpesvirus, scarring and blindness may result. If you wear contact lenses, wash your hands before placing them in your eyes.

Herpes and Pregnancy

If the virus is contracted during the first twenty weeks of pregnancy, there is an increased risk of abortion. If genital herpes lesions are present during the actual birth, the virus can be transmitted to the newborn; for one in four herpes-infected infants, the virus can have fatal complications. Depending on the location of the sores, doctors and midwives will recommend a cesarean section or will cover the lesions for vaginal delivery.

Fortunately, women seem to develop a resistance to herpes toward the end of a pregnancy; only 1 out of every 250 herpes-infected women has an active outbreak at the time of delivery. Interestingly, some babies born to mothers with herpes are endowed with an immunity to the disease.

Herpes Triggers

The first outbreak of herpes lesions is usually the worst. Most people find that outbreaks diminish in occurrence and severity over time. Most people also find that their bodies produce unique symptoms that signal an imminent herpes outbreak. These include tingling, burning, or tenderness in the area of the first outbreak.

New eruptions are most likely to occur when an infected person is experiencing physical, emotional, or immune system stress. These types of stress can be triggered by fatigue, illness, fever, overexposure to sun and wind, an imbalanced diet, poor thyroid function, liver congestion, having multiple sexual partners, or even wearing tight, chafing clothes.

Treatment

There is no cure for herpes. Those who have it must learn to live with it. Natural therapies can be of benefit in preventing new outbreaks and minimizing the severity and duration of outbreaks. They focus on promoting overall good health, strengthening the body's immune system, supporting the nervous system, and expediting the healing of an outbreak.

DIET

Proper diet is essential for minimizing the occurrence of herpes outbreaks. Of particular interest is the amino acid lysine, which has been shown to inhibit replication of the virus. Foods rich in lysine include:

- Beans (especially lima, mung, and soy)
- Cultured foods, such as cheese (preferably made from unhomogenized milk), kefir, nutritional yeast, sauerkraut, and yogurt
- Fish (especially flounder, halibut, salmon, shark, shrimp, and tuna)
- Poultry
- Quinoa and millet
- Red meat (but be sure that it comes from animals that were raised using organic methods and without hormone treatments)

The amino acid arginine has been shown to promote the activity of herpesvirus. Arginine-rich foods to avoid include excess barley, chocolate (though raw cacao is not reported to be a problem), coconut, coffee, nuts, oats, peanuts, and wheat. If you do consume arginine-rich foods, balance their effect by also eating lysine-rich foods. Lysine tends to inhibit the body's absorption of arginine.

Be sure to consume plenty of immune-strengthening foods such as apples, carrots, garlic, green, leafy vegetables (kale, collards, mustard greens, and spinach), onions, and winter squashes. Sea vegetables such as kelp, dulse, wakame, and hiziki also offer excellent support for the immune system, and they improve thyroid function as well. Minimize your intake of high-fat foods, especially those containing hydrogenated oils, which can make the immune system sluggish.

Herbs to include in the diet include basil, cilantro, coriander, and parsley. These green wonders are rich in antioxidants and have strong antimicrobial activity.

An alkaline diet will improve the quality of the blood and make you less susceptible to a herpes outbreak. Wild greens, such as dandelion and lamb's-quarter, can be of great help in alkalizing the blood. Avoid acidic foods such as alcohol, citrus fruits, coffee, hot spices, sugar, and tomatoes.

TOPICAL APPLICATIONS

A multitude of topical treatments have been reported to give relief, fight infection, or speed up the healing process when an outbreak occurs. Most experts agree that a moist herpes lesion should be kept dry and a dry herpes lesion kept moist, so choose from the list below accordingly.

- Aloe vera gel—soothes and dries the lesions.
- Chaparral extract or powder—dries the lesions.
- Comfrey salve—moistens the lesions and promotes wound healing.
- Echinacea extract—dries the lesions and has antiviral activity.
- Geranium essential oil—dries the lesions and has antiviral activity.
- Hyssop essential oil—dries the lesions and has antiviral activity.
- Ice—reduces inflammation, particularly in the early stages.
- Melissa (lemon balm) essential oil—dries the lesions and has antiviral activity.
- Myrrh tincture—dries the lesions and has antiviral activity.
- Osha tincture—dries the lesions and has antiviral activity.
- Propolis—dries the lesions and promotes wound healing.
- Saint John's wort oil—dries the lesions and relieves pain.
- Spirits of camphor—dries the lesions and has antiviral activity.
- Tea tree oil—dries the lesions and has antiviral activity.

- Vitamin E oil—moistens the lesions, promotes wound healing, and helps prevent scarring.
- Wine—promotes wound healing.
- Witch hazel—dries the lesions.

HERBAL THERAPY

Herbs that can help heal herpes lesions and prevent future outbreaks include the following.

Black walnut (*Juglans nigra*). One theory holds that herpesvirus blocks electromagnetic energy from flowing through the nervous system. The leaf and green nut of black walnut, which are high in ellagic acid and manganese, improve energy flow through the nervous system. They are alterative, anti-inflammatory, and antiseptic.

Burdock (*Arctium lappa*). The root improves the function of the organs of elimination and helps purify the blood and lymphatic system. It has an overall cooling effect and is alterative, anti-inflammatory, antiseptic, astringent, demulcent, febrifuge, and nutritive.

Chaparral (*Larrea tridentata*). Take 1 teaspoon of chaparral leaf tincture in 1 ounce of water first thing in the morning for twenty-one days to inactivate the virus at the first sign of an outbreak. The leaf is an alterative, antiseptic, antioxidant, antiviral, bitter tonic, and immunostimulant. Avoid in cases of liver or kidney disease, including cirrhosis or hepatitis, and during pregnancy. Discontinue use if nausea, fatigue, fever, or jaundice occur. Do not use for more than one month at a time. Consult with your health care provider before use.

Echinacea (*Echinacea purpurea, E. angustifolia*). The root stimulates macrophage and interferon activity, making cells less susceptible to viral takeover. It is an alterative, antiseptic, anti-inflammatory, antiviral, astringent, immunostimulant, and vulnerary.

Goldenseal (*Hydrastis canadensis*). The root clears heat and dries dampness. It soothes irritated mucous membranes and stimulates macrophage activity in the immune system. It is an alterative, anti-inflammatory, antiseptic, and astringent. Goldenseal is very bitter, and most people find it easiest to ingest in capsule form. Topical applications of goldenseal tincture or powder can help dry the lesions, but they will stain clothing. Avoid during pregnancy. This herb is endangered in the wild; do not use wildcrafted supplies.

Lemon balm (*Melissa officinalis*). The herb has an overall cooling effect and strengthens the nervous system. It is an antipyretic, antiviral, and nervine.

Licorice (*Glycyrrhiza glabra, G. uralensis*). The root supports the body's production of interferon and soothes irritated mucous membranes. It also helps calm the emotions. It is anti-inflammatory, antiviral, demulcent, and emollient. Avoid during pregnancy and in cases of edema, high blood pressure, or diabetes. Do not use in combination with digoxin drugs. Excessive use can cause sodium retention and potassium depletion.

Oregon grape (*Mahonia aquifolium*). The root contains the alkaloid berberine, which has strong antiseptic properties. It is also an alterative, antipyretic, antiseptic, and immunostimulant.

Peppermint (*Mentha piperita*). The herb is cooling and calming and improves circulation. It is an analgesic, anodyne, antiseptic, and antiviral.

Sarsaparilla (*Smilax* spp.). The root has an affinity for the genitourinary tract, which it helps purify and clear of eruptions. It is an alterative and a tonic.

Tea (*Camellia sinensis*). The leaf is high in tannins that coat the virus cells and can neutralize them. Because this herb also contains caffeine, its use should be limited to an occasional cup of tea. It is an analgesic, antioxidant, antiseptic, astringent, immunostimulant, and nervine.

Yellow dock (*Rumex crispus*). The root is cooling and detoxifying. Like tea, it is high in virus-neutralizing tannins. It is an alterative, antipyretic, antiseptic, antiviral, and astringent.

NUTRITIONAL THERAPY

Nutritional supplements can play an important role in supporting overall good health and making the body resistant to activation of the herpesvirus.

Acidophilus. Acidophilus boosts immune system activity; as a happy side effect, it destroys harmful bacteria. Take 2 capsules three times daily.

Beta-carotene. Beta-carotene is the precursor to vitamin A, which stimulates the production of antibodies and strengthens mucous membranes. Take 25,000 to 500,000 IU daily.

Calcium and magnesium. These two nutrients, which are often combined in a single supplement, nourish the nervous system. Take 1,000 mg of calcium and 500 mg of magnesium daily.

Essential fatty acids. EFAs strengthen cells, making them more resistant to viral infiltration. Fresh ground flaxseed, hempseed, and evening primrose oils are excellent sources of EFAs. Take 3 tablespoons daily.

Lysine. As previously explained, lysine is a potent ally against the herpesvirus. Take 500 mg daily as a preventive. When symptoms of an imminent herpes outbreak appear, increase that dosage to 500 mg three to six times daily for no more than ten days.

Vitamin B complex. Like vitamin A, the B vitamins support the production of antibodies; they also nourish the nervous system. Take 50 mg daily.

Vitamin C plus bioflavonoids. This formula can speed the healing of oral sores and strengthen capillaries. Quercetin, a component of bioflavonoids, has demonstrated antiherpes activity. Take 1,000 mg of vitamin C with 500 mg of bioflavonoids three times daily.

Vitamin E. Vitamin E helps the body make better use of oxygen, thereby supporting immune system function and promoting the healing of herpes sores. Take 400 IU daily.

CHINESE PATENT FORMULA

LUNG TAN XIE GAN PILL. According to traditional Oriental medicine, herpes infection is a condition of damp heat. The Chinese patent formula LUNG TAN XIE GAN PILL, sometimes called LONG DAN XIE GAN WAN or GENTIANA PURGE LIVER PILLS, helps clear damp heat from the body.

HOMEOPATHIC REMEDIES

When the development of herpes matches one of the descriptions below, try the suggested homeopathic remedy. The usual dosage is 4 pellets, or as many liquid drops as the package label recommends, taken under the tongue four times daily. Rather than swallowing the pellets whole, allow them to dissolve slowly.

APIS MELLIFICA. The lesions cause a stinging pain.

ARSENICUM ALBUM. The lesions are deep and bleed when the crusts are removed; they cause a shooting, burning pain. Symptoms are worse at night.

BORAX. The patient is a child.

CALCAREA CARBONICA. The skin ulcerates easily. Symptoms are worse in open air and better in a warm room.

CARBO VEGETABILIS. The lesions are evident on the chin, lips, and face. Glands swell; lesions itch, then burn when scratched.

DULCAMARA. Ulcerations are oozing and moist; they have thick brown crusts with reddish borders and occur in clusters. Symptoms are more likely to be evident during cold and wet weather, during changes in temperature, or around the time of menses.

GRAPHITES. There is a painful or clear oozing from the lesion.

HEPAR SULPHURIS CALCAREUM. This remedy can help control infection and prevent the need for antibiotics. It is particularly helpful for the patient who has tender oral sores located in the center of the lower lip and across the face toward or in the eyes, making them moist and weepy. There may be swelling in the upper lip. The lesions are sensitive to cold air.

MERCURIUS SOLUBILIS. The lesions bleed easily and burn when touched.

NATRUM MURIATICUM. The sores occur in the middle of the upper or lower lip (or both), as well as on the chin and the sides of the nose. The eruptions are moist and itchy. The infection may be stress related; the patient may be a stoic who doesn't express emotions, bears burdens silently, and rejects sympathy even though he or she craves it. This remedy is excellent when used in the early stages of infection, while the upper lip is swollen but vesicles have not yet formed. It is best used in a 200C potency, which can be obtained from a homeopathic practitioner.

NITRICUM ACIDUM. The lesions are in the corners of the mouth and may crack or feel tender. This remedy can also be used for genital outbreaks.

PSORINUM. The patient feels chilled and weak. Application of heat brings relief. Use for chronic cases that cause itching.

RHUS TOXICODENDRON. The outbreak is sudden and includes intense itching and burning. Red, irritated tissue surrounds the sore, from which acrid, crusty, yellow fluid may emerge. The cold sores erupt around the nose, lips, and chin. The patient may be sensitive to cold and dampness. If the herpes is preceded by fever and diarrhea, heat helps relieve the symptoms.

SEPIA. The patient experiences feelings of pressure, itching, constipation, and irritability. In other cases, the lesions may appear inside the nasal cavities, on the lips, and in the corners of the mouth. The face may swell, there may be dark circles under the eyes, and the patient may experience chills, exhaustion, and depression. This remedy is suitable for sores that occur during pregnancy, before menses, or during menopause.

SILICEA. The skin is very sensitive and ulcerates easily.

SULFUR. The patient experiences burning discomfort, often with a secondary infection. Heat may increase the discomfort.

THERAPEUTIC BATHS

To bring relief to a painful outbreak of genital herpes, add one of the following therapeutic formulas to the bath:

- 1 to 2 pounds of sea salt
- 1 to 2 pounds of Epsom salts
- 2 cups of apple cider vinegar
- 10 black tea bags
- 4 or 5 drops of an antiviral essential oil, such as geranium, hyssop, melissa, tea tree, wintergreen, or wormwood

Soak, relax in the warmth, and enjoy.

ACUPRESSURE

The acupressure point known as Urinary Bladder meridian point 63 can help relieve pain and even curtail an outbreak of genital herpes, if used at the first sign. The point is located three thumbs' width forward of the crown of the outer ankle bulge, moving toward the little toe. Apply deep pressure with the thumb. You should feel a twinge of sensitivity. Press this point for twenty seconds, on both feet, four or five times daily.

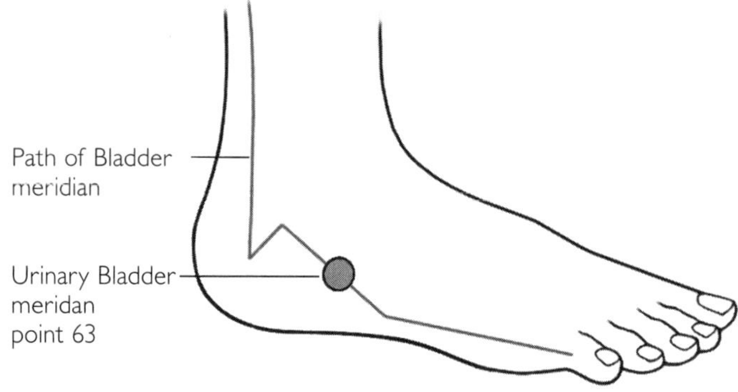

Pressure on Urinary Bladder meridian point 63 can help to prevent an outbreak of genital herpes.

SYPHILIS

Syphilis is caused by the spiral-shaped bacterium *Treponema pallidum.* The disease progresses through four stages: primary, secondary, latent, and tertiary. The primary stage occurs ten days to twelve weeks after exposure and includes the development of a small, hard lesion, known as a chancre. The chancre usually appears on the penis, vagina, or rectum but may also appear on the face or hands. It is painless and may secrete a clear fluid.

The secondary stage sets in several weeks later. Some infected persons do not experience any symptoms at this stage, but if symptoms do appear, they manifest as fever, swollen glands, fatigue, headache, joint pain, and a rash on the hands and feet. Multiple lesions may form in the mucous membranes, such as those of the mouth, throat, rectum, and vagina. The infection is highly contagious during this stage, because secretions from the lesions carry the bacteria.

During the latent stage, the disease seems to disappear. For many infected people, the infection does not progress any further. For others, it resurfaces years later, in the tertiary stage. In this stage, the bacteria spread throughout the body, causing irreversible damage to the brain, spine, heart, eyes, and other organs. It can be fatal.

Until the discovery of penicillin, syphilis was a major killer, causing dementia and a slow, agonizing decline in those who were infected. It does respond readily to antibiotic treatment, however, and its spread has been controlled in most developed countries. Control, however, does not equate to elimination. Syphilis is still present in the population of the United States.

Transmission

Syphilis is spread through direct contact with mucous membranes. It can be transmitted through vaginal, anal, and oral sex, and even kissing. If you spot a genital lesion, suspect that you have syphilis, or have been exposed to syphilis, and cease all sexual activity until you have been properly diagnosed and treated. Proper diagnosis can be made only through a blood test or microscopic examination of fluid from a sore.

Treatment

When detected early, syphilis is treatable. Antibiotic therapy—penicillin is most effective against the bacteria—is called for.

While you are taking antibiotics, add to your diet fermented foods such as rejuvelac, kombucha, plain yogurt, unpasteurized sauerkraut, apple cider vinegar, miso, and tamari. These foods support and replenish the friendly bacteria in the body.

After a course of antibiotic therapy, begin a course of acidophilus therapy to restore the friendly bacteria that are necessary for digestion, elimination, and healthy reproductive organs. Take 1 or 2 capsules three times daily for three to four months.

TRICHOMONIASIS

Trichomonas vaginalis is a parasitic single-celled protozoan. Infection with "trich," as it's called, can lead to trichomoniasis. In women trichomoniasis infects the vagina and cervix and can cause painful urination, genital itching, a green or yellow vaginal discharge that smells unpleasant (like dirty sneakers), and small reddish spots. In men trichomoniasis infects the urethra and can cause painful urination and a whitish discharge. It is often asymptomatic in men and sometimes asymptomatic in women. It frequently occurs in combination with other STDs.

Left untreated, trichomoniasis can result in cervicitis, fertility dysfunctions, urethritis, and prostatitis.

Transmission

Though trichomoniasis is usually transmitted through sexual contact, the parasite can survive for several hours outside the body and be transmitted through the sharing of towels, washcloths, underclothing, sex toys, and similar items.

Treatment

Trichomoniasis can be treated successfully with natural therapies. The therapies focus on strengthening the body's immune system and making the vagina or urethra an inhospitable environment for the protozoans.

Men who suspect they have trichomoniasis should avoid ejaculating, because semen nourishes the protozoans. If the diagnosis is confirmed, continue to avoid ejaculating for a total of ten days.

Women who suspect they have contracted trichomoniasis should begin using an antiseptic suppository until diagnosed. Soak a tampon in a mixture of 2 tablespoons of apple cider vinegar, 1 drop of tea tree essential oil, and 2 cups of warm water. Insert the tampon; do not remove for at least four hours. Skip the suppository treatment on the day you're going to be tested, as it can affect the test results.

HERBAL THERAPY

Herbs that support the immune system, nurture overall health, and fight off infection are especially helpful for treating trichomoniasis.

Calendula (*Calendula officinalis*). The flower increases peripheral circulation and helps dispel infections that are trapped in the body. It is an alterative, antifungal, anti-inflammatory, antiseptic, and vulnerary.

Chaparral (*Larrea tridentata*). The leaf is an alterative, antiseptic, antioxidant, antiviral, bitter tonic, and immunostimulant. Avoid in cases of liver or kidney disease, including cirrhosis or hepatitis, and during pregnancy. Discontinue use if nausea, fatigue, fever, or jaundice occur. Do not use for more than a month at a time. Consult with your health care provider before use.

Echinacea (*Echinacea purpurea, E. angustifolia*). The root has a powerfully stimulating effect on the immune system. It is also an alterative, antifungal, and antiseptic.

Garlic (*Allium sativum*). The bulb contains compounds that help the body resist a wide range of pathogens. It is an alterative, antibiotic, antioxidant, antiseptic, immunostimulant, and vasodilator. Try eating a clove of raw garlic daily. Some people are allergic to garlic. Excessive use can cause emotional irritability and irritation of the stomach and kidneys. Avoid therapeutic doses during pregnancy; also avoid during the first three months of nursing, as it can cause breast milk to become unpalatable for infants. Avoid eating garlic for one week before having surgery.

Goldenseal (*Hydrastis canadensis*). The root is active against a wide range of pathogens and is especially effective for relieving inflammation of the mucous membranes. It is an alterative and an antibiotic. Goldenseal is very bitter, and most people find it easiest to ingest in capsule form. Avoid during pregnancy. This herb is endangered in the wild; do not use wildcrafted supplies.

Licorice (*Glycyrrhiza glabra, G. uralensis*). The root boosts immune system function and soothes irritated tissues. It is an antibiotic, anti-inflammatory, antiviral, and nutritive. Avoid during pregnancy and in cases of edema, high blood pressure, or diabetes. Do not use in combination with digoxin drugs. Excessive use can cause sodium retention and potassium depletion.

Nettle (*Urtica dioica, U. urens*). The leaf is rich in chlorophyll. It builds overall health, inhibits infection, and speeds healing. It is an alterative, circulatory stimulant, and antiparasitic. Contact with the fresh plant will irritate the skin. Use only dried herb. Wear gloves when collecting.

Usnea (*Usnea barbata*). The lichen helps rid the body of infection without killing friendly intestinal flora. It is an antibiotic, antifungal, and immunostimulant.

VINEGAR DOUCHE

A douche made from 2 tablespoons of apple cider vinegar and 4 cups of warm water can help clear the infection. Douche just twice daily; getting overzealous with this treatment can wash away friendly vaginal flora.

SUPPOSITORIES

A garlic clove or 2 capsules of acidophilus can be used as vaginal suppositories to eliminate the infection. See page 250 for instructions. The garlic has an antiparasitic effect; acidophilus supports friendly vaginal flora that compete with *Trichomonas vaginalis.*

SITZ BATHS

Sitz baths increase circulation to the pelvic area, which can bring great relief to people suffering trichomoniasis symptoms. See page 169 for instructions on how to prepare a sitz bath. Add to the tub 1 cup of apple cider vinegar and the juice from 7 cloves of garlic.

PART FOUR

Love and Relationships

WORLD PEACE begins in the bedroom. If you want to do something wonderful for your children, your community, and humanity, focus on building a good relationship with your partner.

Few of us were blessed with healthy relationship role models. We've journeyed long and far in search of the meaning of love, and we've made mistakes—some that we regret, and some that we appreciate—as we've tried to negotiate the mountains and quagmires that stand in front of a good relationship. With luck, we've learned what it takes. That lesson is the most important tool we can give to our children. Strong relationships are gifts of love to the world.

Relationships are like two stones in a tumbler. We can get out of the tumbler. We can stay in and get cracked. Or we can hang in there, tumbling together, polishing our rough edges, and emerge as gleaming gems.

20 The Fine Art of Flirting and Attracting a Mate

SINCE WE ARE NOT usually born knowing who our love-mates are, most of us go through one or more periods of seeking a partner. For those readers who are fortunate enough to have found their mates, think of this chapter as advice to help your single friends who are still questing for their soul's complement. What follows are a multitude of ideas and inspirations to help you make that connection that will lead to true love, or maybe just great sex, or best yet—both!

ABOVE ALL, LOVE YOURSELF

Love is attracted to love. When you shine with tenderness for yourself, others will want to be around you, and to be loved by you. So start by loving yourself. Write down ten qualities you appreciate about yourself. For example, you might note that you are grateful for your vision, your ability to sing, your talent in the garden, your facility with numbers, or whatever else serves you.

Next write down seven aspects of yourself that you would like to improve upon, followed by a dozen things you will do to improve yourself.

Be Positive

Having a positive attitude toward yourself and others will improve your experience of each day—and will draw others to you. Pay attention to what you say. Do you hear yourself saying things like, "I can't," or "I should"? Or "I shouldn't," or "I hope"? If so, turn those mantras around! Try telling yourself and others "I can!" Or "I will." Optimistic suggestions will eventually penetrate your consciousness and disempower any negative thoughts. Even if you don't believe your affirmations at first, continuing to say them will help you realize them even sooner. Better yet, write them down and post them where you will see them often. Either way, it's free!

EXAMPLES OF AFFIRMATIONS

- Every day I am growing more loving and attracting love.
- I consciously make the right choices to attract loving relations into my life.
- Everything I choose to eat adds to my health, beauty, and attractiveness.
- I am good to myself.
- I am good to others.
- I am grateful for all the help and blessings that are in my life.
- My body is beautiful and ageless.
- My mind is alert.
- I appreciate all the help I have in bringing love into my life.

Of course, you can create your own affirmations, depending on what your needs are. Just be sure that they are positively phrased, so that they affirm the self you want to become.

Delight in Your Own Sensuality

Don't save it all for someone else or for when you meet "the one." Wear your beautiful clothes now. Smell flowers today. Enjoy fresh fruit, breath-giving baths, and massages. Enjoy the delights of life for their own sake. Rather than focusing on finding the ideal person, pay attention to being the ideal person. A happy person has a better chance of connecting in a relationship than one who is immersed in negativity. Open yourself to attracting what is positive and for the highest good.

Sensual fabrics might make people want to touch you, such as cashmere, sand-washed rayon, velvet, satin, and soft silk. Go global and wear your true colors in hemp or organic cotton. Cool and comfortable lingerie can make you feel sexy and confident. Wearing ripped, stained underwear can inhibit spontaneity and make you feel less than honored.

Present Your Best Self to Others

Present yourself as capable and knowledgeable. Radiate confidence. Too many people focus only on their outer assets to attract a mate: clothes, car, and career. Remember that a healthy lifestyle and spiritual reflection helps to harmonize your vibration.

It is certainly fair to make yourself look clean, attractive, and sexy, using hair, clothing, and friendliness. Look and feel your best so you are ready to encounter people and don't feel like you need to hide. (I once had a girlfriend who would see the man of her dreams in Whole Foods, then run and hide, because she was in baggy sweats!)

Express yourself! Wear your love like heaven! While on this planet we can be expressions of truth, beauty, and goodness. However we see fit. Colors are rainbow opportunities. Gray, olive green, and brown may be reminiscent of the military or camouflage you. What are your intentions? Wearing red in autumn and winter might make you seem cozy to snuggle up against. If you want to be noticed at night, light colors stand out.

For women (and men too for all they may desire!) jewelry, eye makeup, and hair ornaments are all glimpse-catching. Jewelry adds light and color and can be used to emphasize features. If you like, outline your eyes and highlight your best facial features. It's a time-tested tradition that often gets people to look deeper into your eyes.

For men, look and smell clean. Trim your beard if you wear one to allow lips and cheekbones to be visible. Wear sensuous fabrics like silk, sand-washed rayon, and soft cottons.

HOW TO MEET A GREAT DATE

Make a list of the qualities you want in a partner. Though the list may be long, write everything down. Give each item a number that indicates its importance to you. Roll up the list. Tie it with a red string or ribbon and place it in the relationship sector (farthest right from the door) of your bedroom. (See chapter 8 on feng shui.) Visualize yourself with the person you love.

Read your list out loud three times daily for three days in a row, then burn the piece of paper over a sink, while visualizing you are sending your prayers out into the You-niverse. Don't stand by the smoke detector while doing this.

Pray for someone to love you as much as you love them . . . at the same time (an important clause)! Tell your friends you are available and looking. The more people you meet, the better your chances of finding someone wonderful. Ask your friends how they met. Talk to happily married couples on what some of their success secrets are. Read this book and others!

The Science and Art of Flirting

For many people, flirting has become a lost art. Yet it is a powerful way of signaling to others that you are open to interaction. A playful conversation (whether verbal or nonverbal) can be enjoyed for its own sake and can also lead to someone wanting to get to know you better.

Flirting increases endorphin production and is a great way to delight in your own sexiness. It is an art that shouldn't be too obvious: do it for your own pleasure rather than with a goal in mind. Friendliness is key.

Smile. Even making your mouth into the crescent shape of a smile increases cerebral blood flow and the release of neurotransmitters. When someone else's smile meets yours, the moon circle is complete.

You can't flirt alone in your home. You must go out. Women may find flirting more effective during the first half of their menstrual cycle, before progesterone levels elevate. You could even consult the planetary aspects in selecting the most auspicious times.

Have a business or calling card. You needn't include your address or e-mail (or phone number) and you don't have to have an occupation listed. Always have a pen and paper ready to get or give a phone number. (You never know when you might have an opportunity for a moment of truth!) Initially, it might be best to give only a daytime work number until you are sure of a person's integrity. But do exchange numbers!

Practice flirting with all kinds of people—it's fun! The best place to meet someone to flirt with is at an activity or event that interests you, whether it's an art opening, the gym, church, synagogue, classes, sports activities, or political and environmental group meetings. For others, it could be ayahuasca ceremonies, raves, coffeehouses that serve herbal tea, or exotic restaurants. (*Okay, I admit I met my husband in a bar. But I was with the band!*)

Volunteer for groups that support your philosophy. Show off your best talents. Sing! Play ball! If you only go to women or men's support groups, classes, or gyms you will only meet people of the same sex. (Which is perfect if that is what you are looking for.) Spend time in the coed steam room and whirlpool. Stagger the times you go to the gym, and so forth, so you encounter different people. Check things out.

Ask for advice at hobby and sports stores. Natural food stores and farmers' markets can be good places to meet health-conscious, hip people. At grocery stores, ask someone what to do with an unusual food. Talk to people in video or music stores. Ask them if they've seen a movie you're considering, or if they can suggest something for you. Comment on their choice. Perhaps, "That's a fabulous movie, book, CD!"

Ask someone cute for directions. Carry an interesting conversation piece with you—like a favorite book or an unusual piece of jewelry. Wear a button with a statement on it, interesting enough to provoke a comment (*Make Love Not War*). As Mae West said it so memorably, it's "better to be looked over than overlooked."

If it's a book you carry, have the title visible, which might connect you with someone of similar interests. I know that the *Urantia* book I often carry has gotten the attention of some very interesting folks in my life . . .

When you see someone who looks interesting, seize the moment and make contact. Even say, "I have this feeling we are supposed to meet. My name is . . ."

Extend your hand and introduce yourself. Make the first handshake count. Don't oversqueeze and crush a person's fingers. Radiate vitality and energy as if an electric current were coursing through you. If you really want to get someone's attention while shaking hands, you can reach out and quickly and slightly brush the fingers of their right hand with your left hand. Do this quickly so it is barely noticed.

Don't overdo the eye contact or you can make a person uncomfortable. Use your eyes to register warmth and interest in the person you seek. Make eye contact, then gaze toward their lips or body, and then slowly back to their eyes. Flirting often commences with a smile, a pout, a flash of the eyebrows, and brief eye contact. Slowly proceed to make more eye contact a few times.

Learn to read (and use) body language: if someone is looking at you with raised eyes, lips parted, and a slightly open jaw, toes pointed inward, or a shoulder raised, they might be interested in you! Caressing an object such as a glass or key chain, or unnecessary primping of hair and smoothing of clothing (called *preening*) are often subconscious signs that someone is interested in a person in their vicinity. Men preen by adjusting hats, pulling up socks, or straightening ties or collars. Women preen by straightening their hair or their clothing.

If you advertise in a classified column for singles, do it in the kind of publication the person you would like to meet would read. Personal ads can be more effective if you place your own, getting many responses rather than answering one. Focus on listing what you want in a partner rather than what you don't want. (Of course, when meeting a stranger, stay in public, well-lit places and take your time before giving out too much information.)

Go to parties. Nightclubs and bars can be too noisy for getting to know anyone. When entering a room, do it with pizzazz. Enter and stop. (*This is where I like to take off my black velvet cape.*) Turn around and do a half turn, giving people the opportunity to check you out and slowly look into the room, while looking about a foot lower than people's heads; as you are not yet ready to engage. Take a big breath, give a half smile, and you have just made a dramatic entrance! By being noticed you increase your potential for being seen for who you are.

The best place to stand at a party is to the right of the entrance, as 90 percent of partygoers will veer to the right when entering a room. Be at least ten feet away from the door, though, to give people a chance to acclimate and not feel bombarded. Other choice places to connect are in the back of the room, which is a place of authority, and in smaller rooms where people will have to stand closer together and conversations can be more intimate.

Find something to sincerely compliment. Rather than using a line, say something that is very individual. Instead of asking someone "What do you do?" which often comes across as "How much money you make?" try, "What did you do today?" or "What is your opinion?" or "What was the best part of your day?" Ask questions that you would sincerely like to hear the answers to. At a party, ask someone interesting how they know the host. Mentioning names is okay. It doesn't have to be dropping names of the rich or infamous; when you find out that you have friends in common with someone, it brings you closer.

Use the name of a person you just met three times in conversation so you will remember it and they will feel noticed. Remind your companion of your name.

Dance with anyone that asks. If someone desirable sees you rejecting dance offers, they might not ask you. Dancing is an opportunity to make yourself visible and to express creativity. What's three minutes out of your life? It can be a kind way of making someone's day or week. You get the exercise. Just be sure to excuse yourself after one dance if that is your intention.

Make it clear whom you are flirting with. Approaching an entire group could leave everyone thinking you are after their friend. If in close quarters, gently brush past the one you have your eye on and make contact, placing your hand on his or her arm (considered neutral territory) for a brief moment as you say, "Excuse me." If you are always hanging out with a crowd, it makes you less approachable.

When you have an opportunity to have a conversation with someone you like, put personal problems aside for a while. Better to be the bearer of good news. Talking negatively about a previous love can make a current prospect wonder what you might say about them someday.

Speak softly, so the two of you will have to stand close to each other. Tell him or her a secret (not a real big one you swore to keep) to create a moment of depth and intimacy. (*I'm having brunch with the author Tom Robbins tomorrow!*) When talking, occasionally moisten your lips with your tongue and widen your eyes.

Watch where you put your hands. For both men and women, being patted on the back too early in an encounter can feel patronizing. Touching the face of someone you barely know is often perceived as an attempt to encroach on their personal territory.

Leave them wanting more. By staying too long, your allure dwindles. Flirt, make an impression, and then back off. Try, "I should go talk to my neighbor, but I want to tell you something later." Then make a quick comeback later with less intensity—to get your jacket, or to say good-bye.

Finding the Next Steps

It may be wise to avoid telling a person you are attracted to them, unless you have gotten some hints they feel the same way. This is especially true for women, who need to give men the opportunity to fulfill their ancient hunter instincts of enjoying the chase.

If you get asked out and you are not available for that time, suggest another possibility. If you are asked out and you know there is no potential, it is kinder to say, "I don't think we have enough in common to date, but I'm glad we met." This is kinder than not returning phone calls.

Politeness, honesty, and sincerity will take you far. Be friends first. We tend to like people we frequently see. Find a way to run into your heart's desire more often, if possible make a repeated appearance. Play back details of your previous encounter the next time you meet. "How was the concert you were going to last week?" "How's your mom doing?" This helps forge emotional bonds.

Allowing a person of interest to help and protect you is one of the oldest flirting techniques in the world. Men love to be heroes. Ask him to reach something high up, undo a stuck jar lid, or some other act. Women can be asked to offer help in so many wise ways—healing, feeding, and knowing.

If you're talking with someone you are interested in, mirror his or her movements. Walk in step. Breathe in synch. Match their volume. Sit or stand facing the person you're speaking with, rather than sideways, which creates cutting chi. Lean toward them. When they shift, copy their shift. If they put their hand on the back of a chair, follow suit. This is called mirroring, and it can be followed after a few seconds and does not need to be exact, just similar. Many people do this unconsciously when they are speaking with someone they like. It has a powerful psychological effect and fosters rapport and trust. The listener mirrors the speaker.

Later, after you know each other, you can make touching contact—bare skin to skin is the most effective. If contact gets made let it become more prolonged. Brush hair out of his or her eyes. Brush lint off a jacket. Preen each other. Use two fingers to do a quick walk on someone's arm. Women can cross their legs, squeezing them together to convey excitement.

Early on, stay away from strong sexual comments, which give the impression you are just out to get laid. Many women and men are turned off by rude and crude. Sending out sexual availability messages, then acting shocked or angry when someone makes a pass is unfairly confusing. Be kind.

Dress nicely, especially for a first date. It doesn't hurt at all to always put care into your appearance, even after decades of marriage. On a date, ask questions about the person you are with. How did they get into their career? What was their family like? What brought them to this part of the country? Be a good listener. Nod and say "uh huh" once in a while.

Find something positive to say. Always complaining about the food, band, movie, and so on, can make you seem difficult to please. Before inviting someone to a restaurant, movie, concert, or play, find out if it is worthy. Read reviews and/or talk to friends. Spending time and money for less than enjoyable events can be disappointing. Though of course, sometimes it is inevitable. Our time is precious. Spend it wisely.

The general rule is, whoever did the asking out, pays. After a first date, you can split the bill, take turns, or make dinner for one who has taken you out several times. Have a reasonably clean home with some welcoming snacks to share with your friend. If you always require being taken out to catch a bite, you might just seem too much to keep up with. Subconsciously, your date might think that a life lived in restaurants might have little return in ways of health or savings.

Avoid telling your entire life story too soon. Have some boundaries. Avoid talking about other past relationships excessively early on or openly flirting with someone else on a date. Appearing too eager early in a relationship takes away the thrill of the chase. Avoid, "I want you to meet my parents" on the second date, or "Are you available for New Year's?" when it's only June. In the beginning of a relationship avoid overwhelming someone with too many calls and flowers. If those kinds of things are overdone you can appear too eager and even desperate.

Giving a small gift is okay, but gifts that are too large intimidate. Early on, a single flower can be sweeter than a whole bouquet.

GETTING PHYSICAL

The first time you get intimate with someone, consider stopping after the first kiss, leaving him or her turned on and wanting more. Show you have respect for your partner and self-control. Keep it light and exploratory, sensual and unhurried.

Stay sober. Drink slowly. Never decide to sleep with someone when intoxicated or altered. Decide beforehand, and stick to your decision. Decisions made under the influence are often regretted. Sleeping with someone can cause a hormonal reaction that makes you think you are more in love than you are. Having sex too soon in a relationship can cloud and distort your perception, causing you to feel and expect more than might be appropriate. Getting sexually intimate too soon also connects you to the other person's energy and emotions—which you may later regret. And once you have been sexually intimate, it can be difficult to say no the next time. Make sure you are truly compatible and think there is a possibility for a relationship. Wait at least until the third date, and even longer if that's what it takes. Though I admit, we didn't always follow those rules in the 1960s and '70s.

If you spend the night with someone, no matter how awesome it was, give him or her space to contemplate you and leave him or her wanting more. If you are there for breakfast, lunch, and dinner the next day after your first encounter, they may start thinking about how to get rid of you rather than how to see more of you.

Avoid saying "I love you" too soon as it can cause one to be overly vulnerable and lack credibility. Women who are smart know that giving men a chance to pursue is exciting to them. Women should be careful about taking too much for granted—calling a man your boyfriend when you've only had two dates or making long-term plans can make someone feel trapped. And avoid being taken for granted: if you are always available and always doing the initiating, he will be wanting less, not more, from you. It really is best to let the man show he is interested, otherwise he can feel that too much is being demanded of him and pull away. You might not agree, but knowing this aspect of psychology helps you get the love you desire.

WHAT KIND OF PERSON ARE YOU LOOKING FOR?

An important element to look for in a lover is someone who brings out the best in you. Someone quick to praise, to show appreciation, and be a good listener. Protect your heart by being careful about whom you give it to. Look for warning signals on those first few encounters and get out early if you see things you couldn't live with.

Look for someone who supports a healthy lifestyle. Does the person you have an interest in treat others in friendship and business ethically? Make a living in a respectable manner? Is this person honest? Reliable? Do they have old friends? Are they financially stable? What do their ex-lovers/spouses say about them? How do they get along with their parents?

It's not that you can't work with some of life's difficulties, but if there are many warning signs early on, it probably won't get better without lots of work. People who are addicted to substances, have intense anger issues, hate their families, or have no friends might have lots to work on that you may or may not be able to help with. When someone tells you they are not interested in or deserving of a relationship, believe them. When they proclaim they just want to be friends, need space, or that you are too good for them—take their word. You've been warned.

People who are married, living with someone, just broken up, or sleeping with someone else are usually not looking for a new relationship. Play it cool. They may become available later on.

Learn to read a potential partner. Are they more visual? Auditory? Or feeling-centered? If your partner is mostly attuned to sound, you can spend hours dressing and cleaning, but the sound of your voice and tone is what will really move them. The visual person cares most about how things look. Your looks, home, and food presentation might be of value. The feeling person is affected by how things feel. What kind of vibes are being put out?

It can take up to a dozen relationships to know what it is you do or don't want. It may be safe to assume that many people come from somewhat dysfunctional families. Unconsciously we often find partners that mimic some of the positive and negative behaviors of our parents. This can be an opportunity to heal past circumstances and drama. Unfortunately, many are raised with violence, sexual abuse, abandonment, and addiction. When childhood is over, we often return to similar patterns. Rather than getting stuck and having the same issues, we help change a negative pattern and make the world a better place!

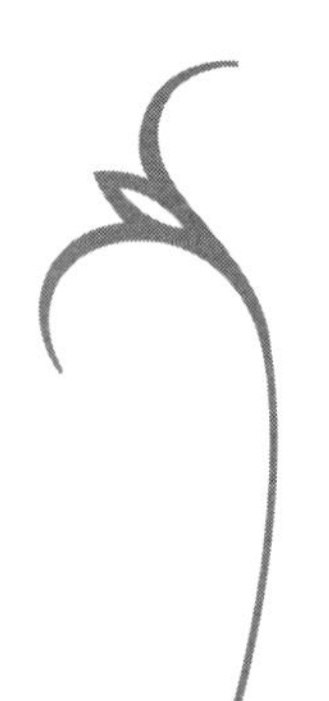

21
Keep Your Love Alive
The Twenty-five Principles of a Strong Relationship

RELATIONSHIPS ARE LIKE PLANTS. They thrive when cared for; they wither when neglected. To maintain a commitment to a lover, we must learn to tend our relationships as if they were gardens, cultivating the flowers of spiritual fulfillment and the fruits of earthly nourishment. How? By following the twenty-five principles listed here.

THE TWENTY-FIVE PRINCIPLES

1. Understand that relationships take work.
2. Make a commitment to daily appreciation.
3. Be kind.
4. Practice romance.
5. Respect each other's sexual energy.
6. Make your relationship a priority.
7. Make time for sex.
8. Allow spiritual energy to imbue your relationship with higher meaning.
9. Keep your voice pleasant.
10. Develop mutual interests. Allow space for individual interests. Help each other with things.

11. Spend time with couples who are positive role models.
12. Evolve together.
13. Make room for quiet time with each other.
14. Communicate.
15. Praise in public; criticize in private.
16. Express, rather than accuse.
17. When having an argument, stick with the issue at hand.
18. Argue from both sides.
19. Be affectionate.
20. Greet each other warmly.
21. If you have children, find a babysitter whom you trust implicitly.
22. If you have children, maintain a united front.
23. Give gifts.
24. Be open to therapy.
25. Be responsible for your own happiness.

1. Understand that relationships take work.

The marriage cliché "This match was made in heaven" is both erroneous and potentially harmful. There are no perfect relationships or even perfect mates. A marriage or committed relationship is made and continually remade by two people who work very hard at it.

Fuel your love with daily expressions of affection, appreciation, and attention. Upon waking each morning, turn to face your partner and remind yourself why you are in love with this person. Be willing to nourish love and to repair it when necessary. Celebrate love! Celebrate life! Keep the magic alive.

2. Make a commitment to daily appreciation.

Never take the love, presence, or daily contributions of a lover for granted. Express appreciation not only for acts that go above and beyond what you might expect but also for the mundane—meals prepared, lawn mowed, car fixed, and so on. Let your lover know every day that he or she is appreciated.

Be generous with compliments not only about the way a partner looks but also about what he or she says and does. Appreciate each other's strengths. Accept each other's weaknesses.

3. Be kind.

Simple acts of kindness can go a long way toward strengthening a relationship. You and your partner should each try to perform at least one act of selfless kindness for each other each day. When your beloved is stressed out, offer to give a back massage or to run a tub so that he or she can take a relaxing bath. If your mate will be out late, leave a light on when you retire to bed. Surprise your mate occasionally by taking care of some of his or her usual chores.

Practice politeness. Being polite to each other, day in and day out, helps you build, support, and express a measure of respect for each other. And when politeness becomes a habit, it can help you maintain civility and remind you of your connection in times of marital strife.

Some conflict is normal in relationships. Everyone is entitled to an occasional bad mood. How you treat each other during these times of difficulty is a gauge of the strength of your relationship.

4. Practice romance.

Find ways to be romantic every day. Remember all those "silly" things you used to do to try to make a good impression when you were courting? Don't stop doing them now, just because you're in a committed relationship. Long-term relations should be given more effort, not less, than courtship.

Go on regular dates, taking turns planning them. Plan for special times and surprises. Dress up for each other. Take walks after dinner. Hold hands. Enjoy nature together. Go on elegant picnics, even in your own backyard. Eat in romantic places—by the shore, fireplace, overlooking the city. Have teatime. Work on a project together, such as starting a garden and preparing the food you grow. Make your home beautiful with candles, art, and music. Obtain a guidebook for your region or town and explore together the local sights and scenes you've never visited. Look at the stars.

Leave love notes for each other. Write poems together. If you have to be away for a few days, leave your beloved a farewell note. While you're away, send home a postcard, even if you'll end up returning home first.

5. Respect each other's sexual energy.

Sexual energy is like the changing Moon. Sometimes we are filled with desire; other times, we would rather lie quietly next to our beloved, enjoying intimacy without sex. No matter how great a relationship is, there will be times of mismatched libido. There are times in life where the ultimate pleasure might be a foot massage!

However, if lovers always waited to have sex until they were both in a high state of arousal, sex would be a rare occurrence. Be patient. You didn't choose to be with each other just so you'd always have someone to have sex with. Give yourselves the space to say no when you're not in the mood.

Make masturbation a part of your sexual repertoire; if you don't feel sexual but your partner does, he or she could masturbate while you hold and kiss him or her. You might also offer to please your beloved orally or manually. And recognize that it is perfectly acceptable for your partner to simply "go for it" once in a while, meeting his or her own needs.

Most important, communicate. It's better to say "no" than to say "yes" and make love with a "no" attitude.

6. Make your relationship a priority.

Your lover should always feel that he or she is more important to you than your job, your parents, your hobby, the television, or anything else. You would never start a business, putting tremendous energy into it for the first few years, and then expect it to thrive without any effort. Should you do less for love?

In the same vein, your lover may occasionally be involved in a project that requires all of his or her attention for a short span of time. During this time, recognize that supporting the relationship is more important than allowing yourself to feel neglected. Find ways to keep yourself occupied rather than adding to the burden by making your lover feel guilty for not paying attention to you. Remind yourself that your job is to keep your relationship strong so that, when the project is finished, your lover can return to you with joy and gratefulness for your support. Thank you, Tom, for all the yerba matés and raw cacao treats while I write.

7. Make time for sex.

Making time for sex is essential for a healthy relationship. Too often sex happens late at night, when you're exhausted, or first thing in the morning, when you have to be at work in an hour. Though these quickies can be lovely expressions of pure physical lust (not every sexual experience has to be long and romantic), saving sex for last indicates that it's your last priority.

Schedule sacred times for making love, such as sunset, evenings of the full moon (open the windows), sunrise (set your alarm clock for an early hour and leave enough time for a nap afterward), solstices, equinoxes, and Sunday afternoons. Build sexual connection into your celebration of the holidays. For example, instead of toasting midnight on New Year's Eve, try making love instead.

Wait two or three hours after eating before having sex. It's difficult for the body to supply chi and blood to both the sexual organs and the digestive system at the same time. Instead of eating before bedtime, save some hunger for your beloved.

8. Allow spiritual energy to imbue your relationship with higher meaning.

Spiritual depth in a relationship lends meaning to life. Find a form of faith, organized or not, that allows spiritual energy to flow through your lives. Pray together. Give thanks for your blessings, including your love. Honor the god and goddess in each other. If you are of different faiths, participate occasionally in each other's ceremonies and services.

9. Keep your voice pleasant.

Voice can be an important factor in attraction. A high voice indicates lower sexual vitality; a low voice indicates greater sexual vitality. Do your best to modulate your voice, avoiding shrill tones, shrieking, and mumbling. If you're not sure what you sound like, record yourself speaking and then play it back.

When you speak to your lover, inject warmth into your voice. Use your beloved's name often, always allowing the name to come softly and lovingly from your lips.

10. Develop mutual interests. Allow space for individual interests.

Don't let children, finances, or other conveniences be the glue that keeps you together. Occasionally do something with your partner that he or she enjoys and you could care less about. Do it with good cheer. Make a practice of finding at least three things you like about it, rather than grumbling or being critical. Enjoy your beloved's enjoyment!

Have friends in common, but also have friends on an individual level.

Give each other space to spend time alone with friends. (And find goodness in at least a few of your partner's friends.)

11. Spend time with couples who are positive role models.

If you only spend time with friends who complain constantly about their relationship, watch out. It could rub off. Instead, surround yourself with positive role models who bring positive energy to your relationship.

Of course, you should certainly be there for your friends when they're struggling with relationship problems. But if they're always telling the same story of trouble and grief, without progress, it may be time to remove yourself from the circle of negative energy.

As for yourself, if you find that you are complaining about marital problems to a friend, resolve that you will spend twice as much time discussing the issue with your beloved.

12. Evolve together.

The only constant in human life is change. Over the course of a long-term relationship, partners will find that they each continue to grow and learn, and not always together or in the same manner. Rather than getting hung up on what's different about each other, partners must learn to appreciate their differences. Recognizing that a person is never the same from one day to the next, see your partner's evolution as an opportunity to learn more about him or her and to grow and evolve yourself.

If your beloved is developing a new passion, learn more about it so that you can support and encourage his or her new dreams. And develop new passions together, such as pottery, yoga, dance, tennis, drawing, massage, and so on. Every once in a while take a class on enhancing relationship and communication skills.

13. Make room for quiet time with each other.

Find at least twenty minutes a day when you and your partner can speak with each other undisturbed, whether to share concerns or just to check in with each other. Do this beyond the reach of the television, the radio, the phone, or the kids. If you find that the only time you have together is in the evening, don't save your twenty minutes for bedtime, when you're exhausted. Instead, put your kids to bed with a lovely story, turn off the television and the computer, and sit down with each other at a reasonable hour.

14. Communicate.

When you communicate with your beloved, do so honestly, openly, and considerately. Share with each other your feelings, hurts, fears, and disappointments. Be supportive of each other. Thank each other for sharing. Don't dismiss your partner's feelings in an effort to help him or her stop crying. Instead, be a good listener. Allow your beloved to express his or her feelings fully and openly. Don't attempt to problem-solve unless you're sure that your partner wants you to; sometimes a person who is upset doesn't want a solution to the problem so much as just a quiet space and a willing listener.

In Oriental medicine, the tongue is governed by the Heart system. How we talk can open or close the heart to love. Rough words are harsh on the heart. When talking, use hand gestures that take in your partner, indicating appreciation. Truly listen when your beloved speaks, rather than planning your response.

15. Praise in public; criticize in private.

In front of others, praise and criticism have significantly greater impact. Therefore, whenever possible, praise in public, building up your beloved in a way that shows your love and support. Reserve criticism for private times, when you can speak kindly and won't embarrass your beloved in front of others.

Above all, be generous with praise and words of love. There will be times when you'll want to criticize your beloved, but make sure that you praise at least three times as much as you criticize.

16. Express, rather than accuse.

Avoid speaking in an accusatory manner. Speaking of your own needs rather than of your partner's lack will neatly remove accusations from your vocabulary. For example, instead of saying "You always . . ." or "You never . . . ," try "I feel . . ." or "I need . . ." Rather than saying "You never help with housework," try "I feel that I am doing all the housework."

Taping a discussion or argument and listening to it later by yourself or together can be an opportunity to evaluate and improve communication skills. You and your partner should both work on being nondefensive. After one partner has expressed a feeling, the listener should mirror back what he or she heard to make sure that the issue is clear. For example, your lover might say back to you, "I hear you saying that the housework is not split evenly between us."

17. When having an argument, stick with the issue at hand.

The golden rule for a healthy argument is "One issue, one argument." Discussing just one issue at a time keeps negative emotions in check and allows you to focus on finding a solution for a particular problem, instead of just getting angry at each other.

When an argument becomes heated, practice using a "talking stick." Pick out a special stick, crystal, rock, or other item and designate it as the talking stick. Only when you are holding the talking stick are you are allowed to speak—and then without interruption, until you are finished. Pass the stick back and forth until the issue has been cleared.

A sincere apology spoken by one or both partners can be a powerful defuser of tension, as can a simple offer such as, "How can I help?"

18. Argue from both sides.

When communication over a problematic issue breaks down, write a letter to your partner, expressing your feelings and point of view. Then write a letter that you believe expresses your partner's feelings and viewpoint. Your partner should do the same. Then trade letters.

19. Be affectionate.

Physical affection is important for maintaining and building emotional affection. It can help smooth over negative emotions lingering after an argument. A light caress on the shoulders lets your beloved know that you're thinking about her as she works at the computer. A kiss on the cheek when your lover walks in the door tells him that you are delighted to see him.

Delight in one another's embrace! There doesn't have to be a reason other than maintaining that heart-to-heart connection. Connect in a loving way daily—through eye contact, kissing, hugging, dancing, massage, caresses, and loving words.

Create your own rituals. Every time my husband and I are walking over a bridge, we stop for a kiss. Every time we are alone in an elevator, we make out.

Try to go to bed at the same time at least a few times a week to ensure more opportunities for connection. If you need to stay up, at least tuck in your beloved and share some talk and cuddling before going back to the television, the computer, or whatever is keeping you up.

20. Greet each other warmly.

Let your relationship be a place to retreat to instead of a place to escape from. When you or your beloved returns home, greet each other warmly. Let each other know that you're pleased by the other's presence. If you're engrossed in an activity, no matter what it is, at least pick up your head, smile, and welcome your lover back to you.

If you happen to be at home awaiting the arrival of your partner, take a few minutes to straighten up the house. It can make for a wonderful reception. It's harder to relax when things are messy. Unclutter countertops and rooms. Sweep up. Empty the dishwasher. Light a candle, and turn on some music. When your lover walks in the door, she or he will immediately feel more relaxed, and very much welcome.

21. If you have children, find a babysitter whom you trust implicitly.

Having a babysitter you can trust allows you to enjoy time away from your kids—which is vital for a healthy relationship—with total confidence. Occasionally, have the babysitter take the kids out so that you can quietly enjoy the pleasures of your own home.

22. If you have children, maintain a united front.

Do not allow children to divide and conquer. It weakens their respect for you, can demoralize the parent who says "no" when the other parent says "yes," and can lead to parental bickering. Instead, discuss in private how to deal with issues related to the kids. Then keep a united front, no matter what sort of begging and pleading you're subjected to.

23. Give gifts.

Giving a gift can be as delightful as receiving one, and unexpected gifts help maintain warmth, laughter, and kindness in a relationship. Gifts don't have to be expensive. Try gift certificates, books, music, your beloved's favorite snack, or other small treats. Roses are nice but also predictable. Have a stash of gifts that you can dip in to when the moment calls for one.

A true gift of love is something you make with your own hands. When I first realized that Tom (now my husband) was my true love, I embroidered a beautiful mandala on a T-shirt for him. It was the same mandala he had as a decoration on his Jeep the night we first met, when he gave me a ride home from a rock concert. More than thirty years later, he still has that T-shirt.

Do not give a gift with an ulterior motive, such as giving your partner a book because you'd like him to read more or a pair of skis because you love winter sports and you wish she did, too.

When you receive a gift from your beloved, accept it graciously and warmly, even if you're not delighted with it. If your beloved keeps picking out gifts that don't suit you, take him or her window or catalog shopping, pointing out a range of items that would appeal to you. If you have a good relationship, your partner will appreciate the advice.

24. Be open to therapy.

When a relationship devolves into difficult patterns, be willing to see a good marriage therapist, and be willing to find a therapist before you have reached the point of no return. Therapists aren't just for couples that are on the verge of divorce. They are facilitators of open discussion; sometimes it can be helpful just to talk through difficult issues with them. Sometimes even one or two sessions can be enough to yield a better flow of energy in a relationship.

Refusal on the part of one partner to see a therapist may indicate that he or she is unwilling to work to improve the relationship. On the other hand, it may also indicate that he or she is skeptical of therapy. One way to convince a skeptical person to see a therapist is to affirm your love but insist that you both could develop some communication skills. Volunteer to go see the therapist on your own for the first session to check it out and return with feedback.

Find a therapist who specializes in marital issues and ask for referrals from friends who have been helped. Often a couple will wait until too much negativity has occurred and there can be little hope for healing. Pledge to stay in the relationship for at least four months during therapy. It's possible that the reasons you seek out counseling may be different from what you end up discussing in a session.

As private therapy can be expensive, know that many hospitals and religious centers provide low-cost marriage counseling. Counseling can also help you break up or divorce in a more peaceful, fair manner. You can't save a marriage that has already ended.

25. Be responsible for your own happiness.

True happiness comes from within, not from an outside source. A relationship can be an anchor in your life, allowing you to grow, change, try, succeed, and fail, always with a stable center to come back to. But it cannot and will not be the true source of joy in life. If you are not grounded within yourself, you will find that you cannot fully develop a healthy, strong, joyous relationship.

Your beloved is not your sole source of joy. He or she can support you, comfort you, encourage you, and challenge you to grow. But in the end, only you can be responsible for your own happiness. Take this lesson to heart, and your joy in life will grow and grow.

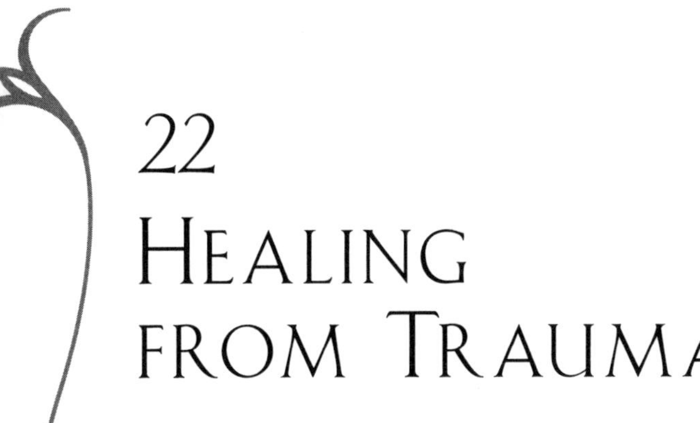

22 Healing from Trauma

SADLY, TOO MANY PEOPLE—women, men, and children—have had some traumatic life experience that causes them to be armored and guarded. I offer this chapter because I know that all the great love and sex on the planet can be less wonderful when one has been traumatized. Trauma may be verbal, physical, psychological, sexual, and/or violent. Rape, incest, miscarriage, abortion, and even fear of pregnancy can all be traumatic. There are way too many forms of trauma that people go through on this planet.

Though women are the most often affected by abuse, it also happens to men. In some cases both partners have been victims of sexual trauma. If abuse issues are never brought up, they can continue to affect current relationships in subtle ways; "The issue is in the tissue." If abuse came from someone of the opposite sex, feelings of hurt, anger, and grief can be transferred to others of that sex. Do counseling even if the trauma occurred years ago. Ask for what you want for your healing.

Talk about your wounds when you can be alone with a trusted friend and undisturbed for at least an hour. Expressing such things may be difficult but can help you release old stored emotions. Speak about your feelings of hurt, anger, grief. Allow the hurt feelings to cleanse out of your body with each out breath. You can let go with sound. Allow yourself to get hysterical, if that needs to happen, or tetanic, or incoherent, for about ten minutes. This helps cleanse all the toxic programming. Remember to breathe. Call on higher powers and angels for your healing. Perhaps take a cleansing salt or lavender bath.

You can benefit by writing about your feelings. Massage, including self-massage over the lower abdomen, or specific sexual favors may be healing. Massage focused near the genitals such as thighs, groin, perineum, and pubic bone are good places to focus in cases of sexual trauma. If emotions get too intense, make sure to stop the massage and simply ask to be held. G-spot work can cause buried sexual emotions to surface and help their release. Having a trusting relationship and working with this sacred spot can be very healing.

Surround yourself with the healing color green. Wear green clothes, sleep on green bedding, eat green foods, have green plants in your midst. Rose essential oil can be inhaled to soothe emotional traumas. Raspberry leaf and schizandra berries are two herbs that can be taken as tea, tincture, or capsules to help heal sexual trauma.

HOMEOPATHIC REMEDIES

IGNATIA helps when sexuality has been altered by grief or trauma. Use if grief causes menses to cease.

FLOWER ESSENCES

Flower essences for trauma include the following:

Hibiscus. For women who have been sexually traumatized.

Mariposa Lily. Helps alleviate trauma from sexual abuse as a child.

Star of Bethlehem. For great physical shock and trauma such as rape, injury, robbery, and accidents.

Rescue Remedy is the Bach Flower Remedy for panic, shock, grief, despair, and other crises. It should be taken in the case of a current crisis situation, as opposed to a past trauma.

By allowing the pain of old emotions to resurface and be cleansed, you can let go of feelings that can get in the way of ultimate love now. Whether you choose to work with a therapist, lover, or trusted friend, see if some of these above ideas can help to heal.

DEALING WITH ANGER

Anger arises when momentum to change meets resistance to change. Excess pressure and lack of recognition can cause anger. Studies show that those with overly disruptive and aggressive behavior often have low levels of serotonin, which transmits nerve impulses from one neuron to another. Exposure to heavy metals such as lead can also contribute to delinquent and angry behavior, while aggression can be traced somewhat to inherited genes.

Anger can put the body through its paces. It is known to contribute to dizziness, high blood pressure, elevated cholesterol levels, tight shoulders, stiff upper back, jaw tightness, eye problems, increased hydrochloric acid production, and ulcers. Clumsiness, irritability, and impatience are also characteristics of anger. Procrastination, "accidentally" destroying an enemy's property, and losing things may also be signs of anger coming to the surface.

Scientists believe that extreme states of anger cause the brain to fill with catecholamines—either adrenaline, noradrenaline, or serotonin. Cortisol and adrenaline triggered by anger stimulate fat cells to release their contents into the bloodstream, which are then picked up by the liver and converted to cholesterol. Sudden anger speeds up one's circulation, while years of anger can block blood flow to the coronary artery.

What is more dangerous than the experience of anger is the repression of it. Pent up angry feelings can be a factor in hemorrhoids, migraine headaches, cancer, rheumatoid arthritis, and heart disease. In a journal, make a list about what aspects of your anger you are accountable for. Focus on what you can do about it. Avoid blaming. In many respects, anger can have its benefits as it contributes to change. Had people not gotten angry, women would still not be able to vote and people of color would still not have the rights they are entitled to. Anger can help change occur.

According to Oriental medical tradition, it is the Liver system that correlates to the emotion of anger. Anger stimulates a contraction of chi that causes stress to the sinews and Liver. An unhealthy Liver can aggravate anger, while excess anger can also injure the Liver. Anger is described in Oriental medicine as ascending chi or Liver yang rising; it is considered a hot emotion. It is interesting that the English word *bilious* refers to someone who is bad tempered as well as to liver problems.

Foods that benefit the Liver and thus mellow the emotion of anger include artichokes, barley, daikon radish, dandelion greens, mung beans, rye, and tart green apples. Dandelion root helps to cleanse emotions of anger stored in the Liver. Excess garlic and onions can be too hot and can aggravate the emotion of anger. Coffee can also make one more likely to fly off the handle.

Herbs that help cool the Liver and thus soothe anger include blessed thistle, bupleurum, cypress, dandelion root, dong quai, gastrodia, licorice root, oatstraw, peony root, and skullcap.

5-HTP (5-hydroxtryptophan) is an amino acid that helps correct neurotransmitter imbalance. Along with behavioral counseling, 5-HTP can help curb anger and violence. Other amino acids that can be helpful for those with extreme anger and/or violent behavior are phenylalanine, leucine, valine, histidine, arginine, lysine, isoleucine, alanine, glutamine, methionine, threonine, and alpha-keto-glutaric acid. Chromium and vitamin B_6 taken with amino acids will help to activate them.

The goal in clearing anger is to reduce heat and move stagnation.

Bodywork helps to soften the Liver and soothe a savage spirit. Yoga will aid in flexibility of mind and body. A folk remedy is to get buried in the sand (with your face uncovered, of course). It is a very calming technique.

HOMEOPATHIC REMEDIES

Homeopathic remedies that can cool fire in the Liver include:

CHAMOMILLA. For angry children or those constantly discontent.

LACHESIS. For outbursts and irrational jealousy. Good for those who are domineering, vicious, suspicious, and talkative.

LYCOPODIUM. For the insecure person who takes anger out on others.

NATRUM MURIATICUM. Aids those unable to express anger.

NUX VOMICA. For the person who is hurried, impatient, and who overemphasizes achievement. Workaholic, annoyed by noise, persnickety, domineering. Can have a violent temper.

MERCURIUS. Sudden anger, fast speech, uncomfortable, violent impulse. Difficulty concentrating.

SEPIA. Critical of partners. Argumentative and pessimistic.

STAPHYSAGRIA. Helps ailments caused by repressed anger. Benefits those that hold their temper until they blow up.

SULPHUR. For the know-it-all person. Haughty, yet philosophical, creative, and impractical. Argumentative for the entertainment of it.

FLOWER ESSENCES

The following Bach Flower Essences assist in the calming of anger.

Cherry Plum. For those who feel that they are about to do something desperate, and for those prone to temper tantrums.

Heather. For those who are easily irritated.

Holly. Can help jealousy and sibling rivalry.

Impatiens. Helps one to be more patient.

Walnut. Protection from outside influences that cause anger. Also helps those who are going through big life changes.

A good calcium/magnesium supplement helps to quell an angry countenance, while essential oils can be used as inhalations, baths, or in other creative ways. Look for basil, cardamom, chamomile, champa, coriander, frankincense, geranium, hyssop, jasmine, lavender, lemon balm, lotus, marjoram, neroli, pine, rose, rosewood, or ylang-ylang.

A person who is balanced in their Liver/Wood element will have good self-esteem. One of the positive aspects of a churned-up Liver is the ability to be creative. Herbalist Michael Tierra often says that "art is toxic discharge." So get out there and use your painting, writing, music, or some other way to express yourself and contribute to your own therapy. Get your "ya yas" out in a healthy way.

If you're one of those people who "sees red" when they're angry, try counting to ten while you visualize the color blue. There may be some occasions where counting to one hundred is what is takes. Hostile experiences can aggravate emotions, resolve nothing, and even put you in peril.

Learn what triggers your anger and try to avoid those situations. Consider writing up a disaster scale and rating the things that make you angry from one to ten. You may find that some of them are not as important. Consider humor a more valuable ally than profanity.

In dealing with anger it helps to affirm that you are angry. Be clear about what it is that is really bothering you. Take a breather and then discuss the conflict. Without attacking, let your feelings be known. Overusing profanity and screaming at another person can impair your ability to be heard. If necessary, remove yourself from a hot situation and return when you can more safely express yourself. If you write a hate letter or vent your anger before your heart rate has calmed down, you may regret it, so collect your thoughts first and then express them. Clear, respectful, and nonaggressive language works best. Avoid "you" statements and stick to "I" statements. Make eye contact with the person you are arguing with. Listen to what he or she has to say without interrupting. Nod or say "yes' to indicate you are listening. Mirror back what you hear. Avoid pointing fingers or using defensive body language such as crossing your arms in front of you. If necessary, do something physical such as pound on a pillow, tear up a phone book, or write down your thoughts. Listen and do your best to understand. Be willing to forgive!

SURVIVING INFIDELITY

Infidelity can cost you a lot: your marriage, custody of children, finances, home, and respect. Think carefully. Sex drive is wonderful, but you can honor the fact that you are attractive to other people—and you can enjoy your own sexual feelings—without acting on them. Thinking clearly and having discipline is always wise. An affair can be evidence that there are problems in the primary relationship. It can also be a partner's attempt to escape intimacy by spreading emotions out, or an attempt to relieve pressure from other problems in life, such as a lack of self-esteem, loneliness, work stress, aging, criticism from one's partner, or mid-life changes. Affairs can be an opportunity to have a relationship without the concerns of bills, children, and chores. Or they can simply be a result of curiosity.

Infidelity is one of the most universally accepted reasons for breakup and divorce. In some cultures, it is legal justification for murder! Some couples have agreements about being able to sleep with others, but mostly it doesn't work and risks the relationship. Many people find creative ways to explore relationships with others, encouraging honesty and openness. Some teach tantra as a gift to the planet.

I am certainly glad that Tom and I never broke up over a few dalliances in our early time together. We communicated, did some therapy, and survived. We are both so glad as love still grows. True pair monogamy is a high goal.

Issues surrounding pregnancy and birth of a child have caused some men to feel deprived of being the main love in their partner's life. Those that are substance abusers or risk takers, have recently lost parents, or are undergoing financial stress might be likely candidates for affairs. If one partner neglects proper hygiene, gains excessive weight, or ceases to be active in the relationship, the other partner may look elsewhere. Lack of communication, appreciation, sexual satisfaction, boredom, and frequent travel by one mate are other common reasons for infidelity. Seek out support of friends and family when going through difficult times rather than seeking outside sexual companionship.

If a partner is having an affair, the one cheated on may want to avoid a confrontation and look the other way. But in order for things to change, confrontation is necessary. Find out why it happened. Is it over? It can be near impossible to make progress in saving a marriage if the affair continues after it has been discovered.

Affairs hurt. However, it does not have to mean the end of a relationship. Improvement in the relationship can come out of this difficult experience. If both people are willing to do the work, look at issues, marriages can indeed be healed, but it may take professional help. Get counseling. Hang in there for at least six months. Be available to solve any underlying problems in the relationship.

An affair can create another demanding person in one's life. If the outside partner had to share in the responsibility of kids, mortgage, and bills, they might not hold a candle to a mate that has hung in there with you. There is no guarantee that life with the person one is having an affair with would be easier or better than with one's mate. Starting over with your current mate can be even better than starting out fresh with a new one.

Monogamy helps provide a setting for trust, safety, and intimacy. To help prevent infidelity give your beloved lots of praise and appreciation. Learn to enjoy sex in a variety of ways. Be willing to try new things and be spontaneous. Keep the romance alive after becoming parents. Rejecting your partner repeatedly can cause him or her to look elsewhere. Be respectful of how much work goes into making money, and avoid being wasteful and frivolous with the money one or both of you earn. Find a multitude of ways to enjoy each other.

Give your beloved space to enjoy what he or she likes. Being overcontrolling, spying, and untrusting can cause resentment and might move a partner to act out what he or she is suspected of. Jealousy has never prevented infidelity. Live life as if you are having an affair with your mate!

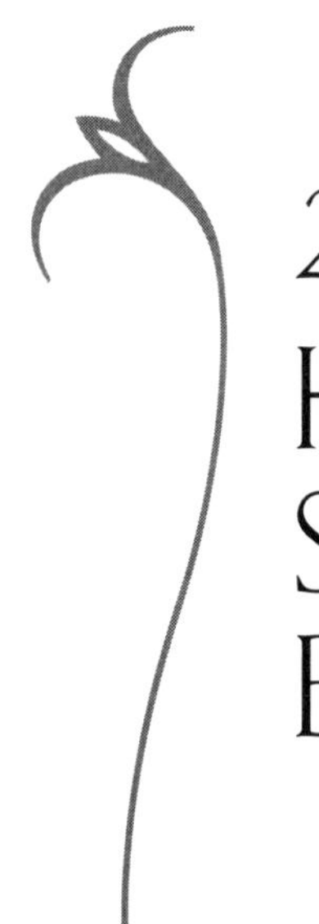

23 Healing the Spirit from a Broken Heart

"What soap is for the body, tears are for the soul."

—Anonymous

IT IS A RARE PERSON who lives without ever experiencing grief. In fact, I might go so far as to say that a life cannot be truly full without the experience of grief. It is a strong and terrible emotion, breaking us open, drilling deep into the nerves of our soul, often unleashing a torrent of emotion that seems impossible to contain.

But without the capacity to express grief, we cannot express love. Grief is the flipside of the coin, the risk we take when we open our hearts to another. It is the cleanser of the broken heart, the cool ocean streaming over the hot and angry sands, the salt that stings the open wound and purifies it.

Experiencing grief is a part of being human. Too often we try to contain it, a study in impassivity, feeling that it shows stronger character to wade through without wincing or crying. In fact, when we don't allow ourselves to experience grief, the sadness is never realized and becomes buried instead like a sticky burr in the soul. We become emotionally numb, distant from friends, family, and other loved ones, never able to fully enter into life.

To live fully, we must love fully and, hence, grieve fully.

EXPRESSING GRIEF

It is healthier to express grief than to repress it. Crying provides emotional release that lowers blood pressure and muscular tension. Crying can also help relieve stress on the central nervous system. The more you grieve, the sooner the heartache will pass.

If tears won't come even though you feel crying would help, here is a technique you can try. Find a safe, quiet space where you will not be disturbed. Place one hand in the middle of your upper chest, on your collarbone. Breathe down only as far as your hand. Then begin to breathe more rapidly. Make a sound of some sort. Hear the feeling in your voice. Go ahead and sound like a crying baby. Give yourself the space to feel the sadness. Think about what's causing the grief, and let the tears flow.

Groaning is another sound that can help dissipate sadness and pain. While groaning, think of your reasons for suffering. When you exhale, visualize sorrow being exhaled from your system.

These breathing exercises are lent extra power when performed in concert with sunrise. Stand facing the rising sun, and let its rays beam on your heart. Visualize the sun healing your grief. Breathe!

AFTER A BREAKUP

Breaking up with a loved one can cause grief similar to the grief felt when a loved one dies. It's also often mixed with anger, frustration, and tremendous disappointment.

When someone breaks up with you, do your best to stay calm; save the freaking out for later. Screaming and throwing things tends to make the person who is departing feel that he or she is justified in leaving, because you're acting like a lunatic. When things simmer down, try writing a letter to your ex, for your eyes only. Use the letter writing as an opportunity to collect your thoughts and express your feelings, getting everything off your chest. Vent venomously! Eventually you may want to send a modified version (without the bad language) to your ex, or you may want to burn the letter. The important thing is to clear your feelings.

Encourage the physical separation; without it, the emotional separation will take longer and be more painful. Put your ex's belongings in a box and return them to him or her with a minimum of drama. If there are mementos you wish to keep, put them in a box and put the box in storage. Clean everything. Feng shui your home. Burn some sage or artemesia to clear the air.

Avoid calling your ex when you are sad, scared, drunk, or depressed. Minimize calling just to "check in." Tell your friends not to give you constant gossip reports about where they saw your ex and who he or she was with. Ask friends who invite you to gatherings to let you know whether your ex will be there, so that you can avoid surprises.

Have a closure ritual. Place a photo of your ex and a sprig of rosemary (for remembrance) in a bowl filled with sand or dirt. Etch a candle with your ex's name, and anoint it with a fragrance that reminds you of him or her. Then place the candle in the bowl with the photo and the rosemary, and light it. Offer a prayer of thanks for the lessons you learned in the relationship. As the candle burns down, reflect upon your relationship, perhaps writing down your thoughts in a journal. It can be therapeutic to remember your "love story." Include memorable dates and events, how you met, and what your feelings and expectations were. Make note of clues that, in retrospect, signaled that the relationship wasn't going to last. Make a list of all the reasons the relationship could not have survived, as well as a list of things you learned from the relationship. Write about what you will look for in a new partner. Be willing to look at any aspect of yourself that may have contributed to the ending, and then let go of it. Give your story a title. Allow the candle to burn itself out. Play "your song" one last time.

Overcoming Grief

Therapy for grief focuses on three aspects:

- Rest
- Positive energy
- Health

Of greatest importance, take care of yourself, and indulge in pampering. The loving support of friends and family members can be a blessing. Ask them to visit; allow them to try to cheer you up. Seek out those who want to see you happy, and avoid people with negative attitudes.

Channeling positive energy into different aspects of your life, such as your career, your children, and your personal growth can help diffuse grief. Develop new talents. Take a class. Read self-help books. Learn a new language. Exercise. Practice yoga. Quit bad habits; overdoing alcohol, drugs, and junk food will only make this time more difficult.

AROMATHERAPY BATHS

Soaking in a bath can encourage muscles and mind to relax and healing tears to flow. Light a candle, blue for calming the emotions or violet for easing grief and raising consciousness. Add 7 drops of a grief-dispelling essential oil, such as cedarwood, clary sage, cypress, geranium, grapefruit, hyssop, lavender, lemon balm, jasmine, marjoram, neroli, orange, rose, rosemary, rosewood, sage, sandalwood, tangerine, or ylang ylang.

When you are done bathing let out the water, and visualize sorrow passing down the drain with the water and being healed by the earth. Then towel dry and apply a massage oil made from one or more of the essential oils mentioned above (8 ounces of coconut oil mixed with 30 drops of the essential oil) over your heart and lungs.

GEM THERAPY

Rose quartz can calm anger, promote love, and help heal grief and emotional wounds. If you sleep with a rose quartz in your hand, your dreams may have a healing effect on your heart. You might also consider wearing rose quartz jewelry.

COLOR THERAPY

The color violet, whether worn or visualized, is good for healing grief. Visualize yourself breathing in a healing violet light. As you exhale, see the somber colors of your sadness departing with your breath.

NUTRITIONAL THERAPY

According to traditional Oriental medicine, grief corresponds to the Metal element and to the Lungs and Large intestine. Eat green- and orange-colored foods, such as violet leaf, dandelion, kale, collards, carrots, and sweet potatoes. These support the Liver, which will help you move through this difficult time. Eat celery to help comfort the pangs of a broken heart. Use pungent condiments such as clove, coriander, and ginger, which move Lung energy. Vitamin B complex, which promotes both calmness and vitality, is always a great ally during times of emotional distress.

HERBAL THERAPY

Herbs can be a great comforter during times of grief.

Hawthorn (*Crataegus* spp.). The leaf, flower, and berry are generally used in herbal medicine to strengthen and improve the physical heart, but hawthorn also benefits the emotional heart. It can aid sleep and establish a feeling of serenity.

Hops (*Humulus lupulus*). The strobile (the conelike fruiting body of the hops plant) quiets the nerves, calms anxiety, and promotes rest. It is an anodyne, muscle relaxant, nervine, and sedative.

Lemon balm (*Melissa officinalis*). The herb, according to some German studies, acts upon the part of the brain governing the autonomic nervous system. It is a nervine and a sedative.

Motherwort (*Leonurus cardiaca*). The herb calms anxiety and hysteria and relieves depression. It can help open the mind to joy after a loss. It is a cardiotonic, hypotensive, nervine, sedative, and vasodilator.

Mullein (*Verbascum thapsus*). The leaf protects the lungs from harm during periods of sadness.

Passionflower (*Passiflora incarnata*). The herb provides precursors to the neurotransmitter serotonin and reduces the rate at which the body breaks down serotonin and norepinephrine. It can induce a mild euphoria and quiet mental chatter. It is especially helpful for those who are weak and exhausted with anxiety, irritability, stress, nervous breakdown, or suicidal tendencies. It is an anodyne and a nervine.

Saint John's wort (*Hypericum perforatum*). The herb has antidepressant properties and can help heal physically damaged nerves. It relieves anxiety, fear, irritability, melancholy, and suicidal tendencies. It is a mild sedative and can be especially helpful for someone who is worn out from sobbing.

Violet (*Viola odorata*). Violet also goes by the name "heartsease"—a good indicator of its use in healing grief. The leaf and flower calm the physical and emotional heart. They are also demulcents.

HOMEOPATHIC REMEDIES

When grief is accompanied by any of the conditions that are described below, try the suggested homeopathic remedy. The usual dosage is 4 pellets, or as many liquid drops as the package label recommends, taken under the tongue four times daily. Rather than swallowing the pellets whole, allow them to dissolve slowly.

IGNATIA. The patient experiences hysteria. He or she sighs frequently and has difficulty sleeping.

NATRUM MURIATICUM. The patient dwells in the past, holds grudges, and rejects sympathy.

PULSATILLA. The patient feels extreme anxiety. He or she is sad, yielding, indecisive, and weepy and needs to be with others.

FLOWER ESSENCES

Flower essences, which have a strong connection to the emotions, can be used in a variety of ways to help heal a broken heart. The usual dosage is 3 drops under the tongue or taken with a glass of water three or four times daily. You can also add flower essences to bathwater, massage oils, and body lotions. Try applying them to the sensitive skin on the inside of the wrists and to the "third eye" at the center of the forehead.

Bleeding Heart. This essence helps foster peace and detachment.

Borage. Borage helps lift the spirits.

Hawthorn. Hawthorn protects the spirit, reminding us of our resiliency during periods of intense grief and stress. It washes negativity from the heart and soothes the pain of emotional separation.

Honeysuckle. For the person who finds it difficult to adjust after the loss of a loved one, honeysuckle can help him or her move out of the past and reintegrate into present life.

Mustard. Mustard helps to dispel deep gloom that comes on strong, then suddenly leaves.

Pear. Pear helps relieve extreme grief that arises from unbalancing emergency situations.

Rescue Remedy. This remedy can be taken to calm the mind in moments of extreme crisis. Take 2 drops under the tongue, as often as necessary.

Star of Bethlehem. Star of Bethlehem soothes the mind when you are having a difficult time coping with the death of a loved one. Dr. Edward Bach called this essence "the comforter and soother of pains and sorrows."

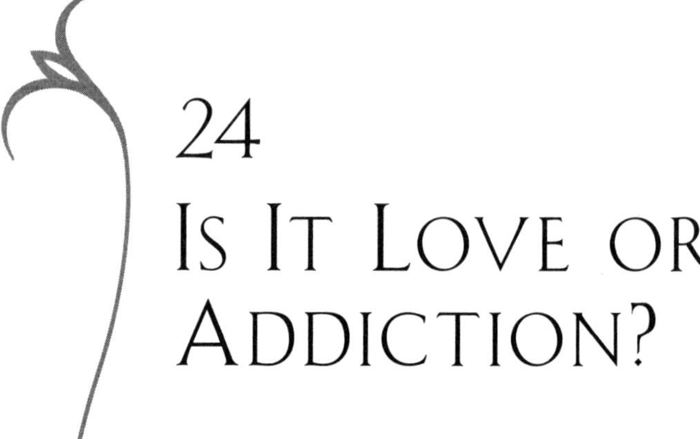

24
Is It Love or Addiction?

BEFORE YOU THINK YOU can't live without that special someone, take a closer look. This may be an opportunity for liberation. Maybe, you are better off without him or her and a more appropriate relationship awaits.

Take some time to think clearly about the relationship you think you want. The person you have loved and lost may not be right for you or may be unable to make a commitment. Perhaps the relationship involved more struggle than pleasure; or perhaps you found yourself engaging in self-destructive behavior. Unless both partners are willing to get professional help, a codependent relationship isn't healthy for anybody. Don't allow fear of change, loneliness, or the opinions of others to get in the way of your forging ahead to find someone more right for you.

Sometimes, however, you may be quite convinced that your relationship needs a second chance. In these cases, it is best to be very patient and proceed with care.

WINNING BACK THE ONE YOU LOVE, BUT LOST

Friends who say, "I would never take anyone back if they had an affair, or did such and such, etc.," are not in your position. Save hysterics for your therapist and friends. To the one that got away, show the cool, calm, and collected you.

Write down your painful feelings to clarify your thoughts and to avoid having the same dialogue run through your brain of things you wish you had said or done differently. When the time is right, you will have organized those thoughts so you will be able to speak more clearly. You can even practice what you will say.

If your ex is constantly calling to check in, tell him or her that it is too painful and that you'd prefer that they not call, until they have something different to offer. You want to keep some distance, though it's a good idea to maintain some contact, perhaps once a week or every ten days. If you are totally out of sight and mind, you can easily be forgotten.

It's okay to not always pick up the phone when your ex calls and to take awhile to return those calls. The chase is part of the play. Wanting and not always being able to have can be a turn-on that fills one with longing. You might say you don't want to play games, but this is part of the age-old dance of yin and yang.

Meet for lunch to catch up and make sure the occasion is pleasant. Don't include your ex's new lover, if there is one, in these meetings. Remind your beloved of the good times. Smells, sounds, and tastes can be powerful messages. Evoke memories that are pleasant. Threatening to commit suicide, using children as pawns, destroying possessions and financial resources is not the way to win back the one you love, but instead reveals ugliness.

Avoid being seen as disheveled, downtrodden, and so available that your ex could have you back at any time. Radiate energy, health, and beauty that they can't be so sure would be available to them. Look and feel better for yourself. If it doesn't work with this person, you will grow in self-esteem and happiness and attract someone else. Helen Gurley Brown said, "Success is the best revenge."

Resist the urge to seduce. If a physical connection happens, let it be your ex's idea. You must be truly willing to forgive past transgressions and not keep bringing them up. Holding on to grudges keeps the relationship strained. Even if you don't win your lover back, what is the worse that can happen? Don't push. Give them room to come to their own conclusions. If it is meant to be, it will happen. Otherwise, let go gracefully.

If you win them back, make it different and better this time. If what broke you up keeps occurring, end the relationship and move forward.

SEX/RELATIONSHIP ADDICTION

If you are a wise person, you will control your sex life rather than allowing it to control you like an addiction. Phone sex, pornography, prostitutes, and autoeroticism can be dangerous to one's health, and expensive. Constantly seeking greater thrills can put you into an addictive relationship—even with children or pets. Sex is sometimes used as a way to disregard emotional pain or depression. Are their other ways for you to feel liked or loved?

Sex is one of the supreme earthly pleasures, and it is best when practiced out of love and desire rather than addiction and compulsion. According to traditional Chinese medicine, sexual energy originates in the Kidneys. Excessive sex can deplete the chi and jing of the Kidneys, leading to premature aging and exhaustion as well as weakened immunity, low energy, impotence, and damage to the genitals. Too-frequent ejaculation can deplete one's chi and the ability to concentrate.

Many sex addicts are trying to escape from boredom in their lives; they are hooked on the endorphins released by the brain during sexual activity. As with many drugs, sexual behaviors can become addicting when we rely on them to calm ourselves. All mood-altering activities tend to produce a sense of euphoria initially. The post-euphoric stage is then followed by a low, which causes the person to seek another episode of activity.

Healthy sex can indeed be a tonic for the body. But if you are finding that sex has become a compulsion for you, take some steps to redirect your energies.

- Establish a daily exercise practice like walking, running, yoga, etc. You can even do these with your partner.
- Take a class or read a book on tantra, and learn how sex can be a transcendent experience. Adding spiritual practice to your sex life can

bring you to higher states of consciousness and bliss and truly satisfy your soul.

- Learn negotiation skills to help you deal with relationships. Try couples counseling, relationship enrichment workshops, and the like.
- Eat less red meat and spices, which will aggravate an overheated condition like sexual addiction or compulsion. Use more cooling foods such as salads and fruit. The herbs hops, vitex, and sage can decrease excessive sexual desire. Essential oils that can help curb excessive sexual desire include lavender and marjoram.

For more ideas on overcoming addictions in general, please check out my book *Addiction Free Naturally* (Inner Traditions, 2001).

THIS HAS BEEN A JOURNEY! I am glad to have learned much in the process and hope this book can be a lifelong companion in helping you love and care for yourself in healthful ways. May you enjoy the best sex ever and find ways to deepen love and get through the bumps in the journey so that we continue to grow as beautiful, healthful, sexy, loving humans! Thanks for joining me on the adventure. May the path grow in truth, beauty, and goodness as you go through life! Enjoy the joy.

APPENDIX ONE

The Chemistry of Love

Here is a small section on the relatively new science of hormones and neurotransmitters; how they affect our health, sexuality, energy, and brain chemistry.

NEUROTRANSMITTERS

Neurotransmitters are chemically analogous to several psychedelic or aphrodisiac chemicals. For example, phenethylamines are related to noradrenaline, the tropanes resemble acetylcholine, and opiates resemble endorphins.

We do know that the hypothalamus, located on a stalk suspended from the brain a couple of inches behind the nose, manufactures hormones and brain chemicals that affect sexuality. All sex hormones are made from cholesterol, which gets converted into a gender-neutral steroid hormone known as pregnenolone—often referred to as a "prohormone."

Acetylcholine

Acetylcholine is an excitory neurotransmitter in the autonomic nervous system. It helps promote efficient memory. Choline is a precursor to acetylcholine and occurs naturally in avocados, broccoli, cabbage, green leafy vegetables, and in flax, sesame, and sunflower seeds.

Dopamine

Dopamine is one of the primary excitory neurotransmitters, produced in the heart and associated with testosterone production. It promotes energy, focus, and motivation. Dopamine is made from l-dopa (associated with libido, erections in men, and orgasmic ability in women) from the amino acids tyrosine and phenylalanine.

Men tend to have dopamine deficiencies. Impulsiveness (acting without thinking), being emotionally unavailable, and boredom with life can be a sign of dopamine deficiency. Being able to make eye contact is a sign of healthy dopamine levels. Dopamine is produced at its peak two hours before midnight to supply the next day—another reason why going to bed early (ideally two hours before midnight) is important (at least most of the time).

Work, sports, action movies, and dangerous activities promote dopamine. You can promote dopamine production in a partner by showing appreciation, trust, and acceptance for who they are. Foods that promote dopamine production include fish, beans, and spirulina. Excessive exercise can lower dopamine levels.

Endorphins

Endorphins are neuropeptides that bind to opioid receptors in the brain and have potent analgesic properties. They are sometimes called "opiates of the mind." They can calm emotions, relieve pain, and reduce anxiety. They also contribute to feelings of happiness. Exercise, physical touch, orgasm, and sitting still all stimulate the brain to release endorphins. Endorphins are also increased when testosterone and oxytocin levels increase.

Serotonin

Serotonin is considered an inhibitory neurotransmitter. It promotes appetite, relaxation, comfort, satisfaction, and optimism and helps us feel assured that things will be okay. The brain produces more serotonin two hours after sunrise. Secure relationships stimulate serotonin.

Women tend to have serotonin deficiencies. Low levels are associated with depression, food cravings and emotional eating, dramatic emotions, needing to constantly talk about concerns, being too giving in relationships, and being unable to feel secure in a relationship. The indoles and tryptamine psychedelics are similar to serotonin.

Stable blood sugar levels and exposure to early morning light helps one maintain good serotonin levels. At high levels, serotonin lowers sexual libido and can inhibit orgasmic ability. A person with low serotonin might be anxious, restless, depressed, and have compulsive habits.

HORMONES

Androgens

Androgens are considered male sexual hormones, although women also produce them in lesser amounts. Androgens include androstenedione, testosterone, androsteniol, DHEA, and DHT (dihydrotestosterone). Androgen precursors are found in alfalfa, celery, fennel, flax, oats, parsley, and rhubarb. Environmental pollutants such as pesticides, phthalates, and bisphenol (used to make plastic flexible) can disrupt estrogen, androgens, and testosterone in the body. Androstenedione is one of the body's two androgens that gets converted into testosterone.

Dehydroepiandrosterone

Dehydroepiandrosterone (DHEA) is the most abundant steroid hormone in the body; it is sometimes called the "mother" sex hormone because many other sex hormones, including testosterone, are derived from it. DHEA is produced mainly by the adrenal glands but also in small amounts by the ovaries, the testicles, and the brain. The body converts DHEA into androstenedione and then to either testosterone or estrone. High levels of DHEA can increase libido. Low levels of DHEA can contribute to weight gain. Most birth control pills decrease DHEA.

DHEA levels are highest from our teens through our twenties and during puberty and pregnancy. They slowly decrease as we age. Practices that increase DHEA include meditation, exercise, stress-reduction techniques, and orgasm.

Before using DHEA as a supplement get tested by your health care practitioner to see if you need it. It is a steroid and should not be used indiscriminately.

Estrogens

Estrogens are a class of hormones that regulate the menses and stimulate the development of female secondary sex characteristics. They are manufactured in the ovaries, testes, fat cells, and adrenal glands and in the placenta during pregnancy. Estrogen improves cognition, performance, mood, vigilance, and reaction time, and contributes to the shapely contours of the female body. It also helps to maintain bone mass and keeps cholesterol levels in check. Estrogen improves the sense of smell and taste, prevents depression, reduces stress, and decreases appetite.

Alcoholism, liver disease, obesity, the first two weeks of the menstrual cycle, intercourse, and high levels of oxytocin can all contribute to elevated estrogen levels. Lack of sex, anorexia, hysterectomy, and menopause contribute to decreased levels of estrogen.

Normal levels of estrogen help prevent osteoporosis and heart disease. Low estrogen levels can make a woman susceptible to these diseases and also diminish her ability to produce vaginal lubrication, which can interfere with sexual pleasure. Low estrogen levels may also cause vaginal atrophy, or thinning of the vaginal walls, which can lead to pain, bleeding, and increased risk of infection. Health care providers often used to recommended that a menopausal woman take estrogen supplements, but these were later discovered to increase certain kinds of cancer risks. Question authority. Use natural lifestyle techniques to improve health before resorting to drugs. It's all a question of balance.

Despite the marketing claims of the pharmaceutical industry, synthetic estrogen and other hormones are not the same as natural hormones. Physiological harmony, the standard-bearer of health, is disrupted when synthetic compounds are thrown into the sanctuary of a woman's (or man's) body. In fact, they are often responsible for causing hormonal imbalance.

There are many natural substances that encourage the body to produce its own estrogen. For example, many herbs are phytoestrogenic, meaning that they simulate or stimulate the production of estrogen in the body. They can also satisfy the body's receptor sites for those hormones so that the body will get the message that it doesn't need to produce excessive hormones. Some of these herbs include alfalfa herb, aniseed, black cohosh root, black haw bark, coffee, cramp bark, dong quai, false unicorn root, fennel seed, fenugreek seed, hops strobile, licorice root, motherwort herb, nettle leaf, parsley leaf, pomegranate seed, red raspberry leaf, red clover flower, rose hip, sage leaf, sarsaparilla root, saw palmetto berry, shepherd's purse herb, vitex berry, wild yam root, willow bark, and yarrow herb.

Foods that promote estrogen production include animal products (meat, eggs, and dairy products—especially from animals raised on synthetic hormones to promote growth and weight gain), apples, beans, beets, buckwheat, carrots, cashews, cherries, corn, dates, eggplant, eggs, fennel seed, garlic, green leafy vegetables, lentils, oats, olives, papaya, peaches, plums, pomegranates, potatoes, pumpkin, rye, sesame seeds, soy foods, strawberries, string beans, sunflower seeds, tomatoes, whole grains (brown rice, barley, oats, and whole wheat), and yams.

Indole-3-carbinol is a phytochemical produced when the body digests cruciferous vegetables (broccoli, cabbage, cauliflower, radish, turnip, rutabaga, and Brussels sprouts). It appears to act as a protective mechanism against carcinogens and elevated hormonal levels by improving the liver's ability to break down hormones. Foods that decrease estrogen levels include berries, broccoli, buckwheat, cabbage, citrus fruits, corn, figs, grapes, green beans, melons, millet, onions, and pineapples, though some of these foods (for example, buckwheat, cabbage, and green beans) can also increase estrogen levels by providing some of the raw material from which the body makes hormones. Excess exercise also lowers estrogen levels.

Xenoestrogens are chemicals that mimic estrogen and bind to estrogen receptor sites. There is evidence that they can contribute to some estrogen-dependent cancers in the breasts, ovaries, and uterus. Sources of xenoestrogens include pesticides, detergents, preservatives such as methyl and propyl parabens, and plastics (think plastic food wrap and water bottles that are producing a terrible amount of plastic pollution).

There are three main types of estrogenic compounds found in the body: estrone, estradiol, and estriol.

ESTRONE

Estrone stimulates the development of breast tissue and, along with estradiol, the buildup of the endometrial lining in the uterus. It is primarily a postmenopausal estrogen, meaning that it doesn't play much of a physiological role until menopause.

ESTRADIOL

Estradiol is secreted by the ovaries and is considered the most potent of the three types of estrogen found in the body. Estradiol levels are highest before menopause. In postmenopausal women, the liver converts estradiol and estrone into estriol.

During a woman's childbearing years, estradiol stimulates buildup of the uterine lining in preparation for a baby, and after childbirth it promotes lactation. It promotes bone health, vaginal moisture and elasticity, and cardiovascular fitness.

ESTRIOL

Estriol, like estradiol, promotes fitness for the vaginal lining and cardiovascular system, but it is specifically beneficial during childbirth and for postmenopausal women. During birth, estriol levels increase by a factor of one thousand; they return to normal two to three weeks after delivery. High levels of estriol are believed to contribute to a lower risk of breast cancer.

Follicle-Stimulating Hormone

Follicle-stimulating hormone (FSH) is produced in the pituitary gland and stimulates development of the follicles in the ovary in preparation for ovulation and stimulates the development of sperm in men.

Luteinizing Hormone

Luteinizing hormone (LH) is produced in the pituitary gland and flows to the ovaries and adrenals. It stimulates development of the corpus luteum in women. LH levels are highest during the first few weeks of pregnancy. It also stimulates structures called Leydig cells in men to make testosterone.

Noradrenaline

Noradrenaline, also known as norepinephrine, is is made from the amino acid tyrosine and produced in the heart. It is considered a sexually inhibiting neurotransmitter that energizes the body during "flight-or fight" situations.

Oxytocin

Oxytocin, sometimes referred to as the "hormone of love" or "cuddle hormone," is an abundant neuropeptide secreted by the pituitary gland and widely distributed throughout the body. It is calming, reducing blood pressure and cortisol levels. Oxytocin is released by both sexes with sexual orgasm. It stimulates the uterine contractions that occur with orgasm and childbirth, increases sensitivity to touch, speeds ejaculation, decreases postpartum bleeding, may contribute to "forgetting" the pain of childbirth, and causes the let-down reflex in a nursing mother who hears her baby (and in some cases other babies) cry. The drug Pitocin, which is often used to stimulate labor, is a form of oxytocin.

Oxytocin plays an important role in encouraging women to care for their children and gather with other women. It stimulates the production of estrogen, testosterone, prolactin, and vasopressin. Oxytocin levels are increased by touch, taste, smell, and other pleasurable activities, especially by intercourse and orgasm. When a woman is offered help, it also boosts her levels of oxytocin. Supplementing the diet with choline may also increase oxytocin levels. Lack of estrogen, lack of touch, and the consumption of alcohol will decrease oxytocin levels.

Pregnenolone

Pregnenolone, also known as a "mother steroid" or prohormone, is the first metabolite of cholesterol, being a primary steroid hormone for women and men. It enhances mental functions.

Progesterone

Progesterone is a precursor of estrogen, testosterone, and corticosteroids. It is both a class of hormones and the name of the specific hormone. Like estrogen, progesterone is instrumental in the ovulation and menstrual cycles. It is produced by the ovaries, corpus luteum, and adrenal glands (as well as by the testes in males). It is also an end-product of the body's metabolization of cholesterol. It is primarily a female hormone; men have only minute quantities.

Progesterone is the dominant hormone in women during the last two weeks of the menstrual cycle and during pregnancy. When it drops sharply before menstruation it stimulates menstrual bleeding and can cause depression, edema, and irritability. A progesterone deficiency can also contribute to bone loss, facial whiskers, and thinning hair.

Progesterone can help normalize libido, though high levels of progesterone decrease sex drive. (It's sometimes given to sex offenders in the form of the drug Provera.) It can cause women to be sexually passive and irritable, as well as more nurturing toward their children. At high levels, it is mildly anesthetic; at low levels, it is sedative. It inhibits uterine contractions, oxytocin sensitivity, and LH production. It helps protect against premature labor in pregnancy and promotes lactation. Progesterone also helps transform fat into energy, is naturally diuretic, and is an antidepressant. It also helps to prevent bone loss.

Progesterone levels increase during pregnancy, nursing, and the premenstrual phase and decrease after menopause.

Phytoprogesteronic herbs include alfalfa, flaxseeds, lady's mantle, sarsaparilla, vitex, wild yam, yarrow, and yucca. It is debatable if the body can transform the diosgenin found in topical progesterone creams into progesterone. Many progesterone creams contain pharmaceutical grade (USP) progesterone, which is readily absorbed through the skin (in areas that have little fat such as the face, upper back, chest, arms, and legs) and utilized by the body. It is not known if herbal creams applied topically using only plant sterol precursors can be converted into an absorbable or utilizable form.

Prolactin

Prolactin is secreted by the pituitary gland. Men need it for the production of sperm, but levels of prolactin that are too high can decrease testosterone production, contributing to erectile dysfunction.

In women prolactin levels peak midway through the menstrual cycle and stay high until the menses begin. If a woman becomes pregnant, prolactin levels remain high, stimulating mammary tissue growth, and, eventually, lactation. Prolactin can decrease libido in men and women and is considered inhibiting to sexual function. The more a mother nurses, the more likely her sex drive will be diminished—perhaps to protect her newborn from having nutritional competition too soon. Prolactin also decreases alertness and sensitivity and can contribute to fatigue and depression. Prolactin levels can be boosted by exercise, stress, nausea, jet lag, nipple stimulation, high-protein meals, opiates, and sleep. They are decreased by meditation.

Prostaglandins

Prostaglandins are fatty acids that perform hormonelike actions in the body. They are produced in the uterus and found in high concentrations in sperm.

In women prostaglandins contribute to the contraction and relaxation of the uterus. Women who suffer from intense menstrual cramps often have elevated prostaglandin levels. Prostaglandins are also thought to trigger labor and orgasm.

Prostaglandin E (PGE) helps regulate uterine tone, protecting against cramps, and can ward off menstrual headaches, edema, breast tenderness, and emotional distress. PGE also helps prevent blood platelets from clumping, thereby reducing the risk of heart attack and stroke.

Raw nuts, seeds, yogurt, and evening primrose, borage, hemp, and flaxseed oils provide the raw materials the body needs to make anti-inflammatory prostaglandins. A diet that is high in animal products (meat, eggs, and dairy products) can contribute to inflammatory prostaglandin production. Bromelain, an enzyme found in pineapple, can decrease prostaglandin production.

Testosterone

Testosterone production begins when nerve cells in the hypothalamus release gonadadotropin-releasing hormone (GnRH). Testosterone is a steroid hormone produced in the adrenals, testicles, and ovaries. It is responsible for producing and maintaining male secondary sex characteristics. For both men and women testosterone is a major factor in determining sex drive and is sometimes referred to as the "hormone of desire." Levels of testosterone fluctuate daily and seasonally, and about 1 percent of a man's testosterone is converted into estrogen. Women have twenty to forty times less testosterone than men.

Aggression, assertiveness, competitiveness, self-confidence, and aloofness are by-products of testosterone. When testosterone levels are elevated, men may become irritable and angry. High testosterone levels have been implicated in episodes of violence and psychotic behavior. However, testosterone is also essential for emotions such as affection, joy, friendliness, and confidence.

Exercise, competition, action movies, pornography (or better yet erotica), and a meat-based diet (it better be organic if you eat it) elevate testosterone levels; excess exercise (such as long-distance cycling or running), stress, vegetarianism, and progesterone decrease them. When a man is asked for help, it encourages his testosterone production. Foods that promote testosterone are high in zinc. Beans, garlic, and animal foods (particularly oysters) are sources that are said to increase testosterone.

Testosterone inhibits the production of prolactin and improves the function of adrenaline and vasopressin.

Vasopressin

Vasopressin is a peptide hormone secreted by the pituitary gland and widely distributed throughout the body. It is sometimes referred to as the "monogamy molecule" or the "bonding hormone," because it discourages extreme sexual and emotional patterns and modulates testosterone activity. It is also a vasoconstrictor and has anti-diuretic properties. Choline can help the body produce vasopressin.

APPENDIX TWO

ANATOMICAL TERMS

FEMALE ANATOMY

Bartholin's glands: Two glands, comparable to the male Cowper's glands, that lie on each side in the lower part of the vagina. They secrete a lubricating mucus.

cervix: The narrow, outer end of the uterus. It is about two inches wide and three inches long, although the visible portion is only about a half-inch. The cervix is shaped like an upside-down pear and is somewhat sensitive to pleasure when stimulated.

clitoral hood: The flap of skin that covers and protects the clitoris. Also called the prepuce.

clitoris: From the Greco-Latin *clavis,* meaning "key." The sole human organ whose only function is to give pleasure! The clitoris is a small shaft of tissue that is rich in nerve endings (it has about as many as the penis) and blood vessels; it is almost twice as sensitive as the vagina. It is hidden under a "hood" of skin at the top of the vagina. When stimulated, the clitoris fills with blood, throbs, becomes sensitive, and moves out from under the hood. Like an iceberg, the visible part of the clitoris is only its tip; a larger mass of clitoral tissue is buried inside the body.

corpus luteum: A mass of progesterone-secreting endocrine tissue that forms from the ruptured follicle in the ovary immediately after ovulation.

endometrium: A blood- and nutrient-rich membrane that forms the lining of the uterus as part of the fertility cycle. If fertilization occurs, the fertilized egg implants in the endometrium. If fertilization does not occur, part of the endometrium is shed during the menses.

fallopian tube: A passageway that transports eggs from an ovary to the uterus.

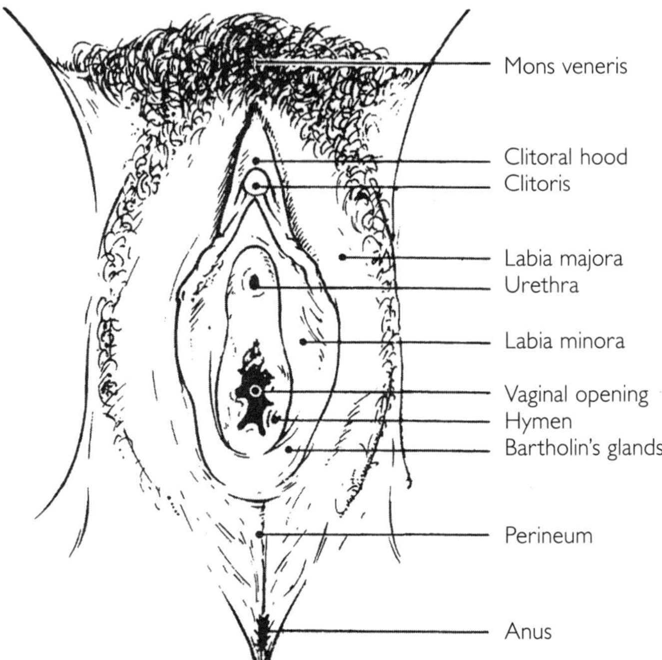

External female anatomy

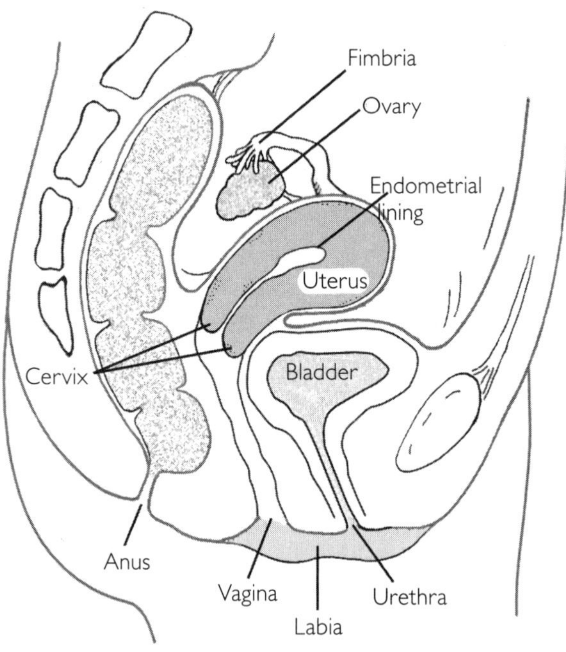

Internal female anatomy

There is one fallopian tube for each ovary. Egg fertilization usually occurs within the fallopian tube.

follicle: One of millions of vesicles containing a germ cell, or egg, in the ovaries.

G-spot: Spongy tissue containing a collection of blood vessels, glands, ducts, and nerve endings surrounding the urethra; it's said to be a source of great arousal for women. It may be easiest to find after a woman's orgasm when it is already somewhat enlarged and sensitive.

hymen: Membrane that partially occludes the vaginal entrance.

labia majora: The outer, larger lips of the vagina, extending from the mound of Venus and tapering to below the vaginal opening. They protect the vagina and urethra and contain sebaceous and apocrine glands. Labia can be smooth or have many folds. One side can be smaller or larger than the other. They are often covered with pubic hair.

labia minora: Hairless inner vaginal lips. When a woman is aroused, the labia minora swell, thicken, and darken. They secrete a sebum that helps lubricate the vagina.

mound of Venus: Loosely translated from *mons veneris* and also referred to as *mons pubis,* this is the fatty tissue mounded over the pubic bone, covered by skin and hair.

ovaries: Two grape-sized organs, located on each side of the uterus, that produce eggs and sex hormones such as estrogen, progesterone, and even small amounts of testosterone. A woman is born with all the eggs she will ever carry already in her ovaries; out of a possible 200,000 to 400,000 eggs, only about 400 ova will be released during a woman's childbearing years.

prepuce: *See* clitoral hood.

urethra: The narrow canal, located in the lower half of the front of the vaginal wall, that carries urine from the bladder and discharges it.

uterus: The womb; an organ for containing and nourishing an egg from fertilization through birth. An empty uterus weighs about 4 ounces; during menstruation, it can weigh 8 ounces.

vagina: The word *vagina* is derived from Latin, meaning "sheath for a sword." A bit warlike, *n'est-ce pas*? The vagina is a three- to four-inch-long tube of muscles and fibers. When relaxed, its thick folded walls, known as *rugae,* touch, so that almost no opening exists. When stimulated, the vagina enlarges, becoming wider and longer. The first layer of the vaginal walls is a mucous membrane that is capable of secreting fluids. Under the mucosa are layers of muscles and connective tissue that are rich in blood and nerve endings. Bacteria keep the moist vaginal climate slightly acidic, helping prevent "unfriendly" bacteria from proliferating.

vestibule: Entrance to the vagina.

vulva: A catch-all phrase that refers to the exterior of the female sexual organs: the vaginal opening, inner and outer labia, clitoral hood, clitoris, urethral opening, and everything else that is visible between the anus and the mound of Venus.

yoni: A term for vagina originating from Sanskrit terminology, meaning "origin" and "source."

MALE ANATOMY

Cowper's glands: Two small glands, comparable to the female Bartholin's glands, found at the base of the penile shaft, lying on either side of the urethra below the prostate gland. Before ejaculation, they produce a clear alkaline secretion that neutralizes any acid remaining in the urethra.

epididymis: A system of long, extensively coiled ducts above each testicle. After sperm is produced, it is stored in the epididymis, where it becomes mature and motile.

foreskin: A fold of skin that surrounds and protects the glans of the penis. It is also called the prepuce and is comparable to the clitoral hood.

frenulum: A connecting fold of membrane on the underside of the penis, where the shaft and glans meet. It is an extremely sensitive spot.

glans: The cone-shaped head of the penis. It has very thin skin and is rich with nerves, which makes it very sensitive to touch.

Leydig's cells: Epithelioid cells of the testes that produce androgens, namely testosterone.

lingam: A term for penis originating in Sanskrit terminology, meaning "pillar of light."

meatus: Any natural body passage. The opening of the glans at the head of the penis is properly called a meatus.

penis: The male organ of copulation, which also serves as the channel by which urine leaves the body. The penis contains spongy tissue, called erectile tissue; when a man is aroused, the tissue becomes engorged with blood and the surrounding muscles contract, causing the penis to become erect. When flaccid, the penis can range in size from 2.8 to 5.6 inches; when erect, the penis is usually 5 to 7 inches long. However, the entire penis and its sensitive nature continues into the body.

prostate: A partly muscular, partly glandular, chestnut-shaped organ located below the neck of the bladder, where the seminal vesicles and urethra join. The prostate secretes a milky, alkaline fluid that is a major constituent of semen.

scrotum: The pouch of skin that encloses the testicles.

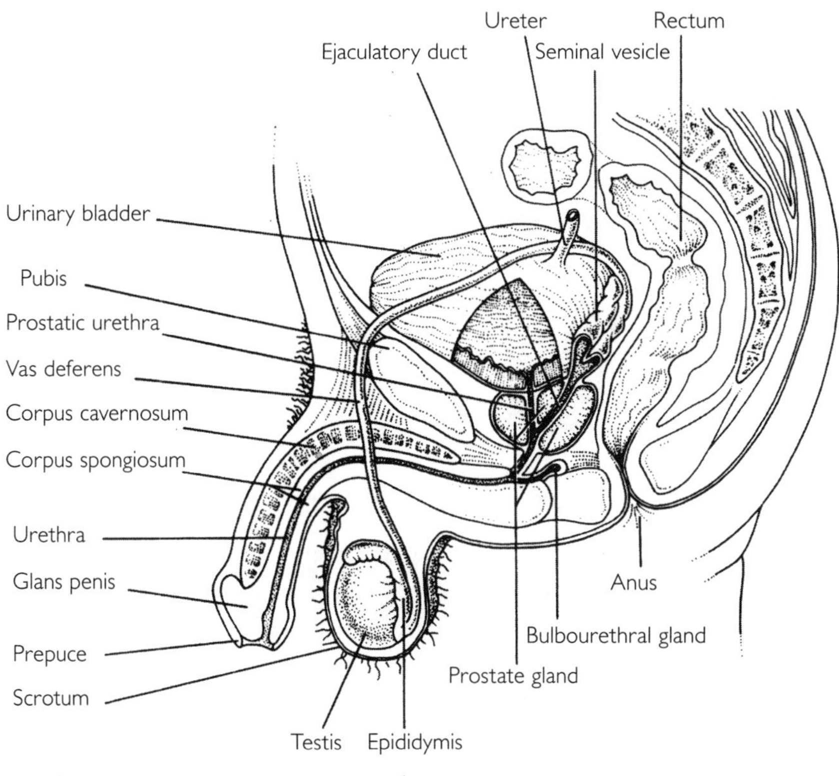

Male anatomy

semen: A milky fluid released during ejaculation consisting of sperm suspended in secretions of accessory glands.

seminal vesicle: A pair of glandular sacs located on either side of the reproductive tract. They produce most of the fluid in semen.

testicles: Reproductive glands that produce sperm. They also produce about 95 percent of a man's testosterone. The testicles are suspended in the scrotum below the penis; being held at a distance from the body allows sperm to stay slightly cooler than body temperature. The word *testicle* comes from the Latin *testis,* which is also the root of *testament* and *testify.* Men used to swear an oath by placing their hands over their testicles.

urethra: The canal that carries urine from the bladder to the meatus of the penis. It also conducts spermatic fluids.

vas deferens: One of a pair of thick-walled ducts that carry sperm from the epididymis to the seminal vesicle ducts.

APPENDIX THREE

HERBAL VOCABULARY

Natural medicines, such as herbs, homeopathic remedies, and flower essences, have a variety of physiological effects. Knowing the vocabulary that describes those effects can help you choose the medicine that best meets your needs.

abortifacient: Capable of inducing abortion.

adaptogen: Increases the body's resistance to stress, working through hormonal response.

alterative: Alters one's condition. Restores body functions. Increases blood flow to tissues, detoxifies, aids assimilation, stimulates metabolism, and promotes waste and excretion.

anabolic: Increases constructive metabolism.

analgesic: Relieves pain.

anaphrodisiac: Curbs sex drive.

anesthetic: Deadens sensation.

anodyne: Lessens pain by diminishing nerve excitability.

antidepressant: Elevates mood and counteracts depression.

antifungal: Inhibits growth of fungal organisms.

anti-inflammatory: Soothes inflammation.

antioxidant: Prevents free-radical damage, which is believed to contribute to cancerous growths.

antiseptic: Prevents bacterial growth, inhibits pathogens, counters sepsis.

antispasmodic: Prevents or eases cramps or spasms.

antiviral: Inhibits viral replication.

aphrodisiac: Increases sexual desire and potency.

aromatic: Is fragrant or pungent; improves flavor of bitter herbs. Often stimulates digestive tract.

astringent: Tightens, tones, and dries.

bitter: Stimulates flow of digestive secretions, as well as those of the pituitary, liver, and duodenum.

cholagogue: Promotes bile flow from the gallbladder.

choleretic: Stimulates bile production in the liver.

demulcent: Soothes irritated tissues, especially of the mucous membranes.

discutient: Dissolves tumors and abnormal growths. Used internally in moderation and also topically.

diuretic: Increases secretion and expulsion of urine by promoting activity of the kidneys and bladder.

emmenagogue: Stimulates uterus to promote menstruation. Normalizes female reproductive system.

euphoric: Produces an uplifting effect, physically and mentally.

galactagogue: Increases the production of mother's milk.

germicidal: Destroys germs, that is, microorganisms causing disease.

hallucinogen: Induces hallucinations.

hemostatic: Arrests bleeding.

hepatic: Strengthens and tones the liver.

hypotensive: Reduces blood pressure.

mucilaginous: Lubricates, soothes, and heals.

nervine: Calms and nourishes the nerves.

nutritive: Supplies nutrients to build and tone the body.

oxytocic: Stimulates the production of oxytocin, a hormone that induces uterine contractions. Can be used to assist or induce labor.

parturient: Assists in labor and delivery.

phytoandrogenic: Provides the raw materials to help the body make its own androgen hormones.

phytoestrogenic: Provides the raw materials to help the body make its own estrogen.

phytoprogesteronic: Provides the raw materials to help the body make its own progesterone.

progesteronic: Aids the body in the production or activation of progesterone.

refrigerant: Cools body temperature.

regenerative: Aids in the repair of bones, flesh, tissue, and cartilage.

soporific: Induces sleep.

rejuvenative: Renews body, mind, and spirit. Can counteract stress and increase endurance.

restorative: Helps rebuild a depleted condition and restores normal body functions.

rubefacient: Increases blood flow to the surface of the skin; draws out deep impurities.

sedative: Slows down body functions. Quiets the nerves.

stimulant: Quickens various body functions and improves circulation.

tonic: Promotes general health and well-being. Builds energy, blood, and chi.

vasoconstrictor: Narrows blood vessels, thus elevating blood pressure.

vasodilator: Expands blood vessels, thus reducing blood pressure.

vulnerary: Encourages wound healing by promoting cellular growth and repair.

RESOURCES

HERBS AND NATURAL PRODUCTS

BodySlant
P.O. Box 1667
Newport Beach, CA 92663
1-888-243-3279
www.ageeasy.com
Offers slant boards, body arches, and other healthful tools.

Essential Living Foods, Inc.
920 Colorado Ave
Santa Monica, CA 90401
310-319-1555
www.essentiallivingfoods.com
Sells excellent superfoods such as sun-cured olives, goji berries, raw cacao, and much more.

Flower Essence Services
P.O. Box 1769
Nevada City, CA 95959
800-548-0075
www.fesflowers.com
Purveyor of quality flower essences.

Foot Reflexology Charts
To order a laminated color version of the foot reflexology chart that appears in this book, e-mail nrflexdiag@gmail.com. The price is $22 plus shipping.

Frontier Herbs
P.O. Box 299
Norway, IA 52318
1-800-669-3275
www.frontiercoop.com
A great mail-order service for herbs.

Gaia Herbs
108 Island Ford Road
Brevard, NC 28712
1-800-831-7780
www.gaiaherbs.com
Maker of liquid extracts and plant-based capsules.

Herbalist and Alchemist
51 South Wandling Avenue
Washington, NJ 07882
1-800-611-8235
www.herbalist-alchemist.com
Purveyor of Western and Oriental herbal formulas.

Herb Pharm
P.O. Box 116
Williams, OR 97544
1-800-348-4372
www.herb-pharm.com
Maker of excellent herbal tinctures.

Horizon Herbs
P.O. Box 69
Williams, OR 97544-0069
541-846-6704
www.chatlink.com/~herbseed
The best source for herb seeds, including many herbs that are endangered in the wild.

Little Moon Essentials
P.O. Box 771893
Steamboat Springs, CO 80477
1-888-273-0683
www.littlemoonessentials.com
Maker of cosmic aromatherapy, bath, health, and sensual products.

Natural Pleasure
58 Charles Street
Cambridge, Massachusetts 02141
717-633-1850
www.naturalpleasure.com
A good source of transdermal arginine creams.

Star West
11253 Trade Center Drive
Rancho Cordova, CA 95742
1-800-800-4372
www.starwest-botanicals.com
A mail-order source for quality herbs.

Sunfood Nutrition
11653 Riverside Drive
Lakeside, CA 92040
(800) 205-2350 or 888-RAW-FOOD
www.sunfood.com
Sells excellent superfoods such as raw cacao, goji berries, body care products, and health books.

SEX TOYS, BOOKS, AND VIDEOS

Eve's Garden
119 West 57th Street, Suite 1201
New York, NY 10019
1-800-848-3837, 212- 757-8651
www.evesgarden.com
Videos, books, and sex toys. On-site retail store and a mail-order catalog.

Good Vibrations
603 Valencia Street
San Francisco, CA 94110
1-800-289-8423, 415- 5225460
www.goodvibes.com
Videos, books, and sex toys. On-site retail store and a mail-order catalog.

Smitten Kitten
3010 Lyndale Avenue S
Minneapolis, MN 55408
612-721-6088
www.smittenkittenonline.com
Progressive sex shop.

EDUCATIONAL RESOURCE GROUPS

American Association of Acupuncture and Oriental Medicine
P.O. Box 162340
Sacramento, CA 95816
916-443-4770
www.aaaomonline.org

Their website offers an up-to-date listing of certified acupuncturists across the United States.

American Association of Sex Educators, Counselors, and Therapists (AASECT)
P.O. Box 1960
Ashland, Virginia 23005-1960
804-752-0026
www.aasect.org

Can provide a list of certified sex therapists in your area.

American Botanical Council
P.O. Box 144345
Austin, TX 78714-4345
www.herbalgram.org
1-800-373-7105

A member-supported education and research organization in the field of herbal medicine. Sells herb-education books and publishes *Herbalgram* magazine.

American Herb Association
P.O. Box 1673
Nevada, CA 95959
530-265-9552
www.ahaherb.com

Complete listing of schools, programs, seminars, and correspondencecourses in the herb category. Excellent newsletter.

American Herbalists Guild
141 Nob Hill Road
Cheshire, CT 06410
Phone: 203.272.6731
Fax: 203.272.8550
www.americanherbalist.com

The only national organization for professional, peer-reviewed herbal practitioners. Offers a directory of members.

Annie Sprinkle, Ph.D.
annie@anniesprinkle.org
www.loveartlab.org

Prostitute/porn star turned artist/sexologist. She offers a variety of workshops, including Super Sex Technologies, and Fun with Ecstasy Breathing & Energy Orgasms. She also offers feminist edu-porn DVDs, sex-life makeovers, and internships.

The Endometriosis Association
8585 North 76th Place
Milwaukee, WI 53223
414-355-2200
www.endometriosisassn.org

This international nonprofit organization provides information about the causes, symptoms, and treatments of endometriosis. It also offers a physician registry and referrals to holistic health care practitioners.

Herb Research Foundation
4140 15th Street
Boulder, CO 80304
303 449-2265
www.herbs.org

A clearinghouse for herb information.

Institute for the Advanced Study of Human Sexuality
1523 Franklin Street
San Francisco, CA 94109
415-928-1133
www.iashs.edu

A graduate-level school for the study of human sexuality.

The National Center for Homeopathy
801 North Fairfax Street, Suite 306
Alexandria, VA 22314
703-548-7790
www.homeopathic.org

This organization offers general information about homeopathy, practitioner referrals, and educational programs.

National Gay and Lesbian Task Force
1325 Massachusetts Ave. NW
Suite 600
Washington, DC 20005
202-393-5177
www.the taskforce.org

A nonprofit agency focusing on advocacy, electoral work, and sociological research.

National Organization of Circumcision Information Resource Centers
P.O. Box 2512
San Anselmo, CA 94979
415-488-9883
www.nocirc.org

A nonprofit educational center for those questioning the necessity of circumcising male and female infants and children.

Parents, Family, and Friends of Lesbian and Gays
1726 M Street Northwest,
Suite 400
Washington, DC 20036
202-467-8180
www.pflag.org

Can provide referrals to local chapters.

Sex and Love Addicts Anonymous
1550 NE Loop 410, Ste. 118
San Antonio, TX 78209
210-828-7900
www.slaafws.org

Provides information on local support groups and resources for those with sex addictions.

Sexaholics Anonymous
P.O. Box 3565
Brentwood, TN 37024
(866) 424-8777, (615) 370-6062
www.sa.org

Provides information on local support groups and resources for those with sex addictions.

Source School of Tantra
P.O. Box 368
Wailuku, HI 96733
808-243-9851
www.sourcetantra.com

Offers tantra workshops.

Truth Book
www.TruthBook.com

Answers questions about the nature of God the Father; Universe Mother; the cosmos; the history of our planet, Urantia; marriage and family life; Adam and Eve; life on other planets; life after death; and much more!

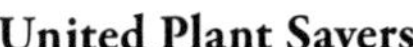

United Plant Savers
P.O. Box 400
East Barre, VT 05649
802-479-6467
www.plantsavers.org

Group that promotes awareness about rare and endangered species of plants. Great newsletter.

HOTLINES

Centers for Disease Control STD and AIDS Hotline
1-800-227-8922 and
1-800-242-2437
In Spanish: 1-800-344-7432
For the hearing impaired:
1-800-243-7889
www.ashastd.org

Provides information and helps people find local resources for emergency housing and medical care.

Domestic Violence Hotline
1-800-799-SAFE

Offers information and referrals for victims as well as a database of shelters, counseling services, and legal services.

Emergency Contraception Hotline
1-800-584-9911

Can provide contact information for health care providers in your area who can supply you with emergency contraception.

Planned Parenthood Federation of America
1-800-230-7526

Provides information on contraception and sexually transmitted diseases.

PMS/Menopause Hotline
1-800-222-4767

Provides informational packets on natural hormone replacement therapy and other women's health issues.

BIBLIOGRAPHY

Aldred, Caroline. *Divine Sex.* San Francisco: HarperSanFrancisco, 1996.

Allardice, Pamela. *Aphrodisiacs and Love Magic.* Dorset, England: Prism Press, 1989.

Anand, Margo. *The Art of Sexual Ecstasy.* Los Angeles: Jeremy P. Tarcher, 1989.

Baker, Jeannine Parvati. *Hygieia: A Women's Herbal.* Berkeley, Calif.: Freestone Publishing, 1978.

Barbach, Lonnie, Ph.D., and David Geisinger, Ph.D. *Going the Distance.* New York: Doubleday, 1991.

Barbieri, Robert, M.D., Alice Domar, Ph.D., and Kevin Loughlin, M.D. *Six Steps to Increased Fertility.* New York: Simon and Schuster, 2000.

Baroni, Diane, and Betty Kelly. *How to Get Him Back from the Other Woman.* New York: St. Martin's Press, 1992.

Beattie, Antonia. *Love Magic.* New York: Barnes and Noble Books, 2000.

Bechtel, Stefan, and the editors of *Men's Health* and *Prevention* magazines. *The Practical Encyclopedia of Sex and Health.* Emmaus, Pa.: Rodale Press, 1993.

Bechtel, Stefan, and Laurence Roy Stains. *Sex: A Man's Guide.* Emmaus, Pa.: Rodale Press, 1996.

Bishop, Clifford. *Sex and Spirit.* New York: Little, Brown & Company, 1996.

Brauer, Alan P., M.D., and Donna J. Brauer. *The ESO Ecstasy Program.* New York: Warner Books, 1990.

Budapest, Zsuzsanna E. *The Goddess in the Bedroom.* San Francisco: HarperSanFrancisco, 1995.

Buhner, Stephan Harrod. *Vital Man.* New York: Penguin Putman, 2003.

Burke, Peggy, and Evan Burke. *The Woman's Gourmet Sex Book.* Canoga Park, Calif.: Malibu Press, 1983.

Cabot, Laurie, and Tom Cowan. *Love Magic.* New York: Delta Publishing, 1992.

Cabot, Tracy, Ph.D. *How to Make a Man Fall in Love with You.* New York: St. Martin's Press, 1984.

Castleman, Michael. *Sexual Solutions.* New York: Simon and Schuster, 1983.

Chang, Jolan. *The Tao of Love and Sex.* New York: E. P. Dutton, 1977.

———. *The Tao of the Loving Couple.* New York: E. P. Dutton, 1983.

Chang, Dr. Stephen T. *The Tao of Sexology.* San Francisco: Tao Publishing, 1988.

Chia, Mantak, *Healing Love through the Tao: Cultivating Female Sexual Energy.* Rochester, Vt.: Destiny Books, 2005.

Chia, Mantak, and Douglas Abrams Arava. *The Multi-Orgasmic Man.* San Francisco: HarperSanFrancisco, 2000.

Chia, Mantak, and Michael Winn. *Taoist Secrets of Love: Cultivating Male Sexual Energy.* New York: Aurora Press, 1984.

Chu, Valentin. *The Yin-Yang Butterfly.* New York: G. P. Putnam's Sons, 1993.

Clapp, Larry, Ph.D., J.D. *Prostate Health in Ninety Days.* Carlsbad, Calif.: Hay House, 1997.

Colgan, Dr. Michael. *Hormonal Health.* Vancouver, BC: Apple Publishing, 1996.

Coleman, Dr. Paul. *The 30 Secrets of Happily Married Couples.* Holbrook, Mass.: Bob Adams Publishers, 1992.

Corn, Laura. *101 Nights of Grrreat Romance.* Tempe, Ariz.: Park Avenue Publishers, 1996.

Cox, Tracey. *Hot Relationships.* New York: Bantam Books, 2000.

———. *Hot Sex.* New York: Bantam Books, 1999.

Crawford, Amanda McQuade. *The Herbal Menopause Book.* Freedom, Calif.: The Crossing Press, 1996.

Crenshaw, Theresa. *The Alchemy of Love and Lust.* New York: G. P. Putnam's Sons, 1996.

Cunningham, Scott. *The Magic of Food.* Saint Paul, Minn.: Llewellyn Publications, 1996.

DeAngelis, Barbara, Ph.D. *How to Make Love All the Time.* New York: Rawson Associates, 1987.

———. *Real Moments for Lovers.* New York: Delacorte Press, 1995.

De Luca, Diana. *Bella Donna.* Sebastapol, Calif.: Bella Botanica Press, 2001.

———. *Botanica Erotica.* Rochester, Vt.: Healing Arts Press, 1998.

Devi, Kamala. *The Eastern Way of Love.* New York: Simon and Schuster, 1985.

Douglas, Nik, and Penny Slinger. *Sexual Secrets.* Rochester, Vt.: Destiny Books, 2000.

Dunas, Felice, Ph.D., and Philip Goldberg. *Passion Play.* New York: Riverhead Books, 1997.

Edell, Ronnie, Ph.D. *The Sexually Satisfied Woman.* New York: Dutton, 1994.

Ellenberg, Daniel, Ph.D., and Judith Bell, M.S., M.F.C.C. *Lovers for Life.* Santa Rosa, Calif.: Aslan Publishing, 1995.

Fellner, Tara. *Aromatherapy for Lovers.* Boston: Charles E. Tuttle Co., Inc., 1995.

Feng Shui Journal 5, no. 1 (Spring 1999). (This is the "Love" issue.)

Feuerstein, Georg, Ph.D. *Sacred Sexuality: The Erotic Spirit in the World's Great Religions.* Rochester, Vt.: Inner Traditions, 2003.

Fisher, Bruce, and Nina Hart. *Loving Choices: A Growing Experience.* Boulder, Colo.: Fisher Publishing Company, 2000.

Fisher, Helen, Ph.D. *Anatomy of Love.* New York: Fawcett Columbine, 1992.

Flatto, Edwin, M.D. *Super Potency at Any Age.* New York: Instant Improvement, Inc., 1991.

Gach, Michael Reed, Ph.D. *Acupressure for Lovers.* New York: Bantam Books, 1997.

Garrison, Omar. *Tantra: The Yoga of Sex.* New York: Julian Press, 1964.

Gibbens, Kalyn Wolf. *Marrying Smart: A Practical Guide for Attracting Your Mate.* Eugene, Ore.: Just Your Type Publishing, 1994.

Gittleman, Ann Louise. *Super Nutrition for Menopause.* New York: Penguin Putman, Inc., 1998.

Gladstar, Rosemary. *Herbal Healing for Women.* New York: Simon and Schuster, 1993.

———. *Rosemary Gladstar's Family Herbal.* North Adams, Mass.: Storey Books, 2001.

Glanz, Larry, and Robert Phillips. *How to Start a Romantic Encounter.* Garden City Park, N.Y.: Avery Publishing Group, 1994.

———. *1001 Ways to Be Romantic.* Boston: Casablanca Press, Inc., 1994.

Gray, John, Ph.D. *Mars and Venus in the Bedroom.* New York: HarperCollins, 1995.

———. *The Mars and Venus Diet and Exercise Solution.* New York: Saint Martin's Press, 2003.

Green, James. *The Male Herbal.* Freedom, Calif.: Crossing Press, 1991.

Haffner, Debra W., M.P.H., and Pepper Schwartz, Ph.D. *What I've Learned About Sex.* New York: Berkeley Publishing Group, 1998.

Hare, Jenny. *Think Sex: The Seven Secrets of Mind-Blowing Sex.* Boston: Element Books, 2000.

Hayden, Naura. *How to Satisfy a Woman Every Time.* New York: Bibliophile Publishing Company, 1982.

Hendrickson, Robert. *Lewd Food.* Radnor, Pa.: Chilton Book Company, 1974.

Hendrix, Harville, Ph.D. *Getting the Love You Want.* New York: HarperCollins, 1988.

———. *Keeping the Love You Find.* New York: Pocket Books, 1992.

Heng, Cheng. *The Tao of Love.* New York: Marlowe and Company, 1997.

Hooper, Anne. *Anne Hooper's Kama Sutra.* New York: Dorling Kindersley, 1994.

———. *The Ultimate Sex Book.* New York: Dorling Kindersley, 1992.

Jensen, Dr. Bernard. *Love, Sex & Nutrition.* Garden City Park, N.Y.: Avery Publishing Group, 1988.

Jillson, Joyce. *The Fine Art of Flirting.* New York: Simon and Schuster, 1984.

Joannides, Paul. *The Guide to Getting It On!* Santa Monica, Calif.: Goofy Foot Press, 1997.

Jonas, Barbara, and Michael Jonas. *The Book of Love, Laughter & Romance.* San Francisco: Games Partnership, Ltd., 1994.

Kelley, Susan. *Why Men Stray, Why Men Stay.* Holbrook, Mass.: Adams Media Corporation, 1996.

Keville, Kathi, and Mindy Green. *Aromatherapy: A Complete Guide to the Healing Art.* Freedom, Calif.: Crossing Press, 1995.

Kilham, Christopher Scott. *Stalking the Wild Orgasm.* San Diego: ACS Publications, 1987.

Kingma, Daphne Rose. *Coming Apart: Why Relationships End and How to Live through the Ending of Yours.* New York: Ballantine Books, 1993.

Kirban, Salem. *How to Win Over Impotence/Frigidity.* Huntington Valley, Pa.: Salem Kirban, 1981.

Kreidman, Ellen. *Light Her Fire.* New York: Villard Books, 1991.

———. *Light His Fire.* New York: Villard Books, 1989.

Lapanja, Margie. *The Goddess Guide to Love: Timeless Secrets to Divine Romance.* Berkeley, Calif.: Conari Press, 1999.

Lee, William H., D.Sc., R.Ph., and Lynn Lee, C.N. *Herbal Love Potions.* New Canaan, Conn.: Keats Publishing, 1991.

Katz, Aaron E., M.D. *Dr. Katz's Gude to Prostate Health.* Topanga, Calif.: Freedom Press, 2006.

Lloyd, J. William. *Karezza.* Hollywood, Calif.: Phoenix House, 1973.

Lozowick, Leo. *The Alchemy of Love and Sex.* Prescott, Ariz.: Hohm Press, 1996.

Masterson, Graham. *How to Make His Wildest Dreams Come True.* New York: Penguin Group, 1996.

———. *Secrets of the Sexually Irresistible Woman.* New York: Penguin Group, 1998.

Meletis, Chris D., N.D. *Better Sex Naturally.* New York: HarperCollins, 2000.

Miller, Light, N.D., and Brian Miller, N.D. *Ayurveda and Aromatherapy.* Twin Lakes, Wis.: Lotus Press, 1995.

Miller, Richard Alan. *The Magical and Ritual Use of Aphrodisiacs.* Rochester, Vt.: Destiny Books, 1993.

Mitton, Mervyn. *Herbal Remedies/Sexual Problems.* Berkshire, England: Foulsham Publishers, 1992.

Moore, Thomas. *The Soul of Sex.* New York: HarperCollins, 1998.

Muir, Charles, and Caroline Muir. *Tantra: The Art of Conscious Loving.* San Francisco: Mercury House, 1989.

Nissim, Rina. *Natural Healing in Gynecology.* New York: Pandora Press, 1986.

O'Hara, Kristen, and Jeffrey O'Hara. *Sex as Nature Intended It.* Hudson, Mass.: Turning Point Publications, 2001.

Oumano, Elena, Ph.D. *Natural Sex.* New York: Plume, 1999.

Paget, Lou. *How to Be a Great Lover.* New York: Broadway Books, 1999.

Peiper, Howard, N.D., and Nina Anderson. *Natural Solutions for Sexual Dysfunction.* New Canaan, Conn.: Safe Goods, 1998.

Pelton, Charles, M.D. *The Sex Book.* Aberdeen, S. Dak.: Family Health Media, 1982.

Ramsdale, David, and Ellen Ramsdale. *Sexual Energy Ecstasy.* Playa Del Rey, Calif.: Peak Skill Publishing, 1991.

Rätsch, Christian. *Plants of Love.* Berkeley, Calif.: Ten Speed Press, 1997.

Reid, Daniel P. *The Tao of Health, Sex, and Longevity.* New York: Simon and Schuster, 1989.

Renshaw, Domeena, M.D. *Seven Weeks to Better Sex.* New York: Random House, 1995.

Rich, Penny. *Pamper Your Partner.* New York: Simon and Schuster, 1990.

Richardson, Diana. *The Love Keys.* Boston: Element Books, 1999.

Roizen, Michael, M.D., and Dr. Mehmet Oz. *You Staying Young.* New York: Simon and Schuster, 2007.

Rose, Jeanne. *Herbs and Aromatherapy for the Reproductive System.* Berkeley, Calif.: Frog, Limited, 1994.

Saint Claire, Olivia. *Unleashing the Sex Goddess in Every Woman.* New York: Bantam Books, 1996.

Saraswati, Sunyata, and Bodhi Avinasha. *Jewel in the Lotus.* San Francisco: Kriya Jyoti Tantra Society, 1987.

Saul, David, M.D. *Sex for Life: The Lover's Guide to Male Sexuality.* Vancouver, BC: Apple Publishing Company, Ltd, 1999.

Selden, Gary. *Aphrodisia.* New York: E. P. Dutton, 1979.

Sellman, Sherrill. *Hormone Heresy.* Tulsa, Okla.: GetWell International, 2000.

Sonntag, Linda. *Great Sex for Life.* USA: Hamlyn Publishing, 1997.

Stiller, Richard. *The Love Bugs.* New York: Thomas Nelson, Inc., 1974.

Stoppard, Miriam, M.D. *The Magic of Sex.* New York: Dorling Kindersley, 1992.

Stubbs, Kenneth Ray, Ph.D. *Women of the Light.* Larkspur, Calif.: Secret Garden, 1994.

Tisserand, Maggie. *Essence of Love.* San Francisco: HarperSanFrancisco, 1993.

Too, Lillian. *Lillian Too's Easy to Use Feng Shui for Love.* London, England: Collins and Brown, 2000.

Tresidder, Megan. *The Secret Language of Love.* San Francisco: Chronicle Books, 1997.

Tseng, C. Howard, M.D., Ph.D., Guilas Villanueva, M.D., and Alvin Powell, M.D. *Sexually Transmitted Diseases.* Saratoga, Calif.: R & E Publishers, 1987.

Urantia Foundation. *The Urantia Book.* Boulder, Colo.: Uversa Press, 2007.

Venus, Brenda. *Secrets of Seduction.* New York: Dutton, 1996.

Walker, Morton, D.P.M. *Foods for Better Sex.* Old Greenwich, Conn.: Devin-Adair Publishers, 1984.

———. *Sexual Nutrition.* Garden City Park, N.Y.: Avery Publishing Group, 1994.

Warburton, Diana. *A–Z of Aphrodisia.* New York: Quartet Books, 1986.

Watson, Cynthia Mervis, M.D. *Love Potions.* New York: Jeremy P. Tarcher, 1993.

Waylor, Susan, Ph.D. *Sexual Radiance.* New York: Harmony Books, 1998.

Wedeck, H. E. *Dictionary of Aphrodisiacs.* London, England: Bracken Books, 1994.

Weed, Susun S. *New Menopausal Years.* Woodstock, N.Y.: Ash Tree Publishing, 2002.

Westheimer, Dr. Ruth. *Sex for Dummies.* Foster City, Calif.: International Data Group Books, 1995.

Wildwood, Chrissie. *Erotic Aromatherapy.* New York: Sterling Publishing, 1994.

Wilson, Dr. Glenn. *Exotic Sex.* London, England: Marshall Cavendish Books, 1992.

Wong, Bruce. *TSFR: The Taoist Way to Total Sexual Fitness for Men.* Princeton, N.J.: Golden Dragon Publishers, 1982.

Yudelove, Eric Steven. *The Tao and the Tree of Life.* Saint Paul, Minn.: Llewellyn Publications, 1995.

ABOUT THE AUTHOR

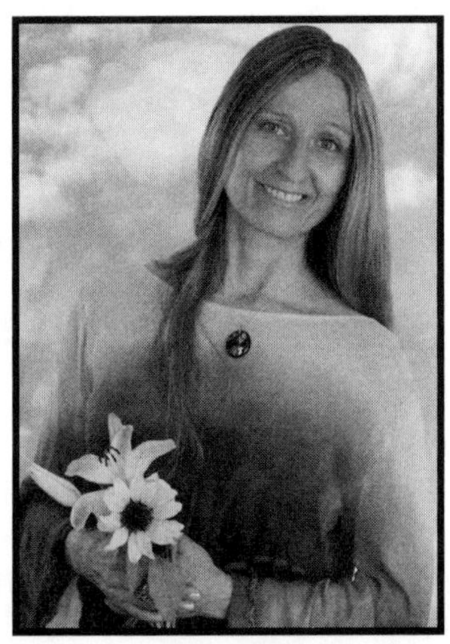

Brigitte Mars is an herbalist and nutritional consultant from Boulder, Colorado, who has been working with natural medicine since the late sixties. She teaches herbal medicine at Naropa University, Boulder College of Massage Therapy, Bauman College of Health and Nutrition, and Omega Institute. She is a professional member of the American Herbalist Guild. She is a mother of two daughters and grandmother of three. She has been with her husband, Tom Pfeiffer, a human design analyst, since 1977. Brigitte Mars is also available for herbal consultations and formulations. For more information, visit her website at:

www.brigittemars.com

OTHER PUBLICATIONS BY BRIGITTE MARS

Books

The Desktop Guide to Herbal Medicine: The Ultimate Multidisciplinary Reference to the Amazing Realm of Healing Plants. Laguna Beach, Calif.: Basic Health Publications, 2007.

Beauty by Nature. Summertown, Tenn.: The Book Publishing Company, 2006.

Healing Herbal Teas: A Complete Guide to Making Delicious, Healthful Beverages. Laguna Beach, Calif.: Basic Health Publications, 2006.

Rawsome!: Maximizing Health, Energy, and Culinary Delight with the Raw Foods Diet. Laguna Beach, Calif.: Basic Health Publications, 2004.

Addiction-Free Naturally: Liberating Yourself from Sugar, Caffeine, Food Addictions, Tobacco, Alcohol, and Prescription Drugs. Rochester, Vt.: Healing Arts Press, 2001.

Dandelion Medicine: Remedies and Recipes to Detoxify, Nourish, and Stimulate. North Adams, Mass.: Storey Books, 1999.

The HempNut Health and Cookbook: Ancient Food for New Millennium, with coauthor Richard Rose. Santa Rosa, Calif.: HempNut, Inc., 2000.

Herbs for Healthy Skin, Hair & Nails: Banish Eczema, Acne, and Psoriasis with Healing Herbs That Cleanse the Body Inside and Out. New Canaan, Conn.: Keats Publishing, 1998.

Natural First Aid: Herbal Treatments for Ailments and Injuries, Emergency Preparedness, and Wilderness Safety. North Adams, Mass.: Storey Books, 1999.

DVDs

Healing Herbs and Wild Food: Herb Walk and Food Preparation. Madison, Wis.: Herb TV.

Rawsome! DVD companion to the bestselling book. Boulder, Colo.: Angel Energy Enterprises, 2007.

Computer Software

The Herbal Pharmacy: The Interactive CD-Rom Guide to Medicinal Plants. Boulder, Colo.: Hale Software, 1998.

Audiotapes

The Herbal Renaissance: How to Heal with Common Plants and Herbs. Louisville, Colo.: Sounds True, 1990.

Natural Remedies for a Healthy Immune System. Louisville, Colo.: Sounds True, 1990.

Index

5-HTP, 446

abstinence, 241
acidophilus, 201, 246, 249–50, 308–9, 329, 398, 411, 416
Aconitum Napellus, 333, 358
acupressure, 163–65, *189*, 414
Acupressure for Lovers, 163
acupuncture, 302–3
addiction, 458–59
after play, 204
Agnus Castus, 141, 391
agrimony, 281, 348
alcohol, 46–47
Aletris Farinosa, 358, 391
alfalfa, 270, 348, 364, 387
alisma, 387
allergens, 13, 252
almond oil, 160
almonds, 28–29
aloe vera, 253
Alpine Lily (flower essence), 376
amber (essential oil), 137
amenorrhea, 344–45
amino acids, 329
anal sex, 202–3
anaphrodisiacs, 48
anchovies, 22
angelica, 262, 296–97, 348, 364, 387
angelica (essential oil), 277, 377, 392
anger, 445–48
anise (essential oil), 357, 377, 392
anise seeds, 41, 348
antibiotics, 246, 248
antifungal teas, 251
antioxidants, 258, 284, 290, 403
antiperspirants, 279–80
Aphrodisiac Formula for Men, 98
Aphrodisiac Formula for Women, 98
aphrodisiacs, 13–14
  beverages, 46–47
  culinary herbs as, 40–45
  See also superfoods
Apis Mellifica, 275, 294, 333, 358, 373–74, 412
apple cider vinegar, 51
apples, 14–15
Argentum Nitricum, 333

arginine, 115, 323, 385–86, 408
Arnica, 269
aromatherapy, 126–39
for endometriosis, 277
for fertility, 392
for menopause, 377
for menstruation, 357
for pelvic inflammatory disease, 291
for STDs, 404
for trauma, 447
for urinary tract infections, 295
for uterine fibroids, 302
for uterine prolapse, 306
Aromatherapy: A Complete Guide to the Healing Art, 136
aromatherapy massage, 267–68, 285
arousal, 178–79
Arsenicum Album, 275, 412
artichokes, 15
asafoetida, 253
ashwagandha, 52–53, 387
asparagus, 15–16, 54–55, 270, 364, 387
Asparagus-Epimedium Tea, 103
Aspen (flower essence), 147
A-spot, 216
astragalus, 281, 297, 310, 387
Atahualpa, 33
Aurum Muriaticum Natronatum, 275, 391
avocados, 16

Bach, Edward, 146
Bach Flower Remedies, 146
bacterial vaginosis, 286
bad breath, 180
bagua, 150–53
Banana (flower essence), 147
bananas, 16–17
barley grass, 253
Bartholin's gland cysts, 246–48
Baryta Carbonica, 247, 333, 391
basal body temperature, 233
basil, 348
basil (essential oil), 357, 392, 447
Basil (flower essence), 147–48
bathrooms, 166–67
baths, 7, 136, 168–69, 256–57, 311, 315, 453. *See also* therapeutic baths
bath salts, 137
bedding, 137
bedroom, 153–57
bee pollen, 329
beets, 17
Belladonna, 247, 275, 285, 333, 358, 374
Bellis, 269
Bells of Ireland (flower essence), 392
benign prostatic hyperplasia (BPH), 327
Berberis, 141–42
Berberis Vulgaris, 294
bergamot (essential oil), 404
berries, 17–18
beta-carotene, 107, 386, 411
beverages, aphrodisiac, 46–47
biotin, 253
Blackberry (flower essence), 277, 392
black cohosh, 262, 270, 281, 297, 304, 307, 348, 364–65
Black-eyed Susan (flower essence), 148
black haw, 348–49, 365
black sesame seeds, 7
black walnut, 253, 410
Bleeding Heart (flower essence), 455
blessed thistle, 262, 281, 297, 349, 365
blood, 269, 296

blue cohosh, 262, 270, 297, 349, 365
blue-green algae, 18
body language, 174
body powder, 137
bodywork, 303–4, 446
Borage (flower essence), 376, 455
Borax, 256, 391, 412
boric acid, 250–51
Brazil nuts, 29
breast-feeding, 220
breasts, 184–85, 201
breathing, 124–25
broken hearts, 450–55
brown algaes, 38
Bryonia, 285, 309, 374
buchu, 292, 330–31
Buddha, 156
bupleurum, 263, 271, 349, 365
burdock, 55–56, 258–59, 271, 281, 286, 297, 349, 365, 402, 410
Butterfly Exercise, 122
butterfly flick, 198

cabbage, 18
cacao, 19
cacti, 152
caffeine, 280
Caladium Seguinum, 142
Calcarea Carbonica, 142, 256, 358, 374, 403, 412
calcium, 112–13, 372, 411, 447
Calendula, 137
calendula, 253, 281, 289, 297, 417
calendula-goldenseal salve, 247
Calendula Officinalis, 403
California Wild Rose (flower essence), 376
candidiasis, 248–57, 285–86
candles, 12, 152–53
Cannabis Indica, 333
Cantharis, 142, 276, 294, 374
carbohydrates, 248, 252
Carbo Vegetabilis, 142, 358, 413
cardamom (essential oil), 128, 447
cardamom seeds, 41
carnitine, 386
carrots, 19–20
cartenoids, 23
castor oil compresses, 267, 275, 290, 302
Cat Stretch, 122
catuaba, 56–57
Caulophyllum Thalictroides, 358
caviar, 22–23
cayenne pepper, 41, 253, 349
cedar leaf (essential oil), 404
ceiling beams, 154–55
celandine, 259, 263, 297
celery, 20
cervical caps, 230–31
cervical dysplasia, 257–61
cervical mucus, 234
cervicitis, 397
chakra anointment, 137
chamomile, 271, 290–91, 297, 324, 349
chamomile (essential oil), 277, 357
Chamomilla, 276, 358, 446
champa (essential oil), 129, 447
chaparral, 253–54, 259, 263, 298, 410, 417
cherries, 20–21
Cherry Plum (flower essence), 447
chia seeds, 29
chickweed, 263, 365
Chimaphila Umbellata, 333

Chinese patent formulas, 68–69, 105, 271, 274, 301, 367, 373, 388, 390, 412
Chininum Sulphuricum, 391
chlamydia, 286, 396–98
chlorophyll, 26, 201, 253, 386
chocolate, 19
choline, 107–8, 274
Cimicifuga Racemosa, 276, 358
Cinchona Officinalis, 142–43, 374
cinnamon, 349
cinnamon (essential oil), 129, 404
cinnamon bark, 41
circulation, 14, 18
circumcision, 313–16
clary sage (essential oil), 129, 357, 377, 392
clay poultices, 247, 291
cleavers, 247, 281, 289, 292, 298, 324, 331, 402
Clematis (flower essence), 148
clitoris, 186–87, 200–201
closets, 156
clothing, 245, 279, 313
clove (essential oil), 130
Clove Anesthetic Balm, 210
clove bud, 41–42
Cocculus Indicus, 358
Coconut-Avocado Love Elixir, 100
coconut oil, 160
coconuts, 29–30
codonopsis, 263, 350
coital alignment technique, 191
cold packs, 318
collards, 26
collinsonia, 298
Colocynthis, 276, 359
colon, 279
color therapy, 156–57, 453
communication, 173–74
condoms, 202, 203, 225, 227, 228–30
Conium, 143, 285, 333, 391
contraception, 227–41, 381
coriander (essential oil), 130, 377, 447
coriander seed, 42
cornsilk, 292, 331
cotton root, 298, 350
couchgrass, 292, 331
Crab Apple (flower essence), 148, 376, 400
crabs, 398–400
cramp bark, 263, 271, 298, 324, 350, 365
cranberries, 329
Crocus Sativus, 374
crying, 204
cryptorchidism, 316–17
crystals, 156
cubeb, 254, 331
culinary herbs, 40–45
cumin (essential oil), 392
cumin seed, 42
cunnilingus, 200–201
curry, 42
cypress (essential oil), 277, 377
cystitis, 291

damiana, 57–58
Damiana Rose Cordial, 97
Dance, Dance, Dance!, 123
dandelion, 259, 263, 271, 281, 286, 298, 350, 365–66, 388, 403
daniana, 387–88
dan shen, 298

Date Parfait, 101
deep breathing, 124–25
Deer Exercise, 119–20
delayed ejaculation, 317
dental dams, 227
Desktop Guide to Herbal Medicine, The, 52
diaphragms, 227, 230–31
diet
  for candida, 251–53
  for fertility, 385
  for fibrocystic breasts, 280
  for healthy menstruation, 347
  for leukorrhea, 286
  for menopause, 363–64
  for STDs, 408–9
  for urinary tract infections, 292
  for uterine fibroids, 296
  for vaginal dryness, 307
dietary imbalances, 212–13
diffusers, 138
DIM (diinodolylmethane), 372
dimethylglycine, 116
Dioscorea, 276
dioxin, 268
disablement, 221–22
diuretics, 330
dong quai, 58–60, 263, 271, 281, 304, 324–25, 350, 366, 388
dopamine, 53, 460
douches and douching, 245, 251, 287, 418
drinking, 322
Dulcamara, 359, 413
dulse, 38
durian, 21
dysmenorrhea, 341–43
ears, 184
Easter Lily (flower essence), 148
echinacea, 254, 259, 282, 286, 289, 310, 318, 325, 331, 397, 403, 410, 417
edible flowers, 12, 45–46
eel, 23
ejaculation, 199–200, 206
  delaying, 208–10
  orgasm without, 210–11
  See also female ejaculation; premature ejaculation
elder, 366
electromagnetic energy, 382
eleuthero, 60–62, 366
Elm (flower essence), 148
Embracing the Uncarved Block, 54
emergency contraception, 232
emotional armoring, 213
endometriosis, 268–77
endorphins, 4, 461
energy levels, 12–13
epididymitis, 318–19
epimedium, 62–63
Equisetum, 294
erectile dysfunction, 7, 16, 32, 319–24
erogenous zones, 183–88
essential fatty acids, 111–12, 284, 308, 342, 412
essential oils. *See* aromatherapy
estrogen, 269, 339, 462–63
estrogenic foods, 329
eucalyptus (essential oil), 295, 404
evening primrose, 254
Evening Primrose (flower essence), 360
evening primrose oil, 372
exercise, 279, 334, 346, 364, 382. *See also* sexercises

Fairy Lantern (flower essence), 360, 376
false unicorn, 263–64, 282, 298, 304–5, 350, 366, 388
fellatio, 197–200
female condoms, 230
female ejaculation, 214–16
feminine hygiene products, 337–38
feng shui, 150–57
fennel, 307, 317, 350, 366
fennel (essential oil), 130–31, 357, 377, 392
fennel seed, 42
fenugreek, 63–64, 366, 388
fermented foods, 246, 250, 252–53, 398, 416
Ferrum Metallicum, 359, 374, 391
Ferrum Picricum, 333
fertility, 378–93
fertility awareness, 233–35
fiber, 252, 330, 342
fibrocystic breasts, 278–85
Fig (flower essence), 392
figs, 21–22
figwort, 264
filberts, 30–31
fish, 7, 22–23
five elements, 4–5
flaxseed, 30, 293, 329
flaxseed oil, 372
flirting, 424–27
flower essences, 146–49, 360–61, 376–77, 392, 444, 455
folic acid, 258
follicle-stimulating hormone, 238
food allergies, 13
footbaths, 138, 168–69
foot powder, 138
foreplay, 165, 182–88, 322–23
foreskin health, 313–16
fraxinus, 264, 298–300
frenulum, 187
fringe tree, 282, 299, 331
fruits, 329–30
Fuchsia (flower essence), 148, 376

GABA, 53
Gach, Michael Reed, 163
Galen, 78
gamma-linolenic acid, 112
gardenias, 152
garlic, 42–43, 250, 254, 286–87, 289, 310, 399–400, 417
Gelsemium, 143, 276
gem therapy, 453
genital massage, 185–88
genital warts (HPV), 400–404
geranium (essential oil), 131, 277, 291, 302, 392, 447
Ghandi, Mahatma, 30
gifts, 440–41
ginger, 43, 264, 271, 282, 299, 351, 366–67
ginger (essential oil), 131
ginkgo, 64–65, 388
ginseng, 66–68, 367, 388
Globe Artichoke, 15
gluten, 24, 252
glycerin, 51
goji berries, 23–24
goldenrod, 293, 331
goldenseal, 254, 259, 264, 282, 289, 299, 310–11, 318–19, 397–98, 410, 417
gonorrhea, 404–6

Grafenberg, Ernest, 215
grains, 24–25
grapes, 25
Graphites, 143, 374, 391, 413
gravel root, 331
Green, Mindy, 136, 137
greens, 7, 26
grief, 450–51, 452–55
G-spot, 203, 215–16

Hahnemann, Samuel, 140
hair rinse, 138
Hamamelis Virginiana, 359
happiness, 442
hawthorn, 282, 299, 367, 454
Hawthorn (flower essence), 455
hazelnuts, 30–31
Heart and Soul Tonic, 103
Heather (flower essence), 447
Helonias Dioica, 276
HempNut Health and Cookbook, The, 31
hemp seeds, 31
Hepar Sulphuris Calcareum, 413
Herbal Ed's Sexy Smoothie, 102
Herbal Salve, 99
herbs and herbal therapy, 12, 49
  for candida, 253–55
  for cervical dysplasia, 258–60
  for cryptochidism, 317
  dosage of, 244
  for endometriosis, 270–74
  for epididymitis, 318–19
  for erectile dysfunction, 323–24
  for fertility, 387–90
  for fibrocystic breasts, 280–84
  for grief, 454
  for healthy menstruation, 347–56
  for leukorrhea, 286–87
  love potions, 97–104
  love tonics, 52–96
  for menopause, 364–70
  for orchitis, 324–25
  for ovarian cysts, 262–67
  for pelvic inflammatory disease, 289–90
  preparations of, 50–52
  for prostate health, 330–33
  for STDs, 397–98, 403–4, 410–11, 417–18
  for urinary tract infections, 292–94
  for uterine fibroids, 296–301
  for uterine prolapse, 304–5
  for vaginal dryness, 307
  for vaginitis, 310–11
  See also culinary herbs; specific herbs
herpes, 405–14
Hibiscus (flower essence), 148, 152, 271, 293, 376, 444
hip circles, 121
histamine deficiency, 212
holidays, 175
Holly (flower essence), 148, 447
homeopathy, 140–45
  for anger, 446–47
  for Bartholin's cysts, 247–48
  for candida, 256
  for endometriosis, 275–77
  for fertility, 390–92
  for fibrocystic breasts, 284–85
  for grief, 454–55
  for healthy menstruation, 357–60
  for menopause, 373–76
  for prostate health, 333–34
  for STDs, 403–4, 412–14

for urinary tract infections, 294–95
for vaginal dryness, 309
Honeysuckle (flower essence), 455
hops, 351, 367, 454
hormones, 4, 462–68
horsetail, 293, 305, 331, 351, 367
ho shou wu, 367
hot flashes, 362–63
hydrangea, 331
hydrogenated oils, 280
hydrotherapy, 166–69
hyssop (essential oil), 277, 357

Ignatia, 143, 359, 374, 455
illness, 221–22
Impatiens (flower essence), 360, 447
infertility, 378–93
infidelity, 448–49
injectable contraceptives, 235
inositol, 274
intellectual distancing, 213
intercourse, 188–94, 288. *See also* sexual positions; techniques
Iodum, 391
Ipecacuanha, 256, 374
iron, 113, 302, 372
isatis, 311

Jamaican dogwood, 272
jasmine (essential oil), 131–32, 137, 302, 357
Jasmine (flower essence), 392
jing, 182
juniper, 293
juniper berry (essential oil), 357

kale, 26
Kali Bromatum, 391
Kali Carbonicum, 359, 374
karezza, 196
kava kava, 69–71, 104
Kegel congress, 195
Kegel exercises, 118–19, 207, 210, 223, 302
Keville, Kathi, 136
kidney infections, 291
kidney rub, 122
Kidneys, 5, 6–7, 23, 183–84, 362
kidneys, 14, 296
kissing, 177–80

labia majora, 186
Lachesis, 276, 285, 359, 446
lady's mantle, 264, 272, 282, 299, 305, 351, 367
latex, 229
lavender (essential oil), 201, 291, 295, 357, 447
Lecheries, 374–75
lemon (essential oil), 295, 306, 404
lemon balm, 411, 454
lemon balm (essential oil), 392, 447
lettuce, 26
leukorrhea, 285–87
libido, 7, 12
licorice, 72–73, 259, 264, 272, 282, 351, 367–68, 389, 411, 418
lighting, 157, 167
linden, 368
lingam, 2, 187–88, *189*
lipase, 16
listening skills, 7
Liver, 5, 23, 339, 343, 362, 445–46

liver, 14, 17–18, 269, 279, 296
lomatium, 260
longan, 307
lotus (essential oil), 302, 447
love, 177–78, 421–22, 460–68
love altars, 152–53, 157
love potions, 97–104
Love Shake, 100
lubricants, 309
Lunelle, 236
Lycopodium, 143–44, 276, 309, 333, 359, 375, 391, 403, 446
lymph, 278–79
lysine, 403, 408, 412

maca, 73–74
macadamias, 31
magnesium, 113–14, 275, 357, 372, 411, 447
Magnesium Phosphate, 276, 359
Male Sexual Vitality Tonic, 102
Male Tonifying Exercise, 120
Mallow (flower essence), 376, 392
mangoes, 26–27
marijuana, 75–76, 351–52
Mariposa Lily (flower essence), 149, 444
marjoram (essential oil), 357, 447
marsh mallow, 254, 293, 332
massage, 158–65, 185–88, 189, 247, 322–23
massage oil, 101, 139, 160
masturbation, 180–82, 212–13, 435
meadowsweet, 352
menopause, 221, 361–77
menorrhagia, 343–44
men's health, 206–7, 312–13. *See also* specific concerns
menstruation, 218–19, 335–61
Mercurius, 446
Mercurius Corrosivus, 276, 294
Mercurius Solubilis, 247, 413
Mercurius Vivus, 276
methionine, 275, 302
metrorrhagia, 345–46
Mimulus (flower essence), 149, 376
minerals, 112–15
mirrors, 157
miscarriage, 219
missionary position, 190–91
molds, 12
mons veneris, 201
morning-after pill, 232
motherwort, 264–65, 272, 299, 352, 368, 454
Mounted Archer, 120
moxa, 317
Mugwort (flower essence), 352, 360, 392
muira puama, 77
mullein, 454
Mustard (flower essence), 455
mustard seed, 43
myrrh, 272, 287, 289, 311

Nasturtium (flower essence), 149
Natrum Muriaticum, 144, 309, 359, 375, 403, 413, 446, 455
natural fibers, 279
Natural Perfumes, 137
neroli (essential oil), 132, 392, 447
nettle, 78–80, 254–55, 283, 293, 332, 352, 368, 389, 403, 418
neurotransmitters, 4, 460–61
niacin, 108, 212–13

niaouli (essential oil), 295, 377, 404
nipples, 201, 207
Nitricum Acidum, 403, 413
nutmeg, 43
nutmeg (essential oil), 132
nutritional therapy, 106–16, 258
  for cervical dysplasia, 267
  for endometriosis, 274–75
  for erectile dysfunction, 323
  for fertility, 385–87
  for fibrocystic breasts, 284
  for grief, 453–54
  for healthy menstruation, 356–57
  for menopause, 371–72
  for pelvic inflammatory disease, 290
  for prostate health, 329–30
  for STDs, 403, 411–12
  for urinary tract infections, 294
  for uterine fibroids, 301–2
  for vaginal dryness, 308
nuts and seeds, 27–34
Nux Vomica, 276–77, 375, 391, 446

Oak (flower essence), 376
oat, 80–81, 368, 389
okra, 34
olives, 7, 35
oral pleasures, 196–201
orchids, 152
orchitis, 324–25
oregano (essential oil), 255, 277
Oregon grape, 255, 265, 272, 293, 299, 311, 332, 352, 411
organic produce, 40
orgasm, 4, 201, 205–16
  inability to, 7, 212–13
  program for intensifying, 206–7
  during sex, 213–14
  without ejaculation, 210–11
ovarian cysts, 261–68
ovulation, 214
oysters, 23

pain, 269
palms of hands, 184
pantothenic acid, 108–9
parsley, 43, 289, 332, 352–53
partridgeberry, 265, 272, 299–300, 353
passion, 178
passionflower, 454
patchouli (essential oil), 133, 137, 404
patience, 207
pau d'arco, 255, 260, 283
peace lily, 152
peaches, 35–36
peanuts, 252
Pear (flower essence), 455
pecans, 31–32
pelvic inflammatory disease (PID), 288–91, 397
pelvic lifts, 121
pennyroyal, 353
peony, 265, 273, 353, 368
peppermint, 353, 403, 411
peppermint (essential oil), 357
perfume, 139
persimmons, 36
perspiration, 279–80
pesticides, 40
Peyronie's disease, 325–26
phenylethylamine, 75
phimosis, 315
Phosphoricum Acidum, 391, 403

Phosphorus, 22, 144, 359, 391
Phytolacca, 285
pine, 82–83
pine (essential oil), 82, 447
Pine (flower essence), 82
pine nuts, 32
pipsissewa, 265, 293, 300, 332
Pirello, Christina, 31
pistachios, 32
Pituitrinum, 391
plantain, 293
Platina, 392
plums, 36
pokeweed, 265, 283, 289–90, 300
Pomegranate (flower essence), 360–61, 377, 392
pomegranates, 36–37
poppy seeds, 32
poria, 368, 389
potassium, 284
pregnancy, 219–20
premature ejaculation, 7, 208–9
premenstrual syndrome (PMS), 339–41
priapism, 326
prickly ash, 255, 265, 273, 300
probiotics, 201, 246, 249–50, 308–9, 329, 398, 411, 416
progesterone, 466
prostate cancer, 328
prostate gland, 203, 216
prostate health, 326–34
prostatitis, 327–28
protein, 323
Psorinum, 413
Pulsatilla, 277, 285, 334, 359, 375, 455
pumpkin seeds, 32–33, 329
pygeum, 332
pyridoxine, 109

quercetin, 25

Radical Resistance Yoni Suppository, 260–61, 267, 274
raspberry, 83–84
red clover, 260, 265, 273, 283, 300, 353, 368, 389
red raspberry, 260, 265–66, 273, 283, 300, 305, 353, 369, 389
redroot, 266, 300
reflexology, 162–63, 185, 393
Rehmann, Joseph, 85
rehmannia, 85–86, 105, 273, 353, 389
reishi, 86–87
relationships
  addiction and, 456–59
  feng shui for, 152–53
  finding a date, 423–29
  getting physical, 429–30
  healing from a broken heart, 450–55
  importance of loving self, 421–23
  twenty-five principles of, 432–42
relaxation, 207
Rescue Remedy, 149, 444, 455
rhodiola, 87–88
Rhus Toxicodendron, 413
rose, 133–34, 353–54, 369
rose (essential oil), 133–34, 302, 357, 392, 447
Rose, Richard, 31
rosemary, 43–44
rosemary (essential oil), 277, 291, 306, 357
roses, 152

Sabal Serrulata, 144, 334, 392
Sabina, 359–60, 375, 392, 404
safe sex, 224–27
Sagan, Carl, 75
sage, 44, 354, 369
sage (essential oil), 377
Saint John's wort, 332, 454
salmon, 22
sandalwood (essential oil), 134, 137
Sanguinaria Canadensis, 375
sarsaparilla, 88–89, 266, 283, 300, 354, 369, 389, 411
Sarsaparilla, 295
saunas, 7, 139
saw palmetto, 89–91, 266, 300, 317, 332–33, 369, 389–90
Scarlet Monkeyflower (flower essence), 149, 377
schizandra, 91–92, 389–90
Scleranthus (flower essence), 377
Sea of Intimacy, 164–65
Sea of Vitality, 163–64
sea palm, 38
sea vegetables, 7, 37
seaweeds, 7, 38, 330
Secale Cornutum, 375
Selenium, 114, 144, 330
self-care, 244
semen, 206
Senecio Aureus, 360
seniors, 220–21
sensate therapy, 321
Sepia, 144–45, 256, 277, 295, 305–6, 360, 375, 404, 413–14, 446
serotonin, 17, 19, 461
sesame seeds, 33
Sets of Nine, 195
sexercises, 117–25
sexual energy, 3–7, 434–35
sexual positions, 189–94, *194*
sexual superfoods. *See* superfoods
sexual vitality, 6–7, 141–45
Shake, Shake, Shake!, 123
shampoo, 139
sharp edges, 155
shepherd's purse, 354, 369
shiitake, 38
Shiva, 75–76, 156
Siberian ginseng, 390
Silicea, 277, 285, 360, 392, 414
sitz baths, 169, 247, 270, 295, 302, 306, 307, 318, 334, 404, 418
sizing differences, 222–23
skullcap, 354
smoking, 322, 383–84
soaking, 28
soles of feet, 184
Solidago Virgaurea, 334
spermicides, 227, 240
spikenard (essential oil), 137
spilanthes, 255
spinach, 26
spirulina, 39
Spleen, 5, 343
Spongia Tosta, 334
sprouted grains, 24–25
Squash (flower essence), 392
squatting, 121
stagnation, 269
Staphysagria, 145, 295, 334, 400, 404, 446
Star of Bethlehem (flower essence), 444, 455
Star Tulip (flower essence), 277, 361

STDs, 225–27, 394–96. *See also* specific STDs
Sticky Monkeyflower (flower essence), 149
storage, 156
stress, 7, 384
Stretching for Partners, 122
sugar, 25, 248, 252
sulfites, 47
Sulfur, 256, 334, 360, 375–76, 404, 414
Sulphur, 447
suma, 369
sun baths, 394
sunflower seeds, 33–34
superfoods, 7, 13–40
superoxide dismutase, 116
supplements, 106–16. *See also* nutritional therapy
suppositories, 250–51, 260–61, 267, 274, 305, 307–8, 311, 418
syphilis, 415–16

tampons, 268, 337–38
tea leaves, 411
teas, 46, 50, 355–56, 370–71
tea tree (essential oil), 404
techniques, 173–74
  anal sex, 202–3
  foreplay, 182–88
  intercourse, 188–94
  kissing, 177–80
  masturbation, 180–82
  oral pleasures, 196–201
  after play, 204
  setting the stage, 174–77
televisions, 157
testicles, 188, 313
testosterone, 220, 321–22, 467–68
therapeutic baths, 256–57, 287, 414
therapy, 441–42
Three-Yin Meeting Point, 164
Thuja Occidentalis, 334, 404
thyme, 290
timing, 174–76
tinctures, 50–51
Tissue-Tonifying Yoni Suppository, 305
toilet paper, 246
tomatoes, 330
touch, 158
toxic shock syndrome (TSS), 337, 338
toxins, 14, 381–82
trauma, 443–49
tribulus, 92–93, 354
trichomoniasis, 286, 416–18
trillium, 266, 300–301, 354
truffles, 39
tuberose (essential oil), 135
tuna, 22
turmeric, 44–45, 255, 266, 273, 301

undergarments, 245
urethral meatus, 187
urethritis, 291
urinary tract infections, 291–95
usnea, 255, 294, 319, 398, 418
uterine fibroids, 295–303
uterine prolapse, 303–6
uva ursi, 294, 333, 354

vacations, 176–77
vaginal dryness, 306–9
vaginal odor, 201
vaginismus, 309
vaginitis, 310–11

valerian, 273
Valeriana, 376
vanilla, 45
vanilla (essential oil), 135
vasectomy, 240–41
vegetables, 329–30
vervain, 266, 283, 301
vetivert (essential oil), 135
Viburnum, 277
Viburnum Opolus, 360
violet, 266, 283, 369, 454
virginity, 217–18
visualization, 207
visual stimulation, 198
vitality, sexual, 6–7, 141–45
vitamins
  vitamin A, 107, 258, 260, 308, 372
  vitamin B, 107, 108–9, 258, 274, 284, 301–2, 356–57, 372, 386, 412
  vitamin C, 109–10, 249, 274–75, 290, 294, 308, 357, 372, 386, 412
  vitamin D, 110
  vitamin E, 110–11, 275, 284, 294, 302, 308, 325–26, 330, 357, 372, 386, 412
vitex, 94–95, 266, 273, 301, 307, 354–55, 369, 390

Walnut (flower essence), 149, 377, 447
walnuts, 34
water, 280, 330. *See also* hydrotherapy
watermelon, 39–40
Watermelon (flower essence), 392
Watson, Sereno, 89
weight, 381
wheat, 13, 24–25, 252
wheatgrass, 201
white willow, 273–74, 355
Wild Duck, 120
wild rice, 7, 24–25
wild yam, 267, 274, 283–84, 301, 355, 369–70, 390
Willow (flower essence), 377
wind chimes, 156
windows, 156
wiping, 245
witch hazel, 370
women's health, 205–6, 245–46. *See also* specific concerns

Xanthoxylum, 360

yarrow, 255, 267, 274, 301, 355, 370
yeast infections. *See* candidiasis
yellow dock, 284, 287, 355, 411
yin and yang, 6
ylang ylang (essential oil), 136, 447
yoga, 123–24
yogurt, 250–51
Yohimbe, 95–96, 145
yoni, 2, 186–87, *190*

zinc, 27, 114–15, 308, 323, 330, 357, 386–87
Zincum Metallicum, 145